A RESEARCH PRiMER

In Occupational and Physical Therapy

The American Occupational Therapy Association, Inc.

Disclaimers

"This publication is designed to provide accurate and authoritative information in regard to the subject matter covered. It is sold or distributed with the understanding that the publisher is not engaged in rendering legal, accounting, or other professional service. If legal advice or other expert assistance is required, the services of a competent professional person should be sought."

—From the Declaration of Principles jointly adopted by the American Bar Association and a Committee of Publishers and Associations

It is the objective of the American Occupational Therapy Association to be a forum for free expression and interchange of ideas. The opinions expressed by the contributors to this work are their own and not necessarily those of either the editors or the American Occupational Therapy Association.

AOTA Director of Nonperiodical Publications: Frances E. McCarrey
AOTA Managing Editor of Nonperiodical Publications: Mary C. Fisk
Designed by Carolyn J. Uhl

ISBN 1-56900-063-8

Printed in the United States of America

Acknowledgments

The author wishes to acknowledge the excellent education she received from her many previous professors including Marilyn Lichtman, Jim C. Fortune, and William F. Seaver. In addition, the author wants to thank students in her research courses who have significantly influenced the final format and content of this book.

Finally, the author wishes to acknowledge the American Occupational Therapy Foundation for its exceptional support and guidance provided to those interested in research in the field of occupational therapy. As a part of this, 25% of the profits from this book shall be donated to the American Occupational Therapy Foundation for funding in research and research training.

—Charlotte Brasic Royeen, PhD, OTR, FAOTA

Assistant Dean for Research
Professor in Occupational Therapy
School of Pharmacy and Allied Health Professions
Creighton University
Omaha, Nebraska

Table of Contents

Foreword

Dr. Charlotte Royeen's book, *A Research Primer in Occupational and Physical Therapy,* provides an introductory "research methodology" handbook that may be useful to the seasoned clinician as well as to the entry-level student in an introductory research class in occupational therapy or physical therapy. Dr. Royeen's purpose is to provide the clinician with the tools needed to demystify and to understand the research that validates clinical practice. The *Research Primer* provides the tools necessary for the clinician to be a consumer of research and to be able to transfer research findings into the clinical practice techniques of the therapist. The *Research Primer* provides the clinician with the basic understanding of the research process needed to translate research findings into the language that the patients and their families may understand. Dr. Royeen's purpose is to enhance the comfort level of the non-research directed student and clinician with the research culture and then to be able to use and apply research data.

Two years ago, I used a photocopied and unedited edition of the *Research Primer* to teach a course in research methods to occupational therapy seniors at Texas Tech University Health Science Center in Lubbock, Texas. The students felt that the text was clearly written and to the point, and that it reduced anxiety in a course that historically generates stress in most students. The use of a conceptual, rather than a mathematical, orientation to statistical analysis is important for students who, as clinicians, are consumers of research rather than producers of research data. Dr. Royeen provides a broad overview of the research process rather than bogging down the students in the intricacies of research jargon and minutiae. She provides a view of the forest, a smell of the trees, without making readers deal with the bears and the wolves of mathematical calculations. This text encourages the student to translate the "foreign language" of research into the everyday language of practice.

Dr. Royeen uses research studies from the occupational therapy and physical therapy literature to describe such esoteric concepts as "quasiexperimental design" or the use of the "nonparametric Kruskal Wallis analysis of variance" to determine differences in several NDT treatment groups. The students will understand the reason for using a nonparametric analysis of variance as opposed to another form of analysis. At this introductory level, the students may know how to perform a specific statistical analysis, but more importantly, they will understand why it should be used and why another analysis would not be appropriate. Furthermore, in a couple of years, when these students may need to review concepts in research design or statistical analysis, they will know where to get the information. They will dig out their copy of Charlotte Royeen's *Research Primer* to get them restarted.

An important analogy made in this book is the strong similarity of the methodology of the researcher and the clinician. When a patient comes to a therapist, the therapist must assess the problem, review how other clinicians have treated similar cases, develop and institute a treatment plan, and assess the patient's progress. The researcher follows a similar process. A research problem develops, the researcher reviews the pertinent research literature to see what previous researchers have done, develops and institutes a research design, and assesses the data that have been collected. After the clinical or research data have been collected, the therapist and the researcher must analyze the meaning, the importance, and the applicability of the treatment or of the research. If either the therapist or the researcher finds an important result, one more obligation must be met. They must disseminate their findings to others in the professions. They must tell their stories so that others may benefit from their findings.

Charlotte Royeen's *Research Primer* addresses an important need for an introductory textbook in research methodology for occupational therapists and physical therapists. This text provides a conceptual understanding of this discipline so that the student may learn to appreciate the professional research literature. It is not meant for graduate or advanced courses in research methodology and design. It is written to "... increase [the] comfort level within the 'research culture,' or to help (the clinician) become cultured in research" (Chapter 1, p. 2). Charlotte Royeen has addressed her mission well and effectively.

Hugh W. Bonner, PhD
Dean
College of Health Related Professions
Health Science Center
State University of New York
Syracuse, New York

CHAPTER 1

Why You Need This Primer

KEY WORDS

Professional literature

Research consumer

Research culture

Research practitioner

Why Every Occupational and Physical Therapy Student Needs This Book

You may never actually publish a piece of research in an academic journal or textbook, but you will undoubtedly use your understanding of research in clinical practice or administration—or, at the very least, during your professional program. To be sure, research will play an integral role in your lifelong activities as an occupational or physical therapist.

It seems, however, that many occupational and physical therapy students—as well as clinicians who are beginning their practices—face a number of hurdles that interfere with their ability to consume research materials. Among the many concerns they cite are

> *"Research is hard to read and understand—that is, if you can stay awake long enough to get through it."*
>
> *"I don't see how research applies to everyday practice."*
>
> *"I wish there were an easier way to understand the complexities of research, especially the use of mathematics and statistics."*

Sound familiar? There are a number of comprehensive textbooks available today for beginning-level research students in occupational and physical therapy. Unfortunately, as educators in these disciplines will tell you, students often find such books intimidating, difficult to comprehend, or not particularly applicable to their interests.

PURPOSE OF THIS PRIMER

I hope to change all that with this book. Unlike many existing texts, this primer is designed to increase your comfort level within the **research culture**, or to help you become cultured in research. Many believe that such training is fundamental for the continued development of the occupational and physical therapy professions. How can occupational and physical therapists become trained in research? Yerxa and Sharrot (1986) define *training* in terms of its Latin origin "...trahere," which means "to pull." Perhaps many of us have feared being pulled or pushed into taking that dreaded research course required in most curricula.

Yet it is not the purpose of this book to pull readers into research competency and turn them into research practitioners. Clearly, it is difficult for students to really assume the role of researcher before they have the fundamental concepts of what research is. Therefore, this text does not assume that you, the reader, will actually execute a piece of research while reading or using the book (even though you may). Rather, the goal of this primer is to teach occupational and physical therapy students and clinicians how to (a) read research, (b) understand the role and "culture" of research, and (c) use or apply research. This text is designed to equip beginning-level research students with the necessary tools.

WHY THIS BOOK IS SPECIAL

Given a clinician's or student's-eye view of the limitations of current textbooks for entry-level research courses, what kinds of approaches might better suit your needs? The following five characteristics, collectively, distinguish this primer from the multitude of other entry-level books on research—in almost any field. This book should

1. develop your basic skills in understanding research, enable you to become an effective **research consumer** and, along with the more traditional approach of developing your research skills, enhance your ability to become a **research practitioner**
2. provide a *conceptual* rather than a *mathematical* orientation to statistics as used in research
3. enable you to apply research concepts by using numerous examples from the **professional literature** in occupational and physical therapy to illustrate research components and processes
4. employ a user-friendly approach that uses nontechnical language whenever possible and technical language only as needed for precision and education
5. offer an inspirational approach that directly links research to each reader's interests and practice.

This last goal is accomplished by including clinicians' views of research and by drawing parallels between the research process and the clinical process whenever possible.

HOW TO USE THIS BOOK

How exactly can this primer teach you to read, understand, and use research in the unique fashion just described? Well, it will require more than merely sitting back and reading the book: it has been my experience that therapists learn best by *doing*. By the end of this textbook, therefore, you should have repeatedly reviewed, dissected, and analyzed research articles and parts thereof. Also included within the primer are a number of written exercises that will allow you to interact with the text to gain a clearer understanding of the basic tenets of research.

The time you invest in studying the text and completing the written exercises and learning activities can give you the tools necessary to be an effective research consumer. Ultimately, this can prove to be highly valuable throughout your academic and professional career. Moreover, the aim of this book is to educate you about research so that it becomes less intimidating and arduous and more applicable to your chosen practice. And believe it or not, once you understand and appreciate its basic concepts and processes, you may even *enjoy* research!

Organization of This Primer

CHAPTER THEMES

Most people seem to learn best by first being introduced to the "forest" (basic concepts or products of research), and then to the "trees" (processes of research). The chapters of this text, therefore, are organized by the so-called forest and tree principles. Chapters 1–5 provide the forest overview. These introductory chapters set the stage for addressing the basic questions of what is research, why is it important in the occupational and physical therapy disciplines, and how is it executed. Chapters 6 and 7 provide you with a foundation for understanding three fundamental tools of research: *sampling, selection,* and *measurement.*

In chapters 8–11, I review and present the most commonly used categories of research found in occupational and physical therapy: *descriptive research, quasiexperimental* and *experimental research, single subject research,* and *qualitative research.* Each category will be defined and illustrated with examples from peer-review journals in occupational and physical therapy, and other user-friendly charts and figures. These examples will help you better understand and apply abstract research concepts throughout the text. The last chapter of this book offers guidelines and suggestions on the numerous ways readers can apply skills learned from this primer. This section describes the many opportunities for professional activities centering on research in physical and occupational therapy.

CHAPTER CONTENTS AND FORMATS

Each chapter first presents content and then provides you an opportunity to apply that content using examples of research and other illustrations. This format includes the following components:

Chapter outline: This section lists the main headings that provide the conceptual organization for the chapter.

Chapter presentation: This is the main content of the chapter.

Examples: These are actual research articles, or sections thereof, from published literature in occupational and physical therapy. Examples may be at the chapter's end or interspersed throughout.

Interpretation: Each research article or section thereof will have an interpretation immediately following it. In the interpretation section, readers will be asked to respond to a series of questions about the research article or illustration.

Answers: Answers to the interpretation questions for each research article presented will be provided. This will allow you to compare your responses with those provided.

References: These are listings of key articles, books, presentations, and other materials readers can refer to for further clarification on the concepts or processes described in the chapter.

Recommended readings: These are three to five useful texts or articles related to the chapter content that can be obtained for independent reading or exploration.

Learning activities: These are activities designed to reinforce and expand the content presented within the chapter.

This primer is designed to give you a step-by-step introduction to reading, understanding, and using research. It should help you directly link the concepts of research and its processes to the professional literature in your discipline. And unlike most research texts, this book will give you a hands-on opportunity to analyze research and compare your analysis with answers that are provided, enabling you to *learn by doing.*

References

Yerxa E. J., & Sharrot, G. (1986). Liberal arts: The foundation for occupational therapy education. *American Journal of Occupational Therapy, 40,* 153–159.

Recommended Readings

Reed, K. L. (1984). Understanding theory: The first step in learning about research. *American Journal of Occupational Therapy, 38,* 677–682.

Strong, J. (1994). Clinical occupational therapists as researchers. *New Zealand Journal of Occupational Therapy, 45,* 4–7.

Wilson, H. S. (1985). *Research in nursing.* Menlo Park, CA: Addison Wesley.

Learning Activities

1. Ask yourself, Does the thought of reading or studying research intimidate me? If the answer is yes, what is it about the topic that concerns you most? Is it the math? The technical or heady language? The format of research articles? Once you identify what intimidates you, determine why you believe it intimidates you.
2. Record on paper all the negative characteristics you associate with research (e.g., course is difficult or unrelated to my interests; research articles are too boring). Share these with the other students in your class or with your professional colleagues, and discuss possible solutions.
3. Set goals related to overcoming these and other roadblocks to reading, understanding, and using research. Consider a time frame for using this textbook in conjunction with achieving these goals.

CHAPTER 2

What Is Research?

KEY WORDS

Data analysis

Hypothesis

Research

Results

Scientific method

Scientific procedures

Research Defined

Science knows only one commandment: contribute to science.

— Bertolt Brecht (1898–1956)

You read it in newspapers or hear it on the evening news every day: Scientists discover a possible genetic link to breast cancer. In the United States, motor vehicle accidents are the number one cause of spinal cord and brain injuries among America's youth. Estrogen-like contaminants found in ordinary cow's milk and other dairy products may cause infertility in women. A new drug shows promising results for autistic children. Americans voice a 53% disapproval rating for the latest occupant of the Oval Office.

These are just a few examples of the multitude of reports we hear or read daily that are products of research. From astronomy to zoology and every imaginable topic in between, each day, around the clock, someone, somewhere, is studying, dissecting, and uncovering answers that contribute to our world's collective body of knowledge. Indeed, no segment of our society engages in this ongoing process more fervently than do researchers in the health disciplines.

As we look beneath the research headlines found in the mainstream media—and even between the pages of our occupational and physical therapy journals—one may ask: What did they do to get to this point? What exactly is research?

Broadly defined, research is one or more activities—based on **scientific procedures**—

executed by scholars, scientists, clinicians, or even laypeople, to gather data and generate knowledge (Jantzen, 1981). **Research** is the process of collecting data and defining the unique categorization of that data. **Scientific procedures** are guidelines or strategies that structure the process of research, and in effect, provide the undertaking with a solid foundation. Just as scientific principles guide intervention strategies used in providing therapy to a client, scientific procedures provide the underpinnings for the research process itself. Thus, research is both a process (how one goes about the task) and a product (the outcome of that process). Again, this is analogous to how treatment is both a process (how you interact with the client) and a product (the functional outcome of the treatment process).

Scientific Method

Let us further explore scientific guidelines or procedures. Scientific guidelines are derived from the **scientific method**, which consists of a process of gathering data to answer questions. In contrast, a nonscientific method allows belief systems rather than data or facts to answer questions. Like a tightly run ship, the scientific method assumes an orderly and sequenced logic, which consists of

1. defining the problem
2. generating **hypotheses**, or best guesses related to the problem
3. gathering the necessary materials to test the hypotheses
4. carrying out procedures designed to test the hypotheses
5. collecting and analyzing the data
6. generating conclusions based on accepting or rejecting the hypotheses.

Do you recall your laboratory experiments in high school? They were all based on information gathered using the scientific method. Note also that the scientific method and the methods of client assessment and intervention planning are very similar.

The Role of Theory

Keep in mind that a critical component in the scientific method is hypothesis generation and testing. Recall that hypotheses are statements of your best guesses to answer the question posed in the problem identification. Going one step further, a researcher's predictions of what will happen often are based on theory. Science gives us a way to obtain knowledge about our world. Yet too much knowledge about our world can overwhelm us, and we are unable to make sense of things. How can we take what we know and organize it in a way that increases understanding and that allows us to use this understanding to predict events? Theory serves this purpose.

In essence, theory allows us to organize and conceptualize known or potential relationships. In other words, it enables us to organize knowledge. At its very core, science is composed of developing theory or testing hypotheses developed from theory (Jantzen, 1981). Theory, therefore, is an integral part of the scientific process. Given this summary of theory, let us take a look at the process of research.

The Research Process

Now, let's look at research in motion.

Figure 2–1 presents research as a circular process, with eight sequential stages. These stages range from recognizing the need for research in a particular area to synthesizing the conclusions from research that relates to the original need. This representation of the

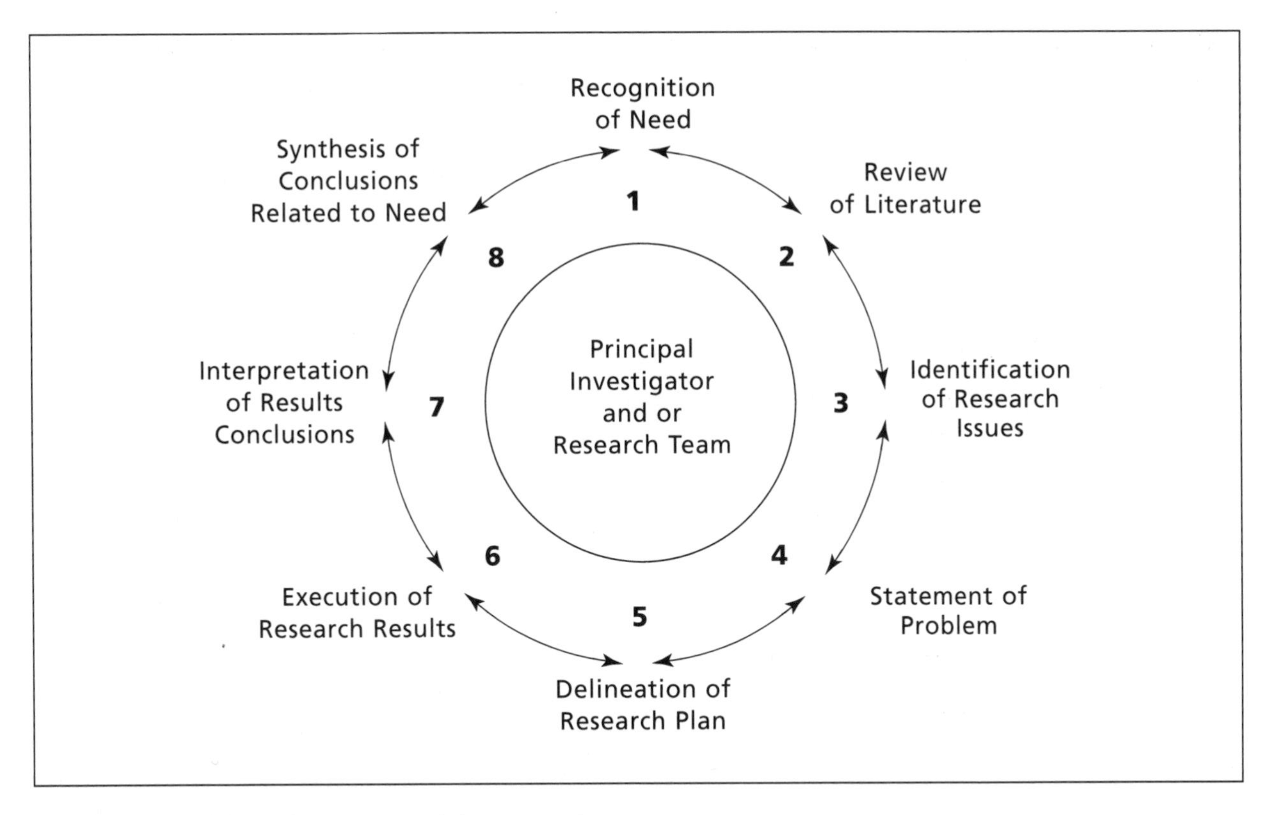

Figure 2–1. Overview of the stages of the Research Process.
Source: Royeen, C. B. (1988). *Research tradition in occupational therapy.* Thorofare, NJ: Slack Publishing.

research process is simplistic and has been executed for teaching purposes. However, research as actually executed is not a process of clearly defined or delineated steps.

Moreover, the stages of research are not mutually exclusive. Like human growth and development, the stages of research are directional, yet they also may overlap. Indeed, a researcher may at times even regress to an earlier stage, represented by the two directions of the arrows in Figure 2–1. The center of the circle in Figure 2–1 contains the principal investigator or research team, which reflects that research can be conducted either by individuals or groups. Often, such groups are termed research teams, with a principal investigator overseeing or managing the research.

Definitions of each of the eight stages of the research process presented in Figure 2–1 follow:

Stage 1: Recognize what research is needed. This may include the need to investigate some phenomenon in clinical practice, to develop or refine instrumentation, or to study aspects of theory or the profession itself.

Stage 2: Review all published material directly and indirectly related to the research need.

Stage 3: Identify the research issues, considering the need for the research in context of the literature review. State the problem by summarizing research issues and focusing on the problem area.

Stage 4: Generate research questions, hypotheses, or both based on the statement of the problem.

Stage 5: Delineate the research plan. This includes providing specifications for directing, interpreting, and coordinating the research.

Stage 6: Execute the research. The steps include conducting the study, verifying and analyzing the data, and organizing and disseminating the results.

Stage 7: Interpret results and conclusions based on disciplinary knowledge, theory, literature, and creativity.

Stage 8: Synthesize conclusions; the synthesis must apply the conclusions to the original need driving the investigation.

Products of Research

The fact that research is a process and not just a product cannot be overemphasized. Yet it is also true that research is a process with results that can be tangible products, such as

- manuscripts
- instruments
- scholarly papers
- presentations
- devices.

Research products may also be intangible, such as research results that change attitudes, alter or modify theories, refine treatment procedures, or change public or private institutional policy. These intangible products of research often take years to manifest themselves. An article by Brooke, Lateur, Diana-Rigby, and Questad (1991) is an intangible product of research. In their study of 10 subjects, they compared three types of interventions for prevention or treatment of shoulder subluxation secondary to hemiplegia. The three treatment conditions tested were a Bobath-type sling, a Harris hemisling, and an armtrough/lapboard attachment to a wheelchair. Using X-rays to measure placement of the humerus with the various interventions, they found the Harris hemisling and the armtrough/lapboard to be superior to the Bobath sling in remediating shoulder subluxation. Though the research is preliminary and needs replication, it does suggest that one type of intervention is preferred over another. Such a finding is an intangible product of research. In all cases, however, sharing these research products and results with targeted audiences constitutes dissemination—the ultimate goal of any and all research.

To understand and learn to use research in the occupational and physical therapy professions, we will further explore a key tool used to disseminate research to the public: the research article. If you glance through the numerous clinical or professional journals available to students in the health care professions, you will find these tangible products of the research process. As discussed earlier, the subjects and results described in research articles are infinite. Studies presented in scholarly journals can be specific or wide-ranging. Research conducted by Corrivieau, Arsenault, Dutil, Besner, Dupuis, Guarna, and Lambert (1992) on intrarater and interrater reliability of a Bobath-based instrument for evaluating a patient with hemiplegia is an example of specific research focused on a narrow range of inquiry. In this case, the restricted range of interest is in determining the specific reliability of the evaluation instrument across raters and by the same rater. This differs from a more wide-ranging approach taken by DeGangi (1994). She examined the effectiveness of short-term neurodevelopmental treatment (NDT) using three case studies. The scope of study in this case is much broader, that is, the relative effectiveness of NDT as compared to the reliability of a specific instrument.

Nevertheless, research articles seen in scholarly journals resemble each other in presentation and format. Typically, they are made up of the following key components:

Abstract. At the beginning of all research articles, just below the title and author(s), a short paragraph called the abstract contains a brief summary of the contents of the article. Not only is the abstract a synopsis of what may be a lengthy, complex article, it is also a useful tool for researchers who often must scroll through dozens of research articles to find one or two that specifically cover their area of interest. Often, when conducting literature searches during the course of researching a particular topic, students use abstracts to help them weed through numerous articles and find the ones that are most suited to their research needs.

Introduction. The introduction section of a research article should include a statement of the nature of the problem being presented, as well as a statement of the problem at the beginning of the investigation. The introduction should also contain a statement of the purpose, scope, and method of the investigation, as well as a review of the pertinent literature.

Method. This section often includes subsections titled Subjects and Procedures. The Subjects section contains a thorough description of the participants in the study and includes the information on participants' ages, demographic data, and any other pertinent information such as diagnosis or socieconomic status (SES). The Procedures section should give the reader a step-by-step description of how the investigation was conducted.

Data Analysis. This section is not always separate from the Methods section, and it describes or delinates exactly what types of analysis were conducted using the data collected in the investigation. Usually, the authors identify what types of statistical analysis they used.

Results. This section presents the findings or results of the data analysis with little or no interpretation. It is simply a report of the facts discovered by the study.

Discussion/Conclusion. This section provides the investigator an opportunity to say what the results mean; this is where he or she interprets the findings as related to the original research problem identified in the introduction.

References. This is a list of all authors cited in the text of the article. No articles should be listed as references that are not cited in the text, and vice versa.

Why Research Is Important

You may now have a better understanding of what research is, and why it exists. The following section may give you a better idea of why research is important in occupational and physical therapy, as well as in other disciplines. In the next section, you can compare your current views on research with those of your peers and with the views of professional researchers.

READERS' PERSPECTIVES ON RESEARCH

First, to better identify your current views, complete the Research Questionnaire. Answer the questions as best you can, taking time to really think about your responses before recording them.

Research Questionnaire

1. What is research?
2. Why is research important?
3. How do you use research?
4. What are your interests regarding research?
5. What do you need to know about research and why?
6. What do you see as the research needs in your field?
7. What is your preferred way to learn about research?
8. What other comments do you have about research in general or research in your field of specialization?

HOW YOUR PEERS VIEW RESEARCH

The following section presents statements other students like yourself have made about research and related issues as addressed in the questionnaire you just filled out. The answers or statements have been collected over the past 5 years from people taking either courses or workshops in research at the undergraduate or master's level. You may find some of the students' responses strikingly similar to your own.

1. What is research? Students of research answered:
   - The collection, collation, and evaluation of data.
   - The organized documentation and observation used to validate hypotheses regarding theories, treatments, and so on.
   - A structured, planned method of logically collecting information to either prove or solve a problem. It is also an organized method by which to study some specific issue or topic.
   - The process of scientific inquiry.
   - A method of studying an area and of expanding our knowledge.
   - The systematic exploration of questions, the answers to which advance knowledge in our respective fields.
   - A systematic look at an idea, a comparison, a frame of reference.
   - Scientific study.
2. Why is research important? Students of research answered:
   - Research is necessary for any endeavor to move forward, expand, change effectively, and benefit society.
   - Research is important because through it we can learn and discover new things.
   - To learn how what we do works, to prove theories, to compare the effectiveness of treatment techniques, to answer questions, to improve the knowledge base on which our professions are based, to provide a basis of normative data, to influence policy decisions, and to affect reimbursement issues.
   - To determine why specific treatment techniques are effective and if they are effective.
   - Because it provides us with validation, or refutes methods, treatments, theories, and so on, on which we base practice.
   - Research is important when the results and conclusions help to answer clinical questions and direct us in our treatment.
   - It is important to gain as much information as possible in a specific area.
   - Research is important for future planning.
   - Research helps us improve our work skills.
   - Gives us reasons or support for practices.
   - To advance and improve on current practice.
3. How do you use research? Students of research answered:
   - I use research to stay current in my field.
   - In treatment planning and in educating parents and the public.
   - I read journals to read results of others' research. This answers some questions in my mind and provides many more.
   - I use research to determine program effectiveness, to best serve our client population, to improve clinical practice, and to influence national policy.
   - I use research as a reference for validating ideas, techniques, or both.

- To provide me with information.
- I use research to better understand the clients I serve.
- I need to be an informed reader of research in order to use research results.
- Up to this point, I have used research mainly in writing term papers!
- For planning and learning better ways to solve problems and do practice.
- In planning programs and giving in-services.
- To improve my overall knowledge of my field and to keep informed of up-to-the-minute information in my field.

4. What are your interests regarding research? Students of research answered:
   - I would like to be able to read, understand, and have an intelligent conversation about research.
   - Just to keep current in my field.
   - I'd like to really understand the data presented and be able to read the statistical analysis.
   - My interests in research are very basic. I want to be able to look at a study and understand it rather than turning the page to get away from it.
   - To get through my professional program!
   - Development of more efficient treatment methods.
   - Interested in a grandiose sense—it sounds great, it's the "right thing to do" among peers at this gathering. I'm stimulated and get charged to do something, but…it's scary, enormous, time-consuming and I wonder if I have the proper brain constructs for it!
   - I feel it is important. There is a definite need to let people know what we do as therapists and why our services are significant.
   - I need to develop skills in knowing what to look for and how to evaluate what I read.
   - Mainly to be able to understand articles in professional publications.
   - I need to read journal articles in a more knowledgeable manner.
5. What do you need to know about research and why? Students of research answered:
   - Mainly, I'll need to know how to use it with a critical eye so I'll know what to incorporate and what to reject.
   - What it really is and how to use it.
   - Everything! I feel totally out of my league in research! I simply want to be able to better understand a research article or report. I want to be able to translate research articles into layman's language for staff and parents.
   - I need to better understand the terms and strategies applied in research. I have not had a statistics course since undergraduate days, if even then.
   - I would like to understand the terminology to improve my ability to read research studies.
   - I would like to learn vocabulary, principles, and processes to read and understand research.
   - I guess to be able to understand what the research studies say.
   - How to read and understand research, interpret data, and draw conclusions.
   - The language used is hard to understand.

- Terminology necessary to read and understand statistical information related to education.
- How to critique research.
- Single case designs.
- How to read research and understand it.
- Everything!
- How to understand terminology!
- How to make sense of the vocabulary and jargon of journal articles.

6. What do you see as the research needs in your field? Students of research answered:
   - I need to get a handle on statistical terms to interpret information. However, I took my last math class in 1968!
   - Relating theory to function in a concrete way.
   - To expand on our already established theory base and get more information.
   - Mainly to understand journal articles and information connected with testing.
   - We need more research on practice.
   - We need to know about research so that we can understand and convey the understanding to others.
   - Since our field is relatively new, more and more information in this area will be helpful.
   - We need research to provide support and ideas for approaches; to improve my own techniques.
   - Research related to the effectiveness of various techniques is needed.
7. What is your preferred way to learn about research? Students of research answered:
   - Something simple, applicable, and precise!
   - Reading in journals.
   - Class discussion and sharing from individual experiences. Evaluating specific research data as a group.
   - Hands on—for example, reading a well-written article so I can identify what I've finally learned. I've read so many and used nothing since I understand very little.
   - Painlessly!
   - Being led by a kind and funny instructor through the intricacies—did you know that people tend to retain information most preceding and just following laughter? Or that some people learn better if they can eat while they learn?
   - Like, I am totally ignorant of what research really is. In other words, slowly.
   - Very slowly, concretely, and easily.
   - To be given information in a systematic way that is understanding, and then when I'm involved to have someone holding my hand along the way as needed, the "TLC" approach to research.
   - I have none.
   - To have someone define and explain jargon terms.
   - By actually doing it!
   - Discussion.
8. What other comments do you have about research in general or research in your field of specialization? Students of research answered:
   - I just want to survive it!
   - I am particularly interested in asking the "So What?" question of research. If one takes time and resources to design a good research project, it must be able to stand up to the questions, Who cares? and Who will benefit from this effort?

- I want it to be applicable to my field.
- Research is intimidating; please try to lessen my insecurities and increase my esteem so that I can do this work successfully.
- I hope I can fill this questionnaire out with more intelligence by the end of this class.
- Why isn't there more emphasis on descriptive and qualitative research?
- Graduate school promotes research but presents it in a totally aversive manner.
- Should be taught more, and brought to the level of the working clinical therapist.
- I've perceived research as being difficult but necessary for our profession. I don't know how to bridge that gap, but I count on it to be applicable to clinical practice and concerns.
- We need more so we can share with others in our own field and credibly share with others outside the field, that is, parents, physicians, educators, and so on.
- I think that many people are put off or feel that research is not something they can do in practice.
- I have a lot to learn.

Were you surprised to read through other students' comments and discover that their feelings and thoughts were similar to your own? It appears that most therapists want to be able to read a research article and have some idea of what it said and how to judge or evaluate it.

Note the last comment in question 8. That student said, "I have a lot to learn." When it comes to research, just like clinical practice, we all have a lot to learn because it is a professional responsibility to continually learn more and increase our expertise. My doctoral-level training was in research methodology and statistics—you would think that would be enough training in research! But like you, I have a lot to learn and am constantly learning more about research methodology. There is no single point in time when one can say, "That's enough! I know about research!" That would be like saying, "I know enough about treatment."

We are in this together—this journey to learn more about research, especially as it relates to the fields of occupational and physical therapy. Let's explore what others—leaders in the fields of occupational and physical therapy—have to say about research. The next section of this chapter presents their responses to the Research Questionnaire.

EXPERTS SPEAK OUT

What you and your peers think about research has been addressed. Now, what do leaders in the field think? The same questionnaire was used as an interview guide with master clinicians, researchers, and research administrators from the fields of occupational therapy as well as physical therapy. The resulting interview summaries, therefore, contain insights and views of therapists whose clinical experience and skills allow them to link research to the real world of your practice.

Mary Joan Delehanty, PhD, PT

Dr. Delehanty was an assistant professor in the physical therapy program, University of Colorado, Health Science Center, Denver, Colorado. Formerly, she served as Associate Director of Education at the American Physical Therapy Association. She earned her certificate in physical therapy from Albany Medical College, her master's degree from Sargent College, and her doctorate from the State University of New York in Albany. She died July 11, 1995.

1. *What is research?*

Research is the organized and documented curiosity about our world.

2. *Why is research important?*

Research is important to pool observations to identify "truths," or at least probabilities.

3. *How do you use research?*

To profit from others' thinking and experience and to improve my own function, to direct my own exploration of the world.

4. *What are your interests regarding research?*

Collaborative research. Quantification of behavioral observations.

5. *What do you need to know about research and why?*

Where to find it. How to evaluate it.

6. *What do you see as the research needs in your field?*

We need outcome-oriented research and measurement. We need better models to address clinical questions.

7. *What is your preferred way to learn about research?*

Reading and abstracts.

8. *What other comments do you have about research in general or research in your field of specialization?*

We are involved in expanding research into all aspects of practice, including the importance of the consumer and of collaboration across and within sites.

Randi F. Jacobson, MA, PT

Ms. Jacobson is a pediatric physical therapist and former President of the Neurodevelopmental Treatment Association (NDTA), Inc. She is currently developing a private practice that includes teaching therapists in the Los Angeles area.

1. *What is research?*

Research is the systematic approach to validating or invalidating ideas, procedures, treatments, concepts, empirical knowledge, and so on. It adds to the established body of knowledge and expands that knowledge. For example, the NDTA, Inc., just published two monographs on research related to NDT.[1]

2. *Why is research important?*

It gives credence and credibility; it asks important questions leading us to ask more questions.

3. *How do you use research?*

I incorporate information gleaned from research articles into my practice and teaching as appropriate to either. Research articles have often made me stop and think and adjust my approach in both arenas.

4. *What are your interests regarding research?*

How, as a clinician, I can substantiate what I do and know empirically so that the medical and educational professionals recognize the depth and breadth of experience of my clinical contributions.

5. *What do you need to know about research and why?*

How to define and isolate a research question so I can begin to write for a journal and participate in a research project.

6. *What do you see as the research needs in your field?*

They are varied and include how the pediatric therapist affects the parent-child relationship while providing therapy to the neurologically impaired infant or child; the role that the family involvement carryover has on outcome of intervention by therapists; what role frequency of therapy plays in progress of an infant and how to separate this from a developmental process that occurs over time, and so on.

1. Royeen, C.B., and DeGangi, G. (1992). A synthesis of the NDT literature 1980–1990, inclusive. Chicago, IL: NDTA, Inc.

7. *What is your preferred way to learn about research?*

By doing it in a step-by-step format.

8. *What other comments do you have about research in general or research in your field of specialization?*

How does an experienced clinician get over the fence of procrastination and begin!

Jane Koomar, PhD, OTR, FAOTA

Dr. Koomar has had a successful private practice in the Boston area for many years. She has completed her doctorate in psychology at Boston University.

1. *What is research?*

Oh, Charlotte! Really, I just won't tackle this one!

2. *Why is research important?*

It allows us to validate our assumptions regarding theory and assess our treatment interventions.

3. *How do you use research?*

To modify my thinking, and evaluation and treatment, and to educate other professionals about my work.

4. *What are your interests regarding research?*

I am particularly interested in research related to sensory integration. Specifically outcome studies, the relationship of sensory integration problems to anxiety, and sensory profiles of adults.

5. *What do you need to know about research and why?*

I need to know how studies are designed and what statistics are used and if they are appropriate for the study so I can evaluate the usefulness of the results.

6. *What do you see as the research needs in your field?*

It is wide open; research is needed in all areas!

7. *What is your preferred way to learn about research?*

Poster presentations at conferences.

8. *What other comments do you have about research in general or research in your field of specialization?*

I would love to see a chapter written on different statistical procedures and the assumptions that cannot be violated regarding sample size, etc.

Shelly J. Lane, PhD, OTR, FAOTA

Dr. Lane is a pediatric therapist with over 15 years of experience. She was an Associate Professor of Occupational Therapy at the State University of New York at Buffalo and is currently Chair, Program in Occupational Therapy, Virginia Commonwealth University.

1. *What is research?*

Broadly defined, research is obtaining an answer to a question. More likely it is the search for answers to questions. It is an acquired skill.

2. *Why is research important?*

The importance of research lies in the expansion of knowledge produced by research. With each new piece of research we learn something more, even if that something more is only a part of the answer being sought. From a clinical perspective, research is important for answers to questions such as, What is the best approach? and What is the optimal length of time for intervention? Research, therefore, provides the foundation for our clinical work.

3. *How do you use research?*

I use research to guide intervention, to plan treatment and programming to meet the needs of the child and family. Research also helps in discussing strengths and weaknesses observed in our clients. Furthermore, research helps us to discuss "expected" or anticipated outcomes while keeping in mind that individual outcomes are always unique.

4. *What are your interests regarding research?*

Developmental problems faced by infants and young children who have a difficult start are my current interests. More specifically, I am interested in the developmental patterns and interaction skills in children drug exposed in utero and in children born prematurely. Once such patterns are identified we will have a better idea of how to plan and program for these children and to better facilitate attainment of quality of life for them.

5. *What do you need to know about research and why?*

One important concept in research is knowing what it means to "control confounding variables," or how to deal with those variables that may be confounding or contaminating your research, but that are out of your control. Poorly controlled studies, or studies that give no consideration to control issues, lack generalizability and, therefore, are not useful beyond the subjects involved in the research.

6. *What do you see as the research needs in your field?*

Study into the effects of our interventions is badly needed in all areas of practice. Such investigations are very difficult to carry out due to control issues, but are critical to our intervention planning.

7. *What is your preferred way to learn about research?*

Wouldn't it be nice to have a book with about a zillion examples of research designs that have worked, along with the statistical analyses, that you could thumb through and find one that matched your own problems? In the absence of such a book, I prefer talking out ideas with colleagues, and then following up on new design or analysis concepts by reading.

8. *What other comments do you have about research in general or research in your field of specialization?*

I think that taking the initial step is the most difficult part of doing research! Getting the first grant written or first proposal put together is the hardest. Once begun, proposal writing can be (almost) enjoyable! It can assist the researcher in refining and organizing his or her thoughts.

Even if you do not need to write a proposal, or do not need funding in order to conduct your research, I would recommend going through this type of process to get your research question refined and your thoughts organized.

The next most difficult part comes when you are seeking funding. Funding is limited. What do you do when the letter from the funding agency comes saying that your idea is good, but not good enough for funding? One thing we must learn is to not take this personally, but to read these rejections with a detached point of view and learn from feedback. A researcher must always keep in mind that money is tight, and to get funded for research you must be better than just good; and you must keep trying!

My third, and final comment is to be truly interested in what you are trying to do. How dreadful it would be to have put all the time and effort into devising a research question, learning the literature, writing the proposal and actually getting funded, only to find yourself collecting data that bores you. Data collection is time consuming, and if you are not really invested in the data, you might become sloppy and slipshod. Think carefully about your project, and be certain it is one on which you can "hang your professional hat"!

Tink Martin, MACT, PT

Ms. Martin is an Associate Professor of Physical Therapy at Indiana University and has over 20 years of experience in pediatrics. She is a past chair of the Pediatric Section of the American Physical Therapy Association, and she is the present Chair, Committee on Sections, American Physical Therapy Association.

1. *What is research?*

The collection of data regarding a subject area. Literature review, case study, and experimental design are included in research. The ability to understand research material is the basis for research.

2. *Why is research important?*

Research is important because we have to be knowledgeable consumers. We have to collect, collate, and disseminate research findings on which to predict theories of assessment and treatment.

3. *How do you use research?*

I use research to exemplify accountability in what we as health care professionals call treatment. I use it to validate theoretical frameworks for my approach to patient assessment and treatment.

4. *What are your interests regarding research?*

Natural history of pediatric disorders and disabilities. Functional skill training, transdisciplinary approaches, and entry-level textbook development.

5. *What do you need to know about research and why?*

Rules of research, types of research, how to frame the research questions—what parameters to measure to assess change that is related to function.

6. *What do you see as the research needs in your field?*

Research related to lifestyle outcomes.

7. *What is your preferred way to learn about research?*

For me, doing is always preferred over reading about. I think collaborating with colleagues and students is fun, but very time consuming.

8. *What other comments do you have about research in general or research in your field of specialization?*

We need to keep it simple for those of us who are not as knowledgeable about statistics, and we need to keep function uppermost in our minds. If possible, forget techniques and try to go after the "meat" or theory of what we do.

Virginia Scardina, OTR/L, FAOTA

Known to many as "Ginny," Ms. Scardina has worked for over 30 years in the areas of sensory integration and occupational therapy. A master clinician, she was an early and key supporter of the research of Dr. A. Jean Ayres.

1. *What is research?*

Research is a systematic experiment or investigation designed to better or more accurately interpret theories or scientific phenomena.

2. *Why is research important?*

Research directs a profession toward more accurate knowledge, practice, and thought-provoking challenges!

3. *How do you use research?*

I use research to improve my clinical practice by (a) gaining a better understanding of the human body functions, (b) advancing skills in evaluating dysfunction in clients, and (c) fostering growth in therapeutic procedures.

4. *What are your interests regarding research?*

Obtaining funds to allow clinical research to greatly increase available resources, allowing clinicians to improve their abilities and critically read research journals, and establishing a center for research in occupational therapy.

5. *What do you need to know about research and why?*

We need to know how to conduct single case study research. We, as clinicians, need to learn methods for controlled research studies. Why should we do this? There are two reasons. First, we need to be able to critique published studies. Second, we need to add to our profession's research database.

6. *What do you see as the research needs in your field?*

There are many. Just some of them are (a) studies regarding the effectiveness of sensory integrative procedures, (b) research involving the theory of occupation in rehabilitation and maintenance of health, and (c) specific studies demonstrating vestibular dysfunction's influences on the ability to cope with stress and maintain wellness.

7. *What is your preferred way to learn about research?*

Having the opportunity to accomplish the task while practicing in a clinic or completing advanced degrees.

8. *What other comments do you have about research in general or research in your field of specialization?*

Research is vital!

The needs are many and so very complex because so few funds are available that I will simply add one statement: I'm optimistic! We have accomplished so very much in the last 8 to 10 years that I know that the occupational and physical therapists of the 1990s will quadruple the number of valid investigations!

Wilma L. West

Wilma L. West has been a primary moving force in focusing and directing the field of occupational therapy toward research. She is a former president of the American Occupational Therapy Association and was, for many years, a high-level administrator in the federal government. She is now retired, living in Reston, Virginia.

1. *What is research?*

A way of discovering knowledge through systematic investigation of a problem.

2. *Why is research important?*

To learn more about how and why treatment works.

3. *How do you use research?*

For literature and historical research: To learn who said what about our profession, its fundamental beliefs, changing trends in practice and education, and emerging theories.

4. *What are your interests regarding research?*

Any and all studies reported in the literature that document efficacy of treatment.

5. *What do you need to know about research and why?*

Different methods and types of research, in order to select the type best suited to investigation of the problem under study; how to design a research study in order to conduct it properly; how to read and interpret a research report in order to apply findings appropriately.

6. *What do you see as the research needs in your field?*

More collaborative research to increase the sample size in specific diagnostic groups under study. More research responsive to requests for proposals to answer specific questions important to therapists versus bits and pieces of unrelated research.

7. *What is your preferred way to learn about research?*

Doing it, first with an established researcher.

8. *What other comments do you have about research in general or research in your field of specialization?*

It needs to include more therapists with a research degree, more faculty qualified to teach research at beginning and advanced levels, more involvement of graduate students in faculty research, more stimulation of academic and clinical therapists to do research, increased identification of researchable problems, the creation of more standardized instruments to measure phenomena of interest to therapists, and greater use of qualitative research methodologies.

Certain key issues emerge after reviewing comments from some of the leaders in occupational and physical therapy. These are

- the use of research in guiding intervention planning
- the use of research to document effectiveness of therapy services
- the use of research as consumers.

These key issues are not so different from what the students of research identified as primary interests in research. And both groups also identified the need for a step-by-step approach to understanding research that is application oriented. *The Research Primer* is intended to give you your own step-by-step process that will put an understanding of research within your reach. Let's begin.

References

Brooke, M. M., Lateur, B. D., Diana-Rigby, G. C., & Qeustad, K. A. (1991). Shoulder subluxation in hemiplegia: Effects of three different supports. *Archives of Physical Medicine and Rehabilitation, 72,* 582–586.

Corrivieau, H., Arsenault, A. B., Dutil, E., Besner, C., Dupuis, C., Guarna, F., & Lambert, J. (1992). An evaluation of the hemiplegic patient based on the Bobath approach: A reliability study. *Disability and Rehabilitation, 14,* 81–84.

DeGangi, G. A. (1994). Examining the efficiency of short term neurodevelopmental treatment intervention using a case study design: Parts 1 and 2. *Physical and Occupational Therapy in Pediatrics, 14,* 71–88(1), 21–61(2).

Jantzen, A. C. (1981). *Research: The practical approach for occupational therapy.* Laurel, MD: RAMSCO.

Recommended Readings

Mosey, A. C. (1992). Theory and basic scientific inquiry (Chapter 6, pp. 109–120), The method of science (Chapter 7, pp. 121–136), Theory and its development (Chapter 8, 137–168). In *Applied scientific inquiry in the health professions: An epistemological orientation.* Rockville, MD: American Occupational Therapy Association.

Learning Activities

1. Discuss the ways in which treatment planning is similar to the scientific method.
2. Talk with an administrator in a clinic, school, or hospital where you study or work. Ask the administrator to identify the types of research needs they see. What research data are needed to address the identified needs?
3. Answer the following questions:

   (a) What is research?

   (b) What are scientific procedures?

   (c) What is the role of theory?
4. Keep a journal over the next two weeks. In it, write down every potential research question that arises from your clinical practice or study.
5. Discuss your answers to the research questionnaire with some of your colleagues, either on the job or off. Discussing your views with others may help you clarify and refine your own thinking about research.

CHAPTER 3

Categories of Research

KEY WORDS

Applied research

Basic research

Data collection

Empirical

Evaluation research

Qualitative research

Quantitative research

Research investigation

Rigor

Scientific procedures

Scientific research

Case Study: Research Redefined?

As we saw in chapter 2, different individuals can—and will—define research differently. If you ask five clinicians how they would intervene with an individual who has suffered a right side cerebral vascular accident, for example, you would likely get five different treatment programs, depending on the therapists' frames of reference and experience, the treatment setting, and the age of the patient. And just as treatment programs for a given dysfunction may vary by therapist, definitions of research may also vary by investigator based on their experience, discipline, and specific training.

Herein lies an important distinction between two prevailing types of research today: scientific and case study research. Someone who is trained in laboratory-based **scientific research** may not consider a clinical case study—a systematic method of **data collection** lacking a formal research design—as "true" research. Yet it can be argued that much of modern psychology is based on clinical case studies; the "research" of Erickson and Freud used clinical case studies as an empirical foundation for theory building (Freud, 1924; Piaget, 1952).

PRESENTATION OF A CLINICAL CASE STUDY

Perhaps the best way to begin to understand research is to review examples illustrating the concepts of loose and more rigorous research. Clinical case study research as presented in the following example is the "loosest" or least rigorous form of research. In fact, many investigators would argue that it is not research at all. In my mind, however, such clinical investigations are research.

ILLUSTRATIVE EXAMPLE 3–1

Reprinted from *American Journal of Occupational Therapy*, July, 1981, pp. 443–450. Used with permission.

Relationship of the Southern California Sensory Integration Tests, the Southern California Postrotary Nystagmus Test, and Clinical Observations Accompanying Them to Evaluations in Otolaryngology, Ophthalmology, and Audiology: Two Descriptive Case Studies

Charlotte Brasic Royeen, George Lesinski, Sharon Ciani, David Schneider

Key words: auditory sequential memory • research • sensory integration • testing procedures • vestibular system

The Southern California Sensory Integration Tests (SCSIT), the Southern California Postrotary Nystagmus Test (SCPNT), and clinical observations accompanying these tests have been developed by Ayres as a method of evaluating sensory integrative dysfunction in learning-disabled children (1, 2). These diagnostic procedures are derived from Ayres' theory of sensory integration as proposed in her book, Sensory Integration and Learning Disorders (3). A few researchers, such as Ottenbacher (4, 5) and DeGangi (6), have attempted to clarify and identify characteristics of sensory integrative dysfunction in children.

Other researchers have begun empirical examinations by correlating the SCSIT to other tests (7). Kimball (8), correlating the SCSIT to the Bender-Gestalt, found that, since the Bender-Gestalt could predict children's performance only for certain components of the SCSIT, the Bender-Gestalt might effectively serve as a screening device for sensory integrative dysfunction if observations of the child's postural mechanisms were included. Some investigators have related the SCSIT, or components of it, to particular disabilities (7). To illustrate, Stilwell and others studied postrotary nystagmus (measured by a procedure based upon the SCPNT) as a function of communication disorders (9). It was found that hyporeactive nystagmus related to disorders of articulation and language. Other researchers, using the SCSIT as a basis for occupational therapy procedures, compared the relationship between occupational therapy and physical therapy test scores (10). They concluded that each discipline's evaluation was important.

With regard to the SCSIT, however, there is an apparent lack of cooperative research among disciplines interested in the learning-disabled child. Consequently, it is often difficult to relate characteristics of sensory integrative dysfunction, measured by the SCSIT, the SCPNT, and clinical observations accompanying these tests, to data from other professionals. Moreover, areas for further research may be defined more clearly with an interdisciplinary approach to the evaluation of sensory integrative dysfunction in the learning-disabled child. Therefore, researchers need to investigate the relationship of results of the SCSIT, the SCPNT, and clinical observations accompanying these tests to the results of other evaluations.

Ayres (11, 12) concluded that particular forms of vestibular system dysfunction, characterized by hyporeactive nystagmus, could be ameliorated by sensory integrative treatment. In consideration of the importance of a diagnosis of vestibularly based sensory integrative dysfunction (as revealed by the SCSIT, the SCPNT, and clinical observations), the medical specialty of otolaryngology should be included in an interdisciplinary evaluation. Otolaryngologists have long been involved in testing of the vestibular system, particularly since Baranay first introduced the spinning test in 1907 (13).

More recently, otolaryngologists use caloric testing with electronystagmography during evaluation of the vestibular system (14). A study by Mathog compared normal and abnormal adult males' performance during caloric and sinusoidal evaluation of the vestibular system (14). He found that use of the sinusoidal test, in addition to caloric testing, revealed a more complete understanding of the vestibular system than caloric testing alone. Therefore, in order to further examine occupational therapy procedures that theoretically examine vestibular system function, the SCPNT and clinical observations of hypersensitivity to movement and gravitational insecurity will be compared to results obtained from an otolaryngological examination.

Rotational stimulation of the horizontal semicircular canal, which occurs during any spinning test, excites neurons in the cat's hypoglossei nuclei and nuclei within the reticular formation near the abducens nucleus: these regions are thought to be important in oculomotor control (15). Since components of the SCSIT evaluate visual perception and some of the clinical observations accompanying the SCSIT evaluate visual-motor integration, ophthalmology could be used to further examine the SCSIT. Therefore, results derived from the SCSIT and clinical observations will be compared to results obtained using an ophthalmological exam.

Audiology is a third area particularly relevant to the SCSIT, SCPNT, and the clinical observations accompanying the test. Ayres (16) used an audiological test, dichotic listening, with the SCSIT to study ear advantage in learning-disabled children. She found that children with low right-left ear ratios were more likely to have language difficulty and less likely to have somatosensory problems (16). In addition, Ayres routinely used the dichotic listening test as a diagnostic tool to supplement the SCSIT, the SCPNT, and clinical observations accompanying these tests (17). Consequently, audiology was the third discipline chosen to assess the results of a sensory integrative evaluation.

Initial investigation into the relationship of the SCSIT, the SCPNT, and the clinical observations accompanying these tests to evaluations in otolaryngology, ophthalmology, and audiology will be explored by studying two descriptive case studies.

Methods

Subjects. Two learning-disabled children were subjects. Subject 1 was referred to occupational therapy because his first-grade teacher felt he was distractible, with problems in visual tracking and language skills. Subject 2 was referred to occupational therapy because a psychological evaluation revealed possible sensory integrative dysfunction. The parents, who had initially sought help when informed, thought that he would not pass fifth grade and felt him to be distractible, passive, and immature.

An occupational therapy evaluation indicating vestibularly based sensory integrative dysfunction was a criterion for subject selection. The subjects' scores on the SCSIT are presented in Table 1. Finally, parental consent to allow their child to participate in extensive and somewhat time-consuming testing was another criterion for subject selection.

Procedure. Subjects were scheduled for evaluations in otolaryngology, ophthalmology, and audiology. Except for occupational therapy, testing occurred over 2 weeks

TABLE 1
SCSIT STANDARD SCORES (S.S.) FOR SUBJECTS

Subject 1 **Age: 6 yr., 11 mo., 21 days**		**Subject 2** **Age: 10 yr., 1 mo., 24 days**	
Test	S.S.	Test	S.S.
Manual Form Perception	–1.5	Standing Balance: Eyes Closed	unable to perform
Crossing Midline	–1.3	Localization of Tactile Stimuli*	below –4.0
Crossing Midline: Crossed	–1.3	Standing Balance: Eyes Open*	–2.5
Localization of Tactile Stimuli	–1.1	Space Visualization	–2.5
Motor Accuracy: Left	–0.9	Design Copy	–1.6
Standing Balance: Eyes Closed	–0.9	Imitation of Postures*	–1.2
Finger Identification	–0.5	Crossing Midline*	–1.1
Graphesthesia	–0.5	Finger Identification*	–1.1
Standing Balance: Eyes Open	–0.2	Graphesthesia*	–0.8
Position in Space	–0.1	Motor Accuracy: Left*	–0.7
Motor Accuracy: Right	+0.0	Bilateral Motor Coordination*	–0.7
Kinesthesia	+0.0	Crossing Midline: Crossed*	–0.5
Bilateral Motor Coordination	+0.0	Figure Ground	–0.4
Space Visualization	+0.0	Kinesthesia*	–0.2
Imitation of Postures	+0.3	Manual Form Perception*	–0.1
Double Tactile Stimuli	+0.5	Right Left Discrimination*	+0.0
Design Copy	+0.9	Motor Accuracy: Right*	+0.1
Figure Ground	+1.2	Double Tactile Stimuli*	+0.2
		Position in Space	+1.0

*Indicates that the score was reported according to how a child aged 8 years-11 months (the ceiling age on these tests) would score; such scores falling in the low average range or below suggest deficit areas in child aged 10 years-1 month.

(subject 1) and 2 months (subject 2) before the testing period. Table 2 presents the specialty area, apparatus used, and method of evaluation.

Limitations of the Study. Since the current study merely initiates preliminary investigation into the SCSIT, the SCPNT, and the clinical observations accompanying these tests, two subjects were used. As such, only tentative conclusions can be made.

Interrater reliability was not computed on the more subjective testing procedures employed by the different examiners. However, each occupational therapy evaluation was performed by a therapist certified in sensory integration, and each of the other discipline's evaluations were performed by licensed professionals.

Analysis of the Data

RESULTS (SUBJECT 1)

Occupational therapy (3/27/79): Inadequate specialization of the cerebral hemispheres was indicated by Space Visualization Contralateral Hand Use Score of 27, lack of agreement for preferred hand and eye, and marginal skill in the preferred hand. Vestibular system dysfunction was indicated by hyporeactive nystagmus (SCPNT s.s. = −1.8), coupled with poor prone extension, and bilaterally involved postural mechanisms. Evidence indicates poor tactile discrimination and poor bilateral integration as well as poor ocular-motor control.

Otolaryngology (8/1/79): There is no significant spontaneous or horizontal gaze nystagmus. Dix-Hallpike and position testing were entirely normal. Hot and cold caloric testing shows no significant reduced vestibular response or directional preponderance. This is usually a normal ENG.

Ophthalmology (8/1/79): There are signs of minimal neurological involvement such as jerky eye tracking, relatively gross tracking, and midline cogwheeling. The right eye has a persistent pupillary membrane, which has created a mild amblyopia. Consequently, the subject cannot use both eyes together well.

Audiology (8/14/79): During 60 trials of the Berlin Dichotic Consonant Vowel Test presented in the simultaneous condition, the subject answered correctly 44 times with 29 right ear responses and 15 left ear responses. The Staggered Spondaic Word Test, the Speech-in-Noise Test, and the Test of Impedance Audiometry were within normal limits. However, the subject displayed total inability to perform during the Wepman and Morency Test of Auditory Sequential Memory.

RESULTS (SUBJECT 2)

Occupational therapy (6/23/79): Developmental dyspraxia was indicated by a below normal score on Imitation of Postures, Design Copy s.s. of −1.6, and marginal skill in use of both hands on Motor Accuracy. Such dyspraxia originated from poor integration of tactile and vestibular information evidenced by the following. Three of the five tactile tests were significantly low and the other two were questionable. Difficulty in processing vestibular information was evidenced by gravitational insecurity, intolerance to spinning during the SCPNT (he would not complete the test after spinning to the left), inability to perform Standing Balance with Eyes Closed, and duration of nystagmus on the SCPNT of 6 seconds after spinning to the left. The subject was tactually defensive, had poor bilateral motor coordination, poor visual spatial skills, poor ocular motor control, and inadequate hemispheric specialization indicated by a Contralateral Hand Use score on Space Visualization of 26.

Otolaryngology (8/9/79): ENG testing shows no significant spontaneous horizontal gaze nystagmus. Standard position testing and Dix-Hallpike position testing were negative. Optokinetics and pendular tracking were symmetrical. Hot and cold caloric testing demonstrated no significant reduced vestibular response or directional preponderance. This was essentially a normal ENG.

Ophthalmology (8/1/79): Normal ocular pursuits were observed. Some skipping of the midline while tracking with the eyes was evident, but this was within normal limits. Mild esophoria was noted, also within normal limits. Difficulty with visual acuity was noted with the Snellen Eye Chart.

Audiology (8/7/79): During 60 trials of the Berlin Dichotic Consonant Vowel Test in the simultaneous condition, the subject answered correctly 48 times with 22 right ear responses and 26 left ear responses, indicating a left ear advantage. The subject could not perform the Staggered Spondaic Word Test, which indicates a problem with competing type stimuli. He performed twice as poorly with his left ear as he did with his right. Speech-in-Noise Test and Test of Impedance Audiometry were within normal limits. The subject was definitely lacking in the ability to perform the Wepman and Morency Auditory Memory Test.

Discussion

Relationship of the SCPNT and Clinical Observations to the Otolaryngology Evaluation. Inspection of the data from the evaluations in occupational therapy and otolaryngology reveals contradictory information. The SCPNT evaluation on subject 1 revealed hyporeactive nystagmus (–1.8 s.s.), whereas the otolaryngology evaluation determined the subject's nystagmic response as within normal limits. Similarly, the SCPNT and clinical observations revealed subject 2 as hypersensitive to movement, gravitationally insecure and demonstrating a questionable nystagmic response (6 sec), while the otolaryngology evaluation and the nystagmic response were within normal limits. Consideration of the tests may give insight (subject 1) and 2 months (subject 2) before the testing period. Table 2 presents the specialty area, apparatus used, and method of evaluation.

Limitations of the Study. Since the current study merely initiates preliminary investigation into the SCSIT, the SCPNT, and the clinical observations accompanying these tests, two subjects were used. As such, only tentative conclusions can be made.

Differences in test mechanics should be considered. The SCPNT, like the Baranay spinning test, stimulates both of the subject's ears simultaneously, but limits caloric simulation to one ear at a time (20). The SCPNT allows for visual fixation with the subject's eyes open and the subject positioned in a light room. Conversely, ENG recorded nystagmus during caloric stimulation allows for removal of visual

TABLE 2
SPECIALTY AREA, APPARATUS USED AND METHOD OF EVALUATION

Specialty Area	Apparatus Used	Method of Evaluation
Occupational Therapy (1, 2, 3, 17)	SCSIT Test Kit SCPNT Spinning Board SCPNT Angle Guide stop watch	Southern California Sensory Integration Tests Southern California Postrotary Nystagmus Test Clinical observations of muscle tone, reflex development, ocular and oral motor control, eyes and hand preference and movement through space Developmental history
Otolaryngology (18, 19, 20)	Electronystagmographic equipment Film projector and films for optokinetic testing Irrigation equipment and temperature controlled water reservoir for caloric stimulation Lights mounted in the ceiling for eye tracking for calibration	Spontaneous nystagmus (eyes open and eyes closed) Standard position testing Dix Hallpike position testing Pendular tracking Optokinetic nystagmus Warm and cold caloric testing
Ophthalmology (21)	Snellen Eye Chart Ophthalmoscope	Snellen Chart of Visual Acuity Ophthalmoscopic examination Clinical observations of eye tracing and convergence History of visual performance
Audiology (20, 22)	Grason Stadler Sudiometer 1701	Berlin Dichotic Consonant Vowel Test Staggered Spondaic Word Test Speech in Noise Test Impedance Audiometry Wepman and Morency Auditory Memory Span Text

fixation by having the subject close his eyes while positioned in a darkened room; this allows for a greater and more easily measured nystagmus (20). The SCPNT has the subject perform no concentration task and therefore allows for central suppression of nystagmus. During otolaryngological examination, in order to minimize central suppression of nystagmus, the subject is instructed to perform a concentration task aloud (20). Consequently, the combination of differences on test mechanics may account for the discrepant results between evaluations in occupational therapy and otolaryngology.

The SCPNT measures duration of nystagmus, whereas electronystagraphy during caloric stimulation measures amplitude of nystagmus. During occupational therapy clinical observations, the subject's physiological and emotional responses to movement are monitored. These aspects are not monitored during the otolaryngological examination. Thus, it may be that during occupational therapy clinical observations of a subject's emotional and physiological responses to movement, different aspects of vestibular system functioning are considered which are as important as the nystagmic response for diagnosis of vestibular dysfunction (23).

Differences in the normative sample must also be considered as possible reasons for differences in the occupational therapy and otolaryngology test results. The results of the occupational therapy evaluation were compared to norms developed by Ayres and replicated by Royeen for children ages five through nine (2, 24). Inspection of some of the research from which otolaryngology derives normative data revealed the youngest subject to be 19 (25). Consequently, the otolaryngological evaluation uses adult norms as a reference, whereas the occupational evaluation uses children's norms. This difference may account for the discrepancy between the evaluation results in occupational therapy and otolaryngology.

Finally, the following statement implies the possibility of caloric-rotational dissociation.

Occasionally, the caloric and rotational test results do not agree. For example, there may be a rotational directional preponderance but not a caloric directional preponderance; or there may be a caloric bilateral weakness but normally intense rotational nystagmus. Animal experiments suggest that such caloric-rotational dissociation may be a central sign. However, this possibility has not been systematically studied in humans. (25, p. 750)

M. H. Stroud found that caloric abnormalities persisted longer than postrotary abnormalities (caloric-rotational dissociation) when brainstem lesions were performed on cats (26).

It is provisionally hypothesized that a similar phenomenon, dissociation or lack of agreement between caloric and spinning tests, may also occur in learning-disabled children and hence, explain why the results were discrepant between the otolaryngology and occupational therapy evaluations.

In additional, it should be noted that the duration of nystagmus as measured by the SCPNT may, in fact, have no direct correlation with the vestibular system. Rather, it may reflect the subject's state of central altering, anxiety, visual acuity, and ability to visually fixate and suppress nystagmus more accurately than it directly measures vestibular system integrity.

The need for continued research in this area is the major conclusion drawn from this discussion regarding the discrepancy between the evaluation results in occupational therapy and otolaryngology. A study with a large enough sample to allow for statistical analysis investigating the correlation between caloric testing and the SCPNT is needed. Also, research investigating the reliability of the SCPNT with a learning-disabled population needs to be conducted in order to determine if central alerting and anxiety of the subject significantly affect the SCPNT's reliability. In conjunction with otolaryngologists, occupational therapy researchers may develop normative data and operationally define procedures for measurement of hypersensitivity to movement (physiological response) and gravitational insecurity (emotional response) to movement. Finally, norms for children tested by caloric stimulation may be further developed.

Relationship of the SCSIT and Clinical Observations to the Ophthalmology Evaluations. Generally, there was agreement between the occupational therapy and ophthalmology evaluation concerning subject 1, and disagreement between the evaluations concerning subject 2, Occupational therapy clinical observations of subject 1 revealed poor ocular motor control as evidenced by his inability to smoothly cross the midline with his eyes. In addition, the ophthalmological evaluation revealed that the subject could not smoothly track an object across the horizontal plane with his eyes, and that the subject was probably amblyopic due to a persistent pupillary membrane in his right eye.

However, consideration of the evaluation results of subject 2 disclosed the following discrepancies between the occupational therapy and ophthalmology evaluations. First, occupational therapy clinical observations revealed that the subject frequently manifested a midline skip while tracking an object with his eyes. Ophthalmology evaluation revealed that the subject manifested a midline skip but aged the problem to be within normal limits. Second, the occupational therapy clinical observations and poor overall quality of the object's eye tracking. The ophthalmology evaluation found the subject's eye tracking ability within normal limits. Third, occupational therapists clinically observed that object 2 had difficulty with eye convergence was within normal limits. Of additional interest was the tentative finding by the ophthalmologist that subject 2's actual acuity was depressed; a full eye examination was prescribed. Upon hearing this, the subject's mother commented, "I'm surprised, he is always the first one to read the road signs." It may be that the subject's very poor visual spatial skills, as indicated during occupational therapy evaluation of a Space Visualization s.s. of –2.5, affected his ability to perform visual acuity tasks as tested by the ophthalmologists. One explanation for the discrepancies in evaluations by the ophthalmologist and occupational therapist can be testing error by the occupational therapist. Or, it may be that the lack of standardized norms and consequent use of clinical judgment by the occupational therapist and the ophthalmologist allowed them to view the phenomenon differently. What one professional considers abnormal may be considered normal by the other. Thus, it may be that in working with a population of learning-disabled children, occupational therapists are evaluating and judging very subtle problems, whereas the ophthalmologist may be evaluating from a reference point of pathology and disease. Additionally, many learning-disabled children are inconsistent in their responses and may vary in performance from day to day. Such fluctuation in performance might account for the discrepancy.

Unfortunately, none of these explanations can be appraised empirically due to the lack of experimental data on the subject. Instead, operationally defined procedures of ocular performance in children may offer more objective meaningful information.

Relationship of the SCSIT, the SCPNT, and clinical observations accompanying these tests to the Audiology Evaluation. Among the auditory tests administered, both subjects performed poorest during the Wepman and Morency Test of Auditory Sequential Memory. Subject 1 could not perform the task at all and subject 2 scored well below minus 1 standard deviation. In consideration of this, and in consideration of the possible vestibular system dysfunction common to each subject, the correlation between vestibular system functioning and auditory sequential memory abilities needs further investigation. The possibility of such a correlation is especially important in consideration of recent research by Fishbein (27). He discovered that young, learning-disabled children with relatively strong auditory memory skills benefited most from an intervention program using braille as a tactual modality for language instruction. Those learning-disabled children not benefiting from such an intervention program might display signs of possible vestibular system dysfunction in conjunction with poor auditory sequential memory.

The other auditory test that was atypical for both subjects was the Berlin Dichotic Consonant Vowel Test, which is a form of a dichotic listening test. Subject one obtained a right-to-left ear ratio of 1.9. This is a very high score that can be considered abnormal (28). Subject 2 obtained left-to-right ear ratio of 1.1, which indicated atypical lateralization of language (17). Results of the Berlin Dichotic Consonant Vowel Test on Subject 2 are similar to the findings of Pettit and Helms, who reported that children with language disorders do not have lateralized cerebral dominance for language (29).

In spite of these findings, the experimental nature of the dichotic listening test must be remembered; however, its possible value as a clinical tool must not be underestimated. This sentiment is summarized as follows:

Although the dichotic listening test is primarily a research tool with little practical application, limited longitudinal testing, and considerable controversy regarding its interpretation, theoretically it provides a measure of asymmetry of ear perception. Dichotic listening represents a new approach for investigating hemispheric specialization and its development in children. (30, p 28)

Again, consideration of the possible vestibular system dysfunction common to both subjects, the correlation between vestibular system functioning and the dichotic listening test, reflecting lateralization of language, needs to be further investigated.

Implications for Occupational Therapy

In reflecting upon the results of the two descriptive case studies, two implications for occupational therapists are evident. First, occupational reports delineating the results of evaluations must necessarily include the specification of the procedures used. Therapists should understand the tests and clinical observations they use, as well as somewhat understand tests used by those in other disciplines. Therefore, when our findings do not corroborate with the findings of other disciplines, therapists can begin to understand why.

Second, therapists need to develop continued collaborative research with other disciplines. Many of the areas targeted for future research may be best investigated by an interdisciplinary team. Only by effective communication and research with other disciplines can occupational therapists achieve their maximum potential.

Summary

This preliminary study investigated the relationship between the results of two SCSITs with the results of evaluations in the areas of otolaryngology, ophthalmology, and audiology. Generally, there was little agreement between the evaluation results of otolaryngology and occupational therapy. Occupational therapists and ophthalmologists were in partial agreement over the results. Considering the results of audiology and occupational therapy evaluations, particular tests in audiology were atypical for both subjects. Reasons for the lack of agreement between evaluations were discussed. Areas of future research to help resolve the discrepancies were delineated. Finally, implications for occupational therapy were presented.

Acknowledgments

Appreciation is extended to Elizabeth Newcomber, OTR, M.Ed., for assistance in testing and data analysis.

References

1. Ayres AJ: California Sensory Integration Test Manual, Los Angeles: Western Psychological Services, 1972.
2. Ayres AJ: Southern California Postrotary Nystagmus Test Manual, Los Angeles: Western Psychological Services, 1975.
3. Ayres AJ: Sensory Integration and Learning Disorders, Los Angeles: Western Psychological Services, 1973.
4. Ottenbacher K: Identifying vestibular system processing in the learning-disabled child. Am J Occup Ther 32: 217–221, 1978.
5. Ottenbacher K, Watson PJ, Short MA: Association between nystagmus and hyporesponsivity and behavioral problems in learning-disabled children. Am J Occup Ther 33: 317–322, 1979.
6. DeGangi GA, Berk RA, Larsen LA: The measurement of vestibularly based functions in pre-school children. Am J Occup Ther 34: 452–459, 1980.
7. Price A, Gilfoyle E, Myers C (Editors): Research in Sensory Integration, Rockville, MD: American Occupational Therapy Association, 1976.
8. Kimball JG: The Southern California Sensory Integration Tests (Ayres) and the Bender-Gestalt: A correlative study. Am J Occup Ther 31: 294–298, 1977.
9. Stilwell JM, Crowe TK, McCallum LW: Postrotary nystagmus duration as a function of communication disorders. Am J Occup Ther 32: 222–228, 1978.
10. Foppe KB, Brooks C, Gersten JW, Maxwell S: The relationship between occupational therapy and physical therapy test scores in children with learning disabilities Am J Occup Ther 30: 163–166, 1976.
11. Ayres AJ: The Effect of Sensory Integrative Therapy on Learning Disabled Children: The Final Report of a Research Project, Los Angeles: Center for the Study of Sensory Integrative Dysfunction and University of Southern California, 1976.
12. Ayres AJ: Learning disorders and the vestibular system. Learning Disabil 11: 18–29, 1978.
13. Krynycky A, Mattuci KF: Electronystomography in the examination of the dizzy patient. Ear, Nose Throat J 58: 41–51, 1979.

14. Mathog RH: Testing of the vestibular system by sinusoidal angular acceleration. Acta Otolaryngol 74: 96–103, 1972.

15. Fukushima Y, Igusa Y, Yoshida K: Characteristics of responses of medial brain stem neurons to horizontal head angular acceleration and electrical stimulation of the labyrinth in the cat. Brain Res 120: 564–570, 1977.

16. Ayres AJ: Dichotic listening performance in learning disabled children. Am J Occup Ther 31: 441–446, 1977.

17. Ayres AJ: Interpreting the Southern California Sensory Integration Tests, Los Angeles: Western Psychological Services, 1976.

18. Ransome J, Holdon H, Bull TR (Editors): Recent Advances in Otolaryngology, Edinburgh and London: Churchill Livingston, 1973. Chapters 7 and 8.

19. Ballinger JJ (Editor): Diseases of the Nose, Throat and Ear, Philadelphia: Lea and Febiger, 1977, Chapter 43.

20. Bradford LJ (Editor): Physiologic Measures of the Audio-Vestibular System, New York: Academic Press, 1975, Chapter 3.

21. Walsh TJ: Neuro-ophthalmology: Clinical Signs and Symptoms, Philadelphia: Lea and Febiger, 1978, Chapters 9, 10 and 23.

22. Keither RW (Editor): Central Auditory Dysfunction, New York: Grune and Stratton, 1977, Chapters 1, 4, 5, and 7.

23. Katz J (Editor): Handbook of Clinical Audiology, Baltimore: Williams and Wilkins, 1972. pp. 480–490.

24. Royeen CB: Investigation of the test-retest reliability of the Southern California postrotary nystagmus test. Am J Occup Ther 34: 37–39: Addendum 34: 215, 1980.

25. Coats AC: Vestibulometry. In Diseases of the Nose, Throat and Ear, JJ Ballinger (Editor). Philadelphia: Lea and Febiger, 1977, pp. 725–755.

26. Stroud MH, Marovitz WF, Leyton OC: Vestibular dysfunction after midline lesions in the brain stem of the cat. Ann Otolaryngol 80: 750–758, 1971.

27. Fishbein HD: Braille-phonics: A new technique for aiding the reading disabled. J Learning Disabil 12: 69–73, 1979.

28. Ayres AJ: Cluster analysis of measures of sensory integration. Am J Occup Ther 31: 362–366, 1977.

29. Petit JM, Helms SB: Hemispheric language dominance of language-disordered, articulation disordered, and normal children. J Learning Disabil 12: 12–17, 1979.

30. Kawar M: The effects of sensorimotor therapy on children with learning disabilities. In Research in Sensory Integrative Development, A price, E Gilfoyle, C Myers, Editors. Rockville, MD: American Occupational Therapy Association, 1976.

Illustrative Example 3–1: Discussion

This clinical case study report was based on findings regarding two subjects. No established research design was used in the investigation. Simply, the case investigators addressed the question, Will the findings on the subjects using the Southern California Sensory Integration Tests (SCSIT; Ayres, 1975), the Southern California Postrotary Nystagmus Test (SCPNT; Ayres, 1989), and accompanying clinical observations agree with the findings from ophthalmology, otolaryngology, and audiology? Two different subjects were tested in all areas and the results compared logically in prose format. Discrepancies in the findings were identified and implications discussed.

The article's lack of statistical analysis is typical of case study investigations. If you are planning on eventually writing a term paper or master's thesis, such a loose definition of research would probably not suffice. In this case, a more rigorous[1] method or procedure to define research may be required.

The following article illustrates research that used a more rigorous standard or definition of research, characterizing the latter view. Note the more systematic method of data collection used in this investigation.

1. This may be defined as tightly controlled.

Reprinted from *American Journal of Occupational Therapy,* January, 1980, pp. 37–39. Used with permission.

ILLUSTRATIVE EXAMPLE 3–2

Factors Affecting Test-Retest Reliability of the Southern California Postrotary Nystagmus Test

Charlotte Brasic Royeen

Key words: sensory integration • test reliability • pediatrics

More effective clinical use of the Southern California Postrotary Nystagmus Test (SCPNT) may result if factors affecting test reliability were known. An experiment, a pilot study involving primary grade students, was designed to assess whether time of day or sex affected the test. The SCPNT was administered at a 2-week interval to 12 boys and 12 girls and subject responses were noted and compiled. Pearson Correlation Coefficients revealed high reliability for all conditions. No significant differences existed for sex or time of retest. Responses to the SCPNT revealed that it was typical for a subject to demonstrate pleasure but not typical to show alarm, threat, or loss of body balance while rotating.

In recent years there has been increasing interest in the vestibular system, the system that perceives movement and gravity. It has profound effects upon physical development, behavior, and learning. The relationship of the vestibular system and equilibrium reactions has been accepted since the 1800s (1). Investigations of the vestibular system's relationship to equilibrium reactions involving locomotion, posture and neck musculature of cats have highlighted the importance of the vestibular system on head and neck control and normal gait patterns (2). Studies of the vestibular system reveal that it has a modulating influence on other sensory systems (3-5). This modulating influence is frequently altered in behavior disorders such as infantile autism (6) and adult schizophrenia (2).

de Quiros (7,8) and Ayres (9) have postulated the importance of the vestibular system in language development and learning. de Quiros suggested that the vestibular system plays a key role in the development of postural control, and that as postural control becomes automatic, cortical levels can be used for higher levels of learning (10). Ayres hypothesizes that the vestibular system is important for learning due to its role in organization of higher levels of the nervous system (11).

Given the possible importance of the vestibular system, how does one test its integrity?

Because of the intricate relationship between the eye muscles and the vestibular system, the eyes are a visual key to the vestibular system. Nystagmus, a rhythmical back and forth motion of the eyes, is an optic reflex in response to spinning. Ayres published a standardized procedure in scoring method for evaluating nystagmic response to spinning in children aged five through nine called the Southern California Postrotary Nystagmus Test (SCPNT) (12).

The nystagmic reflex is a neurophysiologic response susceptible to fluctuating levels of central nervous system excitability. For example, just as blood pressure varies somewhat throughout the course of a day depending upon stress and physical exertion, so too nystagmic responses may vary somewhat, depending upon excitatory levels of the central nervous system. Because of this possible variance, the average of two SCPNT administrations is computed in lieu of reliance upon one test only. It has not been determined, however, whether the second test should be administered at the same time of day as the first test. Consistency in time of retest would ensure an attempt to retest a client at similar levels of central nervous system excitability. For example, a child would likely have lower excitability levels before lunch than after lunch if one considers the stimulation of a noisy lunchroom and an active recess. The present study was designed to assess the effects, if any, of time of retest (same or different) on retest reliability.

SCPNT norms show that girls tended to show a lesser duration of nystagmus than boys (12). Would girls be likely to also have a different retest reliability from boys? If so, fluctuation of SCPNT scores should be interpreted differently for girls than boys. To ascertain the effect of sex on retest reliability, sex (male or female) was used as a factor.

Ayres comments on the following responses to the SCPNT by the children in her sample (12): maintenance of balance upon the cessation of rotation, maintenance of head balance upon cessation of rotation, mild vertigo, slight dizziness, and pleasure. It seemed necessary to observe and record these responses in order to more clearly establish atypical responses to the SCPNT.

Method

Subjects. Twenty-four subjects, 12 boys and 12 girls, aged 6 and 7 were used in this study. All were pupils at a small parochial school, and they were selected on the basis of age.

Research Design and Apparatus. Two independent variables (time of retest and sex) were varied two ways (same time retest or different time retest, male and female) to create four experimental conditions. One SCPNT board, one SCPNT scoring manual, a stopwatch, and an angle guide were used during testing.

Procedure. The test were administered in a quiet room by two examiners. Duration of nystagmus was recorded. Observations were made of the subject's loss of body balance while turning, loss of body balance upon stopping, loss of head position while turning, loss of head position upon stopping, vertigo, dizziness, nausea, alarm and pleasure. These responses were scored three, if not observed; two, if slightly indicated: and one, if definitely noted. Vertigo, dizziness, and nausea were determined by asking the child, "Is the room spinning?" (vertigo), "Does your head feel funny?" (dizziness), and "Does your tummy feel funny?" (nausea). Alarm was noted if sympathetic nervous system reactions were observed and pleasure was noted when smiling, giggling, and a desire to continue spinning were observed.

Subjects were individually tested in the morning and were retested two weeks later. Half of them were retested in the morning the same time of day as the first test, and half were retested in the afternoon at a different time of day from the first test. All testing occurred during regular school hours (8 to 3). Administration of the SCPNT was according to the standardized procedure in the SCPNT manual and as taught by the certification faculty from the Center for the Study of Sensory Integrative Dysfunction (CSSID).

Limitations of This Study

This study was restricted to normal primary school children and no screening procedures were used in selecting the sample.

An interrater reliability coefficient for the scores of the two administrators was not computed. However, standardized procedures were adhered to and both examiners were experienced.

Operationally defined procedures for measuring dizziness, body balance, head control, nausea, pleasure and alarm were not used. Instead, clinical judgment, as formed by the guidelines from CSSID and the SCPNT manual, was followed.

Results

Mean scores for this sample were computed and compared with mean scores of Ayres' sample in Table 1. Because of hypersensitivity, one subject was not able to complete the SCPNT and therefore was excluded when the means were computed.

Observations of the nonnystagmic responses to the SCPNT were compiled. Twenty-three children had a pleasurable reaction to the SCPNT. The child not able to complete the SCPNT was the only child to lose body balance while turning and to exhibit alarm.

Nine of the 24 children experienced transient vertigo. Nine children lost their head balance while turning. Nine children lost body balance when spinning stopped. Ten subjects experienced transient nausea, 14 lost head balance upon cessation of spinning, and 16 experienced dizziness.

Pearson Correlation Coefficients (r's) were computed for retest reliability of all four experimental conditions and for all conditions combined. Twenty-two subjects were used in the correlations; another subject was dropped in order to have equally sized groups for retest conditions, i.e., same time of retest or different time of retest. Coefficients were calculated in three categories: standard score for nystagmus to the left, standard score for nystagmus to the right, and standard score for total nystagmus. These coefficients are presented in Table 2, and show acceptable retest reliability for every condition but especially for correlations of retest total scores (0.8524, 0.8379, 0.8514, 0.8537, 0.8535) across all conditions. The significance of the correlations for retest at the same time and retest at a different time was computed since these two correlations were the most likely to yield significance. The significance was analyzed using Fisher's transformation of coefficients and the test for difference between independent correlations (13). No significant differences were revealed ($z = 1.168$; $p > .05$); therefore, there were no significance differences in retest reliability considering sex or time of retest.

Discussion

Table 1 reveals that the sample for this pilot study shows means similar to the sample in the SCPNT manual. Discrepancy does occur within the category with the smallest number of subjects from this study. Small sample size may account for the discrepancy.

TABLE 1
COMPARISON OF MEAN SCORES OF SAMPLE IN AYRES' SOUTHERN CALIFORNIA NYSTAGMUS TEST MANUAL (*N*=90) AND OF MEAN SCORES OF SAMPLES IN THIS STUDY (*N*=23)

Study	Comparison of Scores							
Subjects (age in years)	Male (6)		Female (6)		Male (7)		Female (7)	
No. Subjects Ayres, 1975	21		24		19		26	
No. Subjects This Study	9		5		3		6	
	Duration of Nystagmus, Mean of Spins to the Left							
		S.D.		S.D.		S.D.		S.D.
Ayres, 1975	10.1	5.3	9.8	4.0	9.2	4.6	8.7	3.7
This Study	9.7	4.2	9.0	3.1	13.3	2.8	9.1	2.9
	Duration of Nystagmus, Mean of Spins to the Right							
		S.D.		S.D.		S.D.		S.D.
Ayres, 1975	10.0	4.0	8.5	3.2	9.4	2.5	7.8	2.6
This Study	10.7	5.2	9.4	3.5	15.6	4.2	8.6	4.0
	Duration of Nystagmus, Mean of Total Spins							
		S.D.		S.D.		S.D.		S.D.
Ayres, 1975	20.1	8.7	18.3	6.9	18.6	6.5	16.5	6.0
This Study	20.4	9.0	18.4	6.0	28.9	5.6	17.7	6.4

TABLE 2
PEARSON CORRELATION COEFFICIENTS

	N = 22	*N* = 10	*N* = 12	*N* = 11	*N* = 11
	ALL SUBJECTS	FEMALES	MALES	RETEST SAME TIME	RETEST DIFFERENT TIME
TEST LEFT/RETEST LEFT	0.8430	0.7999	0.8747	0.8087	0.9050
TEST RIGHT/RETEST RIGHT	0.7284	0.6741	0.7534	0.6072	0.8585
TEST TOTAL/RETEST TOTAL	0.8524	0.8379	0.8514	0.8537	0.8535

Results indicate that for this normal population it is atypical to lose body balance while turning to experience alarm or threat in response to the SCPNT. Moreover, it is typical for the subject to experience pleasure in response to the test.

Table 2 reveals that the 9 Pearson Correlation Coefficients are all high, indicating a dependable test not affected by the factors of time of the test administration or sex of the subject. The reliability scores are indications of even greater test reliability if one considers that reliability scores are regarded as the lower boundaries of test reliability (14).

The lack of significance in retest reliability of boys and girls reveals that the SCPNT is as reliable for males as it is for females.

Conclusions

This pilot study indicates that test-retest reliability of the SCPNT is not affected by the time of retest or sex of the subject. Further research is necessary to determine if these findings are consistent for a learning-disabled population.

The study also indicates that lack of pleasure, the presence of alarm, and the loss of body balance while turning are atypical responses to the SCPNT. Further research is necessary to confirm these findings and refine them into diagnostic indicators for vestibular system dysfunction.

Acknowledgments

This research was conducted to fulfill requirements for a class at the University of Cincinnati. Appreciation is extended to Elizabeth Newcomer, OTR, M.Ed., CSSID certification faculty member, for assistance in administration of the test, to Steven Howe for assistance in statistical design and analysis, and to Virginia Scardina, OTR, M.A., for her guidance.

A special thank you to Sister Edward, the staff, and students of Saint Boniface School, Cincinnati, Ohio.

References

1. Jones CL: *Equilibrium and Vertigo,* Philadelphia: Lippincott and Co., 73-80. 1918
2. Wilson VJ. Marda M: Connections between the semicircular canals and neck motorneurons in the cat. *Neurophysiol:* 37: 346-357, 1974

3. Schilder P: The vestibular apparatus in neurosis and psychosis. *J. Nerv Ment Dis* 78: 1-23, 1933

4. Angyal A, Sherman MA: Postural reaction to vestibular stimulation in Schizophrenic and normal subjects. *Am J Psychiatr* 98: 857-862, 1942.

5. Ornitz EM: The modulation of sensory input and motor output in autistic children. *J Autism Child Schizophrenia* 4: 197-215, 1974

6. Ritvo ER, Ornitz EM, Evitar A, Markham CH, Brown MB, Mason A: Decreased postrotary nystagmus in early infantile autism. *Neurol* 19: 653-658, 1969

7. de Quiros JB: Vestibular and proprioceptive integration, its influence on learning and speech in children. In Proceedings of the 10th InterAmerican Congress of Psychology, Lima, Peru 1966

8. de Quiros JB: Diagnosis of vestibular disorders in the learning disabled. *J Learning Disabil* 9: 39-47, 1976

9. Ayres AJ: *Sensory Integration and Learning Disabilities.* Los Angeles, CA: Western Psychological Services, 1973

10. de Quiros JB: Neurophysiological Fundamentals in Learning Disabilities, San Rafael, CA: *Academic Therapy.* 1978

11. Ayres AJ: *Interpretation Manual of the Southern California Sensory Integration Tests,* Los Angeles, CA: Western Psychological Services, 1978

12. Ayres AJ: *Southern California Postrotary Nystagmus Test Manual,* Los Angeles, CA: Western Psychological Services, 1975

13. Brunning JL, Kintz BL: *Computational Handbook of Statistics.* Glenville, IL: Scott, Foresman and Co., 1968.

14. Nunnally JC: *Psychometric Theory,* Philadelphia: McGraw Hill, 1967, p. 214

Illustrative Example 3–2: Discussion

This pilot investigation looked into the test-retest reliability of this assessment. The investigation was called a pilot because it was small in sample size and had been set up as a preliminary to further investigation into the SCPNT. Factors that could theoretically influence test performance were investigated: time of test on retest and sex of the student being tested.

The investigation was designed to then determine the effect of these factors, or variables, on test performance. Half of the subjects were therefore retested at the same time of day as the initial test (morning) and half retested at a different time of day (afternoon). Even numbers of males and females were used to look at differences in retest performance by sex. This produced four experimental conditions: (1) males, retested at same time, (2) males, retested at different time, (3) females, retested at same time, (4) females, retested at different time.

Correlations were computed to determine how reliably the subjects' first test scores correlated with the second test scores for all experiential conditions. Correlations were found to be high for all four conditions (.80 or higher). The differences between correlations of each condition were tested and no significant differences were found. This means that there were no significant effects of time of test or sex of subject. The results suggest that the test is very reliable and that time of retest or sex of subject does not affect test results.

Do you have an idea of the difference in rigor between the two examples? The first example was a clinical case study, whereas the second was based on a correlational research design, which had a research design underpinning it that you could actually draw or graph out. The research design allowed for more **rigor,** or more understanding of the relationship between variables.

You may have guessed by now that research is not a concrete entity. There are many, many varieties of research. Just as one can reasonably discuss discrepancies between diagnostic categories of clients, one can similarly discuss discrepancies about what is and what is not research. In this book, we will take a middle-of-the-road approach, that is, we will define and accept as research almost any form of data collection that uses some sort of systematic data collection method. To illustrate, if you asked every third person in your class or in your clinic the question, What is research? you would be collecting data in some sort of systematic fashion, or, conducting some sort of research.

Other Categories of Research

Given the variations in defining what is and is not research, you may not be surprised to discover that there are also many ways to categorize research. We are all used to categorizing clients in multiple ways, such as by "patterns of function and dysfunction" or in terms of "disease or pathology." Similarly, there are many ways to categorize or pigeonhole research. One of the most common and best understood categorizations is that of basic versus applied research.

BASIC VERSUS APPLIED RESEARCH

Yerxa (1981) defines **basic research** as that which develops new knowledge. Basic research does not seek to answer clinically relevant questions, but seeks to accumulate knowledge simply for the sake of knowledge. Yet such knowledge may have profound implications for practice at a later date. This is a criterion for basic research. On the other hand, **applied research** is that which has immediate benefits, meaning that it can be immediately applied for practical use. Dunn (1985) and Jantzen (1981) suggest that research is simply a way to find answers to practice-driven questions; they are, therefore, using research to mean applied research.

The previous examples were of applied research. Review these examples again. You can see how information from each article has immediate clinical application. Results of the research done in the first example could be used by clinicians to better understand the measurement of sensory integrative and related processes in children. And the information obtained from the research described in the second example could be used to further justify the reliability of a commonly used test, the SCPNT (Ayres, 1975).

The distinction between basic and applied research can be blurred and somewhat artificial, depending on the actual nature of the research investigation. For further clarification, additional examples of basic research are presented in Figure 3–1.

In Figure 3–1, all the examples are investigations of a phenomenon or behavior (hand strength, motor coordination, play behavior, textural perception). Nothing in the topics of the investigations identifies or implies any clinical application. As previously suggested, there may well be theoretical application or clinical application in the future, but nothing that can be used in your clinic tomorrow morning.

Thus, the studies presented in Figure 3–1 are examples of basic research. Recall that we defined basic research as having no immediate clinical application. But it may well set the stage for future work that will have great clinical application. Research in the areas of motor learning (Schmidt, Lange, & Young, 1990) and occupation science at the University of Southern California are two additional examples of basic science research being done now in the fields of occupational and physical therapy.

Let's now look at some examples of applied research (Figure 3–2). The examples of applied research presented in Figure 3–2 have, as a primary intent, development of knowledge that is directly clinically applicable, that is, you can use it in your clinic tomorrow. For example, the validity study by Fisher, Mixon, and Herman (1988) could enhance your ability to discuss a child's vestibular system problem with his parents. Or you might be better able to predict when your client can realistically return to work based on the study done by Smith, Cunningham and Weinberg (1986). You could try with a female adolescent client the program described and tested by Storer, Bates, McGhee, and Dycus (1984).

FIGURE 3–1. EXAMPLES OF BASIC RESEARCH

Research Investigation	Topic
Bowman and Katz (1984)	Studied hand strength and prone extension patterns in normal children.
Cermak, Ward, and Ward (1986)	Studied the correlation between motor coordination and articular disorders in children.
Kielhofner, Barris, Bauer, Shoestock, and Walker (1983)	Studied play behavior in hospitalized and nonhospitalized children.

FIGURE 3–2. EXAMPLES OF APPLIED RESEARCH

Research Investigation	Topic
Fisher, Mixon, and Herman (1988)	Studied the validity of a clinical diagnosis of vestibular dysfunction.
Smith, Cunningham, and Weinberg (1986)	Studied the ability of the Functional Capacities Scale to predict when a client could return to work.
Storer, Bates, McGhee, and Dycus (1984)	Studied the effectiveness of a program designed to reduce self stimulation in a retarded female.

FIGURE 3–3. EXAMPLES OF PROFESSIONAL RESEARCH

Research Investigation	Topic
Coleman (1984)	Studied development of the profession of occupational therapy in terms of a conflict between populist and elitist viewpoints.
Parker and Chan (1986)	Studied perception of occupational and physical therapists regarding the degree of prestige associated with the professions.
Royeen (1984)	Studied the profile of therapists desiring certification by Sensory Integration International.
Royeen, Koomar, Cromack, Fortune, and Domkey (1991)	Showed the validity of the Sensory Integration and Praxis Competency Exam by differential performance on the exam by group (subjects with no experience, subjects with little experience, and subjects qualified to take the exam).

RESEARCH IN OCCUPATIONAL AND PHYSICAL THERAPY

Another category of research is that which investigates the profession itself. For example, if you wish to know why occupational and physical therapists are predominately female, or if you wish to know how occupational and physical therapists learn best, you could conduct research that examines the profession itself. Examples of research into occupational and physical therapy professions are presented in Figure 3–3.

Figure 3–3 reveals that a range of topics of researchable issues exists in the professions of occupational and physical therapy. We will now consider another category of research.

EVALUATION RESEARCH

Another type of research is that which determines the worth or value of a project or program (Suarez, 1982, pp. 193–215). Whereas other forms of research are, supposedly, value free, **evaluation research** is designed to render a value judgment about whether or not a program or project is working, and whether it is worth the cost. Quality assurance (QA) may be considered to be a specialized type of evaluation research (Joe, 1991). Many new developments in the field of research are blending applied research with evaluation research. Action research, intended to change policy at the level of the institution or at regional, state, or federal government levels, is one such example (Ciechalski, 1990). In the field of occupational and physical therapy, there has been relatively little evaluation research. It is a challenge to do more (Royeen, 1986).

QUANTITATIVE VERSUS QUALITATIVE RESEARCH

Simply stated, **quantitative research** is a "formal, objective, systematic process in which numerical data are utilized to obtain information about the world" (Burns & Grove, 1987). Quantitative research is based on the scientific method and scientific procedures. Categories of quantitative research—descriptive, experimental and quasiexperimental, and single subject—will be addressed in chapters 8, 9, and 10, respectively. **Qualitative research** is the "systematic, subjective approach to describe life experiences and give them meaning" (Burns & Grove, 1987). The qualitative approach does not seek to describe, identify, or quantify, but rather to increase understanding. Qualitative research is further discussed in chapter 8.

References

Ayres, A. J. (1974). *The development of sensory integrative theory and practice.* Dubuque, Iowa: Kendall/Hunt.

Bowman, O. J., & Katz, B. (1984). Hand strength and prone extension in right dominant 6 to 9 year olds. *American Journal of Occupational Therapy, 38,* 367–376.

Burns, N., & Grove, S. K. (1987). *The practice of nursing research: Conduct, critique, and utilization.* Philadelphia: W. B. Saunders.

Cermak, S. A., Ward, E. A., & Ward, L. M. (1986). The relationship between articulation disorders and motor coordination in children. *American Journal of Occupational Therapy, 40,* 546–550.

Clark, F. A., Parkham, D., Carlson, M. E., Frank, G., Jackson, J, Pierce, D., Wolfe, R. J., Zemke, R. (1991). *American Journal of Occupational Therapy, 45(4)* 300–310.

Ciechalski, J. C. (1990). Action research, the mann-whitney u, and thou. *Elementary School Guidance and Counseling, 25,* 54–63.

Coleman, W. (1984). The study of educational policy setting in occupational therapy: 1918–1981 [Microfilm # 8421435]. Ann Arbor, MI: University Microfilms International.

Dunn, W. (1985). Occupational therapy's challenge: Caregiving and research. *American Journal of Occupational Therapy, 39,* 259–264.

Fisher, A. G., Mixon, J., & Herman, R. (1986). The validity of the clinical diagnosis of vestibular dysfunction. *Occupational Therapy Journal of Research, 6,* 3–20.

Freud, S. (1924). A short account of psychoanalysis. In the standard edition of the complete psychological works of Sigmund Freud (vol. 19) London: Hogarth Press.

Jantzen, A. C. (1981). *Research: The practical approach for occupational therapy.* Laurel, MD: RAMSCO.

Joe, B. E. (1991). Quality assurance in occupational therapy. Rockville, MD: *American Occupational Therapy Association.*

Keilhofner, G., Barris, R., Bauer, D., Shoestock, B., & Walker, L. (1983). A comparison of play behavior in nonhospitalized and hospitalized children. *American Journal of Occupational Therapy, 37,* 305–312.

Parker, H. J., & Chan, F. (1986). Prestige of allied health professions: Perceptions of occupational and physical therapists. *Occupational Therapy Journal of Research, 6(4),* 247–250.

Piaget, J. (1952). *Origins of intelligence.* New York: International University Press.

Royeen, C. B. (1980). Factors affecting test-retest reliability of the Southern California Postrotary Nystagmus Test. *American Journal of Occupational Therapy, 1,* 37–39.

Royeen, C. B. (1984). Initial profile of therapists seeking certification of the sensory integration and praxis test competency exam. *Journal of Occupational Therapy Research, 11,* 1–9.

Royeen, C. B. (1986). Evaluation of school-based occupational therapy programs: Need, strategy and dissemination. *American Journal of Occupational Therapy, 40,* 811–813.

Royeen, C. B., Koomar, J., Cromack, T., Fortune, J. C., & Domkey, L. (1991). Evidence for content and discriminant validity of the sensory integration and praxis test competency exam. *Journal of Occupational Therapy Research, 11,* 1–9.

Royeen, C. B., Lesinski, G., Ciani, S., & Schneider, D. (1981). Relationship of the Southern California Sensory Integration Tests, the Southern California Postrotary Nystagmus Test, and clinical observations accompanying them to evaluations in otolaryngology, ophthalmology, and audiology: Two descriptive case studies. *American Journal of Occupational Therapy, 35,* 443–450.

Schmidt, R., Lange, C., & Young, D. E. (1990). Optimizing summary knowledge of results for skills learning. *Human Movement Sciences, 9,* 325–348.

Smith, S. L., Cunningham, S., & Weinberg, R. (1986). The predictive validity of the functional capacities evaluation. *American Journal of Occupational Therapy, 40,* 564–567.

Storer, K., Bates, P., McGhee, N., & Dycus, S. (1984). Reducing the self stimulatory behavior of a profoundly retarded female through sensory awareness training. *American Journal of Occupational Therapy, 38,* 510–517.

Suarez, T. M. (1982). Planning evaluation programs for high-risk and handicapped infants. In C. T. Ramey & P. L. Trohanis (Eds.). *Finding and educating high-risk and handicapped infants* (pp. 193–215). Baltimore: University Park Press.

Yerxa, E. J. (1981). Basic or applied: A "developmental" assessment of occupational therapy research in 1981. *American Journal of Occupational Therapy, 35,* 820–921.

Recommended Readings

Mosey, A. C. (1992). *Applied scientific inquiry in the health professions: An epistemological orientation.* Rockville, MD: American Occupational Therapy Association.

Royeen, C. B., & DeGangi, G. (1992). Use of neurodevelopmental treatment as an intervention: Annotated listing of studies 1980–1990. *Perceptual and Motor Skills, 75,* 175–194.

Stein, F. (1989). *Anatomy of clinical research: An introduction to scientific inquiry in medicine, rehabilitation and related health professions.* Thorofare, NJ: Slack.

Learning Activity

1. Select an issue of a professional journal you receive. For each article, categorize it in terms of (a) basic versus applied research and (b) qualitative versus quantitative research.

CHAPTER 4

Quality in Research

KEY WORDS

Critical flaw

Critical issues

Evaluating research

Interpretation criteria

Peer review

Pilot testing

Research competence

Given the discussion of categories of research, how does one ascertain quality in research? Usually, quality in research is discussed in highly technical terms most beginning-level students of research cannot really use. Therefore, this chapter will address what makes an investigation a piece of high-quality research; I use a "common sense" approach, and include an easy-to-use tool for evaluating research. This evaluation tool will be used throughout the book.

Using Common Sense in Evaluating Research

Evaluating research in some manner is important because "every study, no matter how sophisticated or well done, has some flaws or limitations" (Polit & Hungler, 1985 p. 32). This is often a difficult concept and fact for beginning-level research consumers to accept. In my experience, many students categorically reject almost all research once they learn that it isn't perfect. As flaws or limitations are inevitable in any study, how can the beginning-level research student evaluate it? It may be helpful at this point to identify what constitutes quality in research, and use this identification as a foundation for constructing a way to evaluate research.

Little in life is perfect. Why should research be any different? When reading and using research, one should start with the assumption that all research is flawed in some way. What is important is to determine whether the imperfections in the research are acceptable and if the research is still essentially sound and the findings valid in spite of the imperfections.

Quality in Research

Quality in research is related to the research design decisions the investigator makes before implementing the study (Polit & Hungler, 1985). It also relates, however, to the judgement-based decisions the investigator makes during the study about other aspects of the research. For just as the occupational therapist and physical therapist must make judgment decisions that determine quality of treatment, such as appropriate intervention strategies and monitoring of outcomes, the research investigator has to make judgment decisions regarding a variety of components of the investigation. It is the appropriateness of the research investigator's decisions that determines the quality of research.

The question remains, however, What is quality research? There are a minimum of six components to consider when evaluating the quality of any given research:

- critical issues
- comprehensiveness
- competence
- creativity
- cost effectiveness
- critical flaw(s).

CRITICAL ISSUES

When evaluating clinical research in physical and occupational therapy, one should consider whether the research addresses a **critical issue**: Is the research question or issue important? Or is the research investigating something not of particular significance to the field? The problem here is that significance, like beauty, is in the eye of the beholder. One has to assume a rather broad viewpoint and look beyond personal areas of interest to judge if, considering the professions of occupational and physical therapy overall, a particular piece of research addresses a critical issue. That is, does it investigate something pertinent to the field, even if it is not your special area of interest?

Kirchman (1986) reported on an investigation into measuring the quality of life as enhanced by occupational therapy services. Her research most certainly addresses a key and critical issue confronting therapists: What do our services do? She has begun preliminary investigation into documentation of how occupational therapy services enhance the quality of life, given the presence of disease or loss. Her research, therefore, exemplifies research addressing a critical issue.

COMPREHENSIVENESS

A second factor to consider when evaluating the quality of research is whether the review, synthesis, and analysis of the literature pertaining to the issue or problems under investigation are comprehensive. Has the investigator demonstrated a thorough and thoughtful understanding of the literature pertaining to the field of inquiry? Are there omissions or misinterpretations of key articles or research directly related to the investigator's study? An example of a comprehensive literature review can be found in an investigation by Mathiowetz, Roger, Dowe-Keval, Donahoe, and Rennells (1986). In their investigation of norms for the Purdue Pegboard Test, they present an appropriately detailed yet limited review of the literature pertaining to their investigation. The argument presented in the literature review is developed from broad concepts to very specific ones and is logically constructed. It is clear to the reader how the literature presented relates to the investigation and frames the research endeavor discussed.

COMPETENCE

A third consideration is that of **competence**. This is a rather broad category pertaining to the technical soundness of the research regardless of methodology, quantitative or qualitative, that was used. In quantitative research, are the research questions and hypotheses clear? In qualitative research, are the questions under investigation or purpose of the study clear? Is the plan for how the research was conducted clear and logical? Is it methodologically sound? Are the conclusions warranted and related to the research issue or question? Is the investigation competently related to a theory or a set of theories?

An example of competently executed research is one by Oakly, Kielhofner, Barris, and Reichler (1986). In an investigation related to the theory of occupational behavior, they presented the development of an instrument designed to measure factors, in the case roles, pertinent to occupational behavior theory. The steps of the research are clearly presented, that is, the reader can easily figure out what the researchers did and why. The research methodology used is appropriate and well executed. Thus, one can answer "yes" to questions posed about the competency of research.

CREATIVITY

A fourth consideration of quality in research is that of creativity. This is not a euphemism for making changes in data to guarantee significant findings or making interpretations not supported by the data. Rather, it refers to using a unique perspective. For example, it is often difficult to investigate a certain problem due to methodological limitations. Does the research creatively solve that problem?

Or research results can be looked at in a new way that allows for significant theory development or modification. Creativity, therefore, can apply to the research design or research interpretation. One can ask, Does the investigator offer insightful and creative interpretations? An investigation by CooperFraps and Yerxa (1984) is an example of creative research. In this case, a creative interpretation was put forth and logically justified. These investigators studied the social and sexual competence of burned, disfigured adults and found a surprisingly high level of social competence in certain subjects. To explain their unanticipated findings, they posed a creative explanation based on the psychological mechanism of denial. They suggested that denial may allow some severely disfigured burn victims to function at high levels of social competence. This is a novel way to explain their unexpected findings and demonstrates that they interpreted research results in an insightful manner.

COST EFFECTIVENESS

It may be inappropriate to evaluate research funded by large federal grants as one would evaluate research conducted by clinicians on their own time and money. It has been my experience that people often expect the same standards of research for studies funded by external agencies with large amounts of money as for smaller, nonfunded studies. This is a disservice to our fields.

Traditionally accepted research designs and procedures may be beyond the budget of most occupational and physical therapy researchers. And given the cutback in federal funding in general, it may be beyond the budget of more and more researchers. Consequently, it is not reasonable to judge a nonfunded or minimally funded study by standards of research appropriate for large-scale funded studies. Therefore, a standard of quality research to consider involves the financial resources available and whether the researcher has made the most of these resources and obtained valid results.

Paired investigations by Giesel, Lange, and Niman (1984a, 1984b) illustrate cost-effective research. Using the same control populations of children with and without Down's syndrome, they investigated two distinct, yet related, areas: tongue movements and chewing cycles. This was cost effective because they did not have to obtain two separate samples. Yet two preliminary sets of data were obtained on these distinct functions by using the same sample twice.

CRITICAL FLAWS

Absence of a **critical flaw** is the final component of quality research. As previously stated, no research investigation is perfect. Imperfections and limitations in a study, however, should not constitute a critical flaw that is, in fact, fatal to the validity of the investigation. What are critical flaws? They are something, anything, that so seriously effects the conduct or outcome of the study that it renders the conclusions invalid. Such errors critically flaw the study. In my experience, the most commonly occurring fatal flaws are

- data collected cannot answer the research question as posed
- data is overinterpreted
- standardized tests are used inappropriately
- information is lacking on instrument used for measuring change
- subjects are inappropriate
- faulty assumptions underly conduct of the investigation.

An effective way to prevent critical flaws in research is to participate in **peer review** at all stages of research (Dunn, 1985). Submitting one's work for others' review and comment, or peer review, does not guarantee that fatal flaws will not occur. It does assure, however, that work has been reviewed by a more objective person, and allows for insight into possible problems before they are irrevocable.

As previously stated, almost all research contains flaws or imperfections. Nevertheless, flawed research may still be valid and justified in terms of conclusions drawn. Examples of flawed but basically sound research are in Figure 4–1.

Imperfections in research, like fatal flaws, are varied and common. Discrimination between fatal flaws and imperfections in research is basically a judgment call. It is a matter to be decided by the research investigator and, most important, by the research reader and consumer.

Evaluating Research

Combining the components of quality research just presented with the more traditional ways to evaluate research will give the beginning-level research consumer a commonsense way to **evaluating research.** The synthesis of different approaches is presented in Figure 4–2.

The questions posed in Figure 4–2 will be used as the guide for analyzing research articles discussed in the following chapters.

Research is a varied process that, generally defined, consists of the systematic collection of data to answer some specific question. There are numerous ways to classify research ranging from qualitative or quantitative to basic or applied. Most important, this chapter presented the beginning-level research consumer with a way to evaluate research.

[1]This is a form of peer review.

FIGURE 4–1. IMPERFECT BUT ESSENTIALLY SOUND RESEARCH

Research	Purpose	Imperfection
Royeen (1984)	Identify frequency of atypical vestibular functioning in behavioral disordered children.	Principal investigator served as evaluator of the subjects, and examiner bias was introduced.
Royeen (1985)	Modify existing instrument development methodology for use with children.	Pilot testing of items for language comprehension was executed with children from a private school when the instrument itself was for use with public school children. Validity of the test items for use with public school children was potentially jeopardized.
Royeen (1987)	Gather preliminary data on a questionnaire for tactile defensiveness in preschoolers.	A smaller number of teachers rated a large number of subjects with resulting artificial increase in internal consistency of the scale.

FIGURE 4–2. COMMON SENSE EVALUATION OF RESEARCH

1. What is the purpose of the research?
2. Does the literature review provide you an understanding of how and why this investigation is important?
3. Do you think the investigation is important? Why or why not?
4. What is the theoretical or conceptual basis of the investigation?
5. How was the research conducted?
6. What type or kind of research is it and why?
7. What were the research questions or hypotheses?
8. What are the variables or phenomena under study?
9. Who were the subjects or units of study? How many were there?
10. How were the subjects or units of study obtained?
11. What information or data were collected?
12. If specific evaluation tools were used, what were they? Was information on the reliability and validity of the evaluation tools provided?
13. How was the information or data collected?
14. Will data collected be able to answer or address the research question or problem under study?
15. How was the information or data analyzed?
16. What were the criteria for interpreting the data?
17. What were the findings?
18. What were the limitations of the study? Was there a critical flaw?
19. Were the conclusions of the study warranted?
20. How can these research findings be used in occupational and physical therapy?

References

CooperFraps, C., & Yerxa, E. J. (1984). Denial: Implications of a pilot study on activity level related to sexual competence in burned adults. *American Journal of Occupational Therapy, 39,(4)* 259–264.

Dunn, W. (1985). Occupational therapy's challenge: Caregiving and research. *American Journal of Occupational Therapy, 39(4),* 259–264.

Giesel, E. G., Lange, K. J., & Niman, C. (1984a). Tongue movements in 4- and 5-year-old Down's syndrome children during eating: A comparison with normal children. *American Journal of Occupational Therapy, 38(10),* 660–665.

Giesel, E. G., Lange, K. J., & Niman, C. (1984b). Chewing cycles in 4- and 5-year-old Down's syndrome children during eating: A comparison of eating efficiency with normals. *American Journal of Occupational Therapy, 39,* 666–670.

Kirchman, M. M. (1986). Measuring the quality of life. *Occupational Therapy Journal of Research, 6(1),* 21–32.

Mathiowetz, V., Roger, S. L., Dowe-Keval, M., Donahoe, L., & Rennells, C. (1986). The Purdue Pegboard: Norms for 14- to 19-year-olds. *American Journal of Occupational Therapy, 40,* 174–179.

Oakly, F., Kielhofner, G., Barris, R., & Reichler, R. K. (1986). The role checklist: Development and empirical assessment of reliability. *Occupational Therapy Journal of Research, 6,* 157–170.

Polit, D. F., & Hungler, B. P. (1985). *Essentials of nursing research.* Philadelphia: J. B. Lippincott.

Royeen, C. B. (1987). TIP: Touch inventory for preschoolers—A pilot study. *Physical and Occupational Therapy in Pediatrics, 7,* 29–40.

Royeen, C. B. (1985). Adaptation of Likert scaling for use with children. *Occupational Therapy Journal of Research, 5(1),* 59–69.

Royeen, C. B. (1984). Incidence of hypoactive nystagmus among behaviorally disordered children. *Occupational Therapy Journal of Research, 4(3)* 159–160.

CHAPTER 5

Reading, Actually Understanding, and Evaluating Research

KEY WORDS

Analysis of covariance
Chi square
Correlation coefficient
Discriminant analysis
Experimental hypothesis
Factor analysis
Hawthorn effect
Independent *t* test
Kendal Tau
Kruskal Wallis analysis of variance
Mann Whitney *U* Test
Nonparametric data analysis
One-way analysis of variance
Paired *t* test
Parametric data analysis procedures
Post hoc multiple comparisons
Probability value
Regression
Research design
Spearman Rho
Statistical hypothesis
Statistical significance
Student *t* test
Test statistic
Type I error
Type II error
Variables
Wilcoxon Matched Pairs Signed Ranks Test

Why Is Research Boring and Hard to Read?

The boring nature of reading research is a common complaint from clinicians and students who are learning to read research literature. And truthfully, it is also a complaint from quite a few experienced individuals who participate in research for their livelihood. In fact, as an undergraduate student, I can recall lamenting, "This is boring" and "This is so hard to read." Thus, the issue of why research is boring and hard to read will be addressed in this chapter.

We can break the question into two separate parts:

1. Why is research boring?
2. Why is research hard to read?

To answer these questions, we must consider their relationship. Research can be very boring if you cannot understand what it is saying. And one cannot understand what it is saying because it is hard to read. The reasoning is a bit circular, but you get the general idea.

Reading Research as a Foreign Language

This brings us to the question, Why is research hard to read? Think back to high school: Did you take a foreign language class? I studied German, but it doesn't matter which language it was. Recall what it was like trying to read prose in that foreign language. Was it ever difficult! Reading research is a lot like learning to read a foreign language. Only we may teach foreign languages better than we teach reading research. (Then again, maybe we don't, because I certainly cannot read German anymore.)

At any rate, the analogy that reading research is like reading a foreign language provides us with a way to better understand the difficulties in learning to read, understand, and use research.[1] When learning a foreign language you must first learn a basic vocabulary, learn tenses and verbs, and learn how to construct sentences in that language. Learning to read and understand research can be facilitated by a similar three-step process:

1. learning the vocabulary
2. learning the tenses and verbs
3. learning the "sentences" of research.

Figure 5–1 shows the similarities between learning to read a foreign language and learning to read research. Without fundamental skills and abilities, reading research can be like reading a foreign language—very boring indeed!

Basic Concepts for Understanding Research

Just as you must first learn vocabulary when studying a foreign language, you must first learn basic words and concepts when studying research. In the next section of this chapter, I will discuss the basic vocabulary and concepts needed to read research; my discussion will include an example of each concept. This section will be somewhat difficult and will require memorization of facts. There is simply no way to make it easy. You have to start somewhere, and mastery of these fundamental ABCs of research will give you a foundation for reading the language of research.

Experimental hypotheses. These are statements about the anticipated relationships between two or more variables, or the effect of one or more variables on another variable. They

1. The analogy of learning to read research being like learning to read a foreign language is built upon the idea in Chapter 1, "Data terminology: The 'Foreign Language'" from *Research: The practical approach for occupational therapy,* (1981), A. C. Jantzen, Laurel, MD: RAMSCO Publishing Co.

FIGURE 5–1. SIMILARITIES BETWEEN LEARNING A FOREIGN LANGUAGE AND LEARNING TO READ RESEARCH

Step	Foreign Language	Research
1	Learn vocabulary	Learn basic words and concepts
2	Learn tenses and verbs	Learn to conceptually understand common statistical procedures used in quantitative research
3	Learn to construct sentences and verbs	Understand data analysis and interpretation

are guesses about the nature of these relationships. Examples of experimental hypotheses (H) would be

(H_1) Performance of ambulation in post-cerebrovascular accident (CVA) adults is significantly and positively correlated to the number and duration of neurodevelopmental treatment (NDT).

(H_2) Tactile defensiveness in elementary school-aged boys is significantly and negatively correlated with social adjustment.

(H_3) Sensory integrative treatment of adolescent schizophrenics is more effective than traditional group therapy.

An experimental hypothesis should clearly reveal what the nature of the guess is and have clear implications of what is to be measured. For example, in Hypothesis 1 (H_1), the variables needing to be measured are ambulation in adults after CVA and the number of NDT sessions received. In Hypothesis 2 (H_2), the variables to be measured are tactile defensiveness and social adjustment. And in the last hypothesis (H_3), the variable to be measured is effectiveness of two different treatment interventions by looking at performance of schizophrenics.

Statistical hypotheses. These are statements of the relationships between variables that are always stated in the negative or the null so that they can be contrasted or compared to the statistical test results. In a sense, the experimental hypothesis is the substantive or content-laden guess, and the statistical hypothesis is always a negative or null statement of the relationships or effects. A null hypothesis is necessary to logically compare the outcome of the statistical analysis to this statement.

Based on the previous examples, the null (H_0) hypotheses for the previous experimental hypotheses would be

(H_0) There is no significant correlation between performance of ambulation in post-CVA adults and the number and duration of NDT treatments.

(H_0) There is no significant correlation between tactile defensiveness in elementary school-aged boys and social adjustment.

(H_0) There is no significant difference between schizophrenics treated with sensory integration and those treated with group therapy.

Hawthorne effect. This occurs when subjects in an experiment behave differently simply because they are being studied, not because of experimental treatment. By virtue of being in an investigation people may change their behavior. Thus, it may be this effect, and not the treatment effect, that accounts for or causes a behavior change. Research studies need to be controlled for this effect.

An example of the Hawthorne effect would be the following: In qualitative research, when one goes into a classroom or clinic to observe, the required time for observation is long—it should occur over time. In the initial stages of observation, the Hawthorne effect may be in action; that is, student, client, or staff behave differently simply because they are being observed (I know I was always just a bit sharper when the principal or another outsider was going to observe my treatments). Over time, the Hawthorne effect dissipates. This is one reason why any qualitatively based study using observation requires long-term commitment.

In quantitative research, subject groups who do not receive the actual treatment being studied often receive some sort of noncomparable intervention to account for or mitigate potential Hawthorne effects. In such a case, all subjects receive some sort of intervention that can make them feel "special," and the potential Hawthorne effect is distributed across all subjects because all subjects are having something done with them.

Nonparametric data analysis. This is a category of statistical data analysis procedures that have fewer and less stringent assumptions underlying their appropriate use. Usually the only assumptions are of continuous-level data and a symmetrical distribution of the data (Royeen & Seaver, 1986). I will present examples of nonparametric data analysis procedures later in this chapter.

Variables. Variables are the phenomena under investigation in a research study. There are three main types of variables: the independent variable, the dependent variable, and the confounding variable.

Independent variable. This may also be called the x variable. The independent variable is the variable whose manipulation or condition effects change in the dependent variable. In an investigation into the effects of therapy, the type of therapy provided (sensory integrative or group in the earlier hypothesis) is the independent variable. In occupational and physical therapy research, the independent variables are most often subject characteristics, treatment offered, or some combination thereof.

Dependent variable. This may also be called the y variable. This variable changes due to manipulation or conditions of the independent variable. In the earlier hypotheses, the independent variable (treatment condition) affected the level of schizophrenia (dependent variable). The dependent variable is usually a construct or concept. How that dependent variable is measured is the dependent measure. A review of the NDT research literature revealed the following types of NDT-related dependent variables (Royeen & DeGangi, 1992):

- motor
- language
- environmental interactions
- economy of movement
- daily living skills
- EMG and behavioral observations of balance
- muscle tone

- read-only memory
- developmental skills.

Remember that these are the dependent variables. They each must be assessed in some way to provide the measure of the independent variable.

Confounding variable. These are variables that are not controlled for in a research study, and can affect the dependent variable. The Hawthorne effect could be a confounding variable. Typically, in occupational and physical therapy research, confounding variables may be

- different levels of severity within a single diagnostic category (cerebral palsy, CVA, etc.)
- effects of maturation or "natural recovery" on subjects receiving intervention
- categorization of individuals with substantially different levels of performance into one diagnostic category (cerebral palsy, CVA, etc.)
- lack of knowledge about interaction effects of therapist belief and behavior with therapy interventions.

Research design. This refers to the blueprint or plan for how the research is to be conducted. There are numerous types of existing research designs (Campbell & Stanley, 1963; Kerlinger, 1973). Most traditional designs, however, have been developed for use with large samples. In the fields of occupational and physical therapy, as in other service-oriented disciplines, people are developing innovative research designs to meet the unique needs of the discipline (PSI, 1989).

Parametric data analysis. This is a category of data analysis procedures that reflect "the characteristics of a sample (statistics) in order to make inferences about the characteristics of a population (parameters) from which the sample was drawn" (Royeen & Seaver, 1992, p. 192). Stringent assumptions such as normal distribution of the variables and interval level of measurement underlie their appropriate use (Hinkle, Weirsam, & Jurs, 1979; Seaver, 1979). Parametric statistics will be discussed later in this chapter.

Type I error. This is an error committed when an investigator concludes that there is an effect from the experimental treatment when, in fact, there is none.

> An example of a Type I error is rejecting a true null hypothesis. This would be rejecting the null stated as, "There is no significant relationship between test-test reliability and duration of interval between test and retest." Let's say that this null hypothesis is true. So that one, in effect, accepts that there is a significant relationship between these two variables (by rejecting a true null) when there really is none. The outcome of a Type I error is making changes when they may not be warranted. For example, one may inappropriately design reliability investigations without considering a potential confounding variable, that is, length of time interval between test and retest.

Type II error. A Type II error is the reverse of a Type I error. It is committed when the investigator concludes there is no effect from the experimental treatment when, in fact, there is an effect. Or the experimenter may fail to reject a false null hypothesis. Such an error leads to not making change when change is appropriate.

> The following is an example of a Type II error. Let's say the following null hypothesis is false: "There is no significant effect from sensory integrative therapy on hyperactive students." The investigator, however, fails to reject it. By failing to reject the false null, the researcher cannot recommend appropriate action, that is, recommend that

sensory integrative therapy be used for hyperactive students.

We have covered the ABCs for understanding the words of research. Now let's move on to learning how to string those words together. Tenses and verbs are the action of a language. In research, the action is usually data analysis. And past experience suggests that it is data analysis that really confuses most beginning-level students. This appears to be due to the fact that the majority of data analyses in research articles are quantitatively oriented and use statistical procedures. And most beginning-level research consumers have forgotten the majority of the statistics they once knew; they become overwhelmed with the test statistics and probability values used to report outcomes from quantitative studies.

Hence, the next section of this chapter will provide you with a conceptual overview of the most commonly used types of statistical analysis used in occupational and physical therapy research. We will first look at a group of parametric data analysis procedures and then a group of nonparametric procedures. Learning about data analysis procedures is analogous to giving you the tenses and verbs of a foreign language.

Data Analysis Procedures for Occupational and Physical Therapy Research

NONPARAMETRIC DATA ANALYTIC PROCEDURES

These nonparametric data analytic procedures were selected for review based on what are the most commonly used procedures in the occupational therapy literature.[1] Nonparametric data analytic procedures are a class of statistical procedures that do not require the same assumptions as must be met when using parametric statistics.

Correlation analysis. This refers to a statistical procedure used to determine the magnitude and direction of the relationship between two variables. Correlations portray magnitude or degree of relationship only. They in no way illustrate cause and effect. The nonparametric version is either the **Kendal Tau** or the **Spearman Rho.** Spearman Rho is used when the data are not measured at the interval level, or when the data are not normally distributed. The Kendal Tau may be used if both variables are measured at the ordinal level (Burns & Grove, 1987). These may also be called rank correlation because they are based, in part, on ranks assigned to the data.

A Spearman Rho is equivalent to the Pearson r but instead of interval level data, it uses ranks and average ranks (Conover, 1980). Additionally, it can be used for data that is not linearly related; that is, the relationship between x and y is not the same for all values of x and y. Let's assume we are studying aging and are interested in the relationship between number of car accidents per year and age of drivers over 65. Let's assume we have access to the Division of Motor Vehicles (DMV) records for a state and for each person over 65 in that state we are able to correlate age with number of accidents reported to the DMV for each month of the calendar year 1991. We could determine (a) if there was a correlation between age and frequency of car wrecks, and (b) if there was a trend of increased accidents with age.

Kruskal Wallis Analysis of Variance. This tests whether the median score of three independent groups significantly differs, and like the nonparametric correlation, it is based on ranks of scores (Burns & Grove, 1987). It is a nonparametric equivalent to an analysis of variance, and

1. It is assumed that by covering these procedures, the bulk of the data analytic procedures found in the physical therapy literature will also be reviewed.

hence, the name is in its title. And it is nearly as powerful as the parametric analysis of variance, that is, it is nearly as able to discern real differences between groups.

> An appropriate use of the Kruskal Wallis' Analysis of Variance would be the following hypothetical example. Say you were conducting research into pay scales of speech-language pathologists (SLP), physical therapists (PT), and occupational therapists (OT) in your state. And assume that you had information provided on therapists from the respective state associations. You would run this nonparametric analysis of variance on the groups (SLP vs. PT vs. OT) to determine if there is a significant difference in salaries by group.

Mann Whitney U Test. This test analyzes whether two independent or uncorrelated means significantly differ. It is an effective way to determine whether or not two samples are the same or different. You may consider it to be a nonparametric alternative for the independent *t* test (Burns & Grove, 1987).

> The following hypothetical examples illustrate the use of the Mann Whitney *U* Test. Assume that you wish to compare normal children and children with some recognized diagnosis on some aspect of performance. The groups are clearly not related. You may wish to compare duration of nystagmus between normal and hyperactive children or degree of tactile defensiveness between normal and hyperactive children. In each case, the Mann Whitney *U* Test would be appropriate.

The Wilcoxon Matched Pairs Signed Ranks Test. This is a nonparametric test used with dependent samples that are in some way related to each other, that is, matched pairs. The relative rank of the values of the differences between each set of the two groups of scores is considered. It will tell you whether or not there is a significant difference in the two sets of scores. This test can be used with paired or matched data. These data may be from pretest and posttest scores or from subjects matched to each other on some variable (Burns & Grove, 1987). In a study of children with rheumatoid arthritis, the subjects with rheumatoid arthritis were paired or matched with control subjects without rheumatoid arthritis (Giannini & Protas, 1992). The investigators used the Wilcoxon Matched Pairs Signed Ranks Test to test whether or not the groups of matched pairs (normal and those with juvenile rheumatoid arthritis) differed in the amount of exercise they could perform. Not surprisingly, the investigators found that the control subjects were significantly better able to perform than the subjects with juvenile rheumatoid arthritis.

Chi Square. Various forms of the Chi Square exist. The most common form of the test allows us to look at categories of events in terms of frequencies within categories compared with chance. That is, we can determine whether what did happen is the same as what was expected to happen if the categories or variables were really independent.

> The Chi Square could be used as follows. In an investigation of depression and rheumatoid arthritis in 82 adults compared to a control sample of 150 university employees, Frank, Chaney, Clay, and Kay (1991) used the Chi Square to test whether or not subjects with arthritis taking steroids were more or less likely to be depressed. Essentially, they were testing whether or not depression was independent of steroid use for this sample of subjects. They found, among other things, that patients taking steroids were significantly related to the diagnosis of depression, that is, that steroid use and depression were not independent.

PARAMETRIC DATA ANALYTIC PROCEDURES

The following parametric procedures have also been selected because of their frequency in the literature (Royeen, 1986). Parametric data analytic procedures are a class of statistical procedures calculated to "reflect the characteristics of a sample so that one can make inferences about the characteristics of populations (parameters) from which the sample was drawn" (Royeen & Seaver, 1986, p. 62).

Correlation analysis. This refers to a statistical procedure used to determine the magnitude and direction of the relationship between two variables. The parametric version is the Pearson Product Moment Correlation, designated by *r*. Correlations portray magnitude or degree of relationship only. They in no way illustrate cause and effect.

> An example of the use of the Pearson Product Moment Correlation can be seen in the following hypothetical situation. Let's assume we wanted to investigate the validity of a certification exam or process. We could correlate the number of years of experience as a therapist with total scores on the certification test. One would expect a significant and positive correlation between these two variables.

Independent t test (t). This test can determine whether two group means of nonrelated or independent groups are significantly different from each other. Say a therapist wished to know whether a resting splint or a cock-up splint was more effective in reducing pain in women with certain types of arthritis in the hand. The independent *t* test could be used to compare the mean score of pain reported by the group of women using the resting splint to the mean score of women using the cock-up splint. In this test the groups are not related in any way—they are independent.

Paired t test. This test can determine whether two group means of related or correlated groups are significantly different from each other. In the previous example of exercise with normal subjects and subjects with juvenile rheumatoid arthritis, the paired, or correlated, *t* test was also used to test the significance of performance of the two groups on duration of exercise. Not surprisingly, the nonjuvenile arthritis group performed significantly poorer in duration of exercise (Giannini & Protas, 1992).

Student t test. This test can determine whether a sample mean is significantly different from the population mean. A Student *t* test would be used in the following experiment. Let's assume you have a group of subjects of a diagnostic category. You wish to know if they perform significantly differently than the normative population. You may compare their mean score to the mean score of the normative population determined by standardized testing.

One-way analysis of variance (ANOVA). This test can determine whether the mean score of three or more groups significantly differs. Adler, Wright, and Ulicny (1991) used an ANOVA to determine if condition of appeal effected donation to those with disabilities. They had four conditions of solicitation (four groups) compared on the amount of money the subjects reportedly were willing to donate to a hypothetical organization. They found no differences between the four groups.

Post hoc multiple comparisons. If an ANOVA is found to significantly differ by group, a post hoc multiple comparison is run to determine which group means are significantly different. For example, one way to establish validity of a test is to administer it to three different groups of individuals (novice, experienced, and master level). Theoretically, the novice group should score significantly less than the master level group. The ANOVA would reveal whether or not the scores between the groups differ significantly. But a post hoc analysis would determine which groups differed significantly.

Analysis of covariance (ANCOVA). This tests the significance of the difference between group mean scores after controlling for the effects of a variable such as pretest scores. In a study of the neuropsychological functioning of first episode persons with schizophrenia, Hoff, Riordan, O'Donnell, Morris, and DeLisi (1992) used an ANCOVA to control for subject age and educational level in analyzing subjects' performance on a variety of neuropsychological tests. That is, they were able to compare the scores taking the factors of age and education level out of consideration.

Regression. This procedure is based on correlation and allows one to predict the value of y (the dependent variable) based on the value of x (the independent variable). Do you remember taking the Standardized Achievement Test (SAT) to apply to college? Because SAT scores are a good predictor of grade performance in college, SAT scores (x) can predict college grades (y) using regression analysis.

Discriminant analysis. This statistical procedure can (a) predict membership in a category, (b) classify observations into two or more groups, and (c) determine what combination of variables best discriminates between two known groups. Cross and Donaldson (1992) used discriminant analysis to determine whether patients perceived the physical or psychological aspects of therapy as most important after 6 weeks of physical therapy. Using 40 subjects on 20 variables, they reported no statistically significant results.

The next section of this chapter will provide a short summary of how test statistics are calculated, and how they are used to determine whether or not they reveal a significant finding. These three sets of information considered collectively (nonparametric statistics, parametric statistics, and calculation and use of test statistics) give you the beginning-level ability to understand "sentences" in the foreign language of research.

Test Statistics

Test statistics, as used here, refer to the arithmetic outcome from putting data into the formula for one of the previously identified statistical procedures (correlation, analysis of variance, etc.), and calculating the answer using the formula for that statistical procedure. Different statistics have different formulas for calculation. And different statistics have different symbols to represent them. Figure 5–2 presents the symbol notation for the most commonly encountered statistics in occupational therapy and physical therapy literature. Figure 5–3 presents you with an example of a test statistic calculation. This should give you a conceptual understanding of how test statistics are calculated.

FIGURE 5–2. SYMBOLS USED IN RESEARCH

n	number of subjects or scores
Σ	summation
s	standard deviation for a sample
s^2	variance for a sample
r	Pearson Product Moment Correlation
H_o	null hypothesis
t	Student t statistic
df	degrees of freedom
F	F statistic
T	T score
$\overline{x}$	sample mean
x^2	Chi-square statistic
z	z score

Based, in part, upon "Glossary of Symbols," p. 490–491, R. L. D. Wright, Understanding statistics, (1976). NY: Harcourt Brace.

FIGURE 5-3. ILLUSTRATIVE EXAMPLE OF CALCULATION OF A TEST STATISTIC

The nonparametric statistical test of the Kruskal Wallis test (nonparametric version of analysis of variance) has been chosen because of its ease of calculation. Let us assume that you have grade point averages for four groups of students and wish to ascertain whether the groups are equivalent. Further, assume that group designation is based upon the specific course of prerequisites that students had to take prior to entering the professional program. You wish to see if the grade point averages of the groups in the professional curriculum are the same regardless of prerequisite courses taken. Thus, the null hypothesis is:

H_0: The four groups are equivalent.

The groups and corresponding scores are below:

Step One

Group 1	Group 2	Group 3	Group 4
3.406	3.487	3.053	3.418
2.650	3.256	3.343	3.675
3.265		3.440	
3.755			
3.103			
3.390			

The first step is to assign a rank (R) to each score. One must therefore start with the lowest score and assign that rank "1." The next score is rank "2," and so on. This is presented in Step Two.

Step Two

Group 1	Rank 1	Group 2	Rank 2	Group 3	Rank 3	Group 4	Rank 4
3.406	R8	3.487	R11	3.053	R2	3.418	R9
2.650	R1	3.256	R4	3.343	R6	3.675	R12
3.265	R5			3.440	R10		
3.751	R13						
3.103	R3						
3.390	R7						

Step Three

Then, for each group, rank scores are summed together.

R	Σ R1=37	Σ R2=15	Σ R3=18	Σ R4=21

Note also the number of observations or subjects for each group:

n	6	2	3	2

while the total number of observations or subjects is 13=*n*.

Step Four

Now, you use the formula for the Kruskal Wallis to calculate the value of the test statistic. The formula is as follows:

F1 $$\text{Test Statistic}=T= \frac{12}{N\,(N+1)} \sum_{i=1}^{k} \frac{R_i^2}{n_i} - 3(N+1)$$

You then "plug in" your numbers into the formula!

F2 $$\frac{12}{13(13+1)} \left(\frac{37^2}{6} + \frac{15^2}{2} + \frac{18^2}{3} + \frac{21^2}{2} \right) -3(13+1)$$

And, then solve the equation:

F3 $$= .0659341\ (228.16667 + 112.5 + 108 + 220.5) - 42$$

$$= 2.120915$$

Using Table A.2 from Conover (1980), it is determined that the closest critical value for the Kruskal Wallis for this situation (four groups, or k–1=3 degrees of freedom) is 4.108 with an approximate p value of .750. Since the obtained test statistic (2.120915) is less than the critical value for the derived test statistic (4.108) whose corresponding p value is .75, the probable p value is $< .25$.

Thus, $T = 2.120915$, $df = 3$, $p < .25$

We fail to reject the null hypothesis.

And, we conclude that all four groups performed equally well on grade point averages regardless of prerequisites taken prior to the professional program!

Conover, W. J. (1980). *Practical nonparametric statistics.* Second Edition. New York: John Wiley and Sons. (pages 229–239, page 432).

It is beyond the scope of this book to fully address computation of the various statistical formulas. But we will address it enough for you to understand what they are about. In the past, all statistical analyses were done by hand. Recent advances in computerization, however, have resulted in a big change. Now everyone does statistical procedures by computer. Because of this, students in research classes often become confused by test statistics—not having calculated a simple formula to completion, they often don't realize where test statistics come from.

REPORTING TEST STATISTICS

Let us now look at how results of statistical analysis are usually reported as a test statistic, value of the test statistic, and other type of related information. First, how does one read such notation?

- F refers to the test statistic calculated using the statistical procedure of analysis of variance.
- df is degrees of freedom. Degrees of freedom are an essential component of any statistical calculation but differ in calculation for almost every statistic. The mathematical theory behind degrees of freedom is complex. Suffice it to say, they are part of every statistical formula calculation.
- p refers to "the probability of making a Type I error, or the probability that the result occurred by chance" (Cohen, 1988). A p of .001 means that the probability of a Type I error is less than 1 chance out of 1,000. This is a significant finding.

We now need to look further at statistical significance and probability values.

STATISTICAL SIGNIFICANCE AND HOW IT IS REPORTED

Testing for statistical significance is the process of determining whether the phenomenon under investigation is a function of chance as compared to some predetermined probability. Thus, evaluation of significance is really a form of gambling, or evaluating events by their probability or odds. By custom, most researchers commonly use p = .05 as the predetermined level of probability. The level of significance against which a researcher will compare his or her results is the predetermined **probability value** (p value).

The proper interpretation of p values are:

p = .01 The probability is 1 chance in 100 that the observed event is due to chance.

p = .05 The probability is 5 chances in 100 that the observed event is due to chance.

p = .001 The probability is 1 chance in 1,000 that the observed event is due to chance.

We are, consequently, not dealing in black-and-white absolutes but in probabilities of events. And you thought research was cut and dried.

If the probability value of a calculated test statistic is less than the predetermined level, for example, p = .001 when the level of significance was predetermined at p = .05, then we can reject the null hypothesis and accept the research hypothesis. Restated another way, if the calculated test statistic is associated with a p value that is less than the one preset by the investigator, one has a statistically significant finding.

Here are some examples to illustrate these concepts.

$p > .05$ This is, again, the most commonly used preset level of significance. If this result were calculated, the probability value is greater than 5 chances out of 100. Thus, this is not a significant finding.

$p < .05$ This reads as the probability is less than 5 chances out of 100. These odds are beyond chance and, therefore, the finding is significant.

p = .10 This reads as the probability is equal to 10 chances out of 100. If the predetermined p value was p = 05, then this is not a significant finding. But, if the predetermined p value was p = .25, then this is a significant finding.

p = .50 This reads as the probability is equal to 5 out of 10 chances. This is a chance event and therefore not a significant finding.

READING STATISTICS IN RESEARCH LITERATURE

Many beginning-level students of research become confused when reading statistics research articles. I will therefore go over numerous examples of statistical reports taken directly from the published literature in occupational and physical therapy.

Example 1. paired t test, $t = -4.957$, $df = 29$, $p < .05$. (Giannini & Protas, 1992).

The probability of a Type I error is less than 5 chances out of 100. This is a statistically significant finding, that is, the event is not the result of chance.

Example 2. "No reliable differences were found between groups in the amount of money subjects were willing to donate to the hypothetical organization serving people with disabilities, $df = (3, 139)$ $F = 1.02$, n.s.)."

The statistical test was not signifcant. Therefore, the investigator concluded that there were no differences between groups.

Example 3. In a study of first-episode schizophreniform patients, the following results were reported on a test of spatial memory:

Group A Mean score for chronic schizophrenics = −1.60

Group B Mean score for first-episode schizophrenics = −1.22

Group C Mean score for third group = 0.00

An ANOVA (F = 11.59, df 2/78; p = .00004) revealed that the probability of chance events accounting for group differences was 4 out of 100,000. The group differences, therefore, were not because of chance but because of group characteristics. Performance on a test of spatial ability differed significantly by group. A Tukey post hoc test was conducted to determine which groups differed from each other. Groups A and C differed as did groups B and C ($p < .05$).

Evaluating Research

You have just finished a crash course in the fundamentals of research and data analysis. Now it is time to construct some sentences in the foreign language of research. Using the knowledge you have just learned, let's read through some actual examples in the literature. To guide our reading, we will use the "Common Sense Guide to Evaluating Research" presented in chapter 4.

I developed this evaluation tool over the past 5 years by working with individuals like yourself. I have found that most methods of evaluating research assume a technical level of expertise that beginning-level researchers simply do not have—and therefore most guidelines are simply not useful. These guidelines, however, were designed so that everyone from the beginning level to the advanced student of research can use and apply them.

Given this preliminary discussion, let us go through each question in the "Common Sense Guide" in Figure 5–4 step-by-step so that you can understand the rationale for using it as a research evaluation guideline.

Skim through the next section once. Then, reread it for more understanding. Finally, for a third and fourth read, try to understand each example and the corresponding explanation. Believe it or not, experience suggests that once you have mastered this section, you will be able to read and understand more research than many first- and second-year graduate students.

FIGURE 5–4. A COMMONSENSE GUIDE FOR UNDERSTANDING RESEARCH

1. What is the purpose of the research?
2. Does the literature review provide you an understanding of how and why this investigation is important?
3. Do you think the investigation is important? Why or why not?
4. What is the theoretical or conceptual basis of the investigation?
5. How was the research conducted?
6. What type or kind of research is it and why?
7. What were the research questions or hypotheses?
8. What are the variables or phenomena under study?
9. Who were the subjects or units of study? How many were there?
10. How were subjects or units of study obtained?
11. What information or data were collected?
12. If specific evaluation tools were used, what were they? Was information on the reliability and validity of the evaluation tools provided?
13. How was the information or data collected?
14. Will data collected be able to answer or address the research question or problem under study?
15. How was the information or data analyzed?
16. What were the criteria for interpreting the data?
17. What were the findings?
18. What were the limitations of the study? Was there a critical flaw? If so, what was it?
19. Are the conclusions of the study warranted?
20. How can these research findings be used in occupational and physical therapy?

You may find it helpful to use the following article as an example as the evaluation questions are being explained and discussed. First, the article will be presented. Then, the article will be discussed using the questions from Figure 5–4.

Reprinted from *Physical & Occupational Therapy in Pediatrics,* Vol. 7, Number 3, Fall, 1987.

ILLUSTRATIVE EXAMPLE 5–1

Test-Retest Reliability of a Touch Scale for Tactile Defensiveness

Charlotte Brasic Royeen

Abstract. A touch scale for evaluation of tactile defensiveness in elementary school aged children has been developed and, in the current study, the test-retest reliability of the scale was investigated. Twenty-six children, thirteen males and thirteen females aged five to twelve, were administered the scale by a research assistant and then retested two weeks later. A Pearson Product Moment Correlation Coefficient was calculated and found to be significant in terms of variance shared between the first and second testing sessions (r=.5883, p=.001). The results suggest acceptable test-retest reliability for the touch scale, especially considering, (1) the limited variance of the response format upon which the reliability coefficient is based, (2) a two-week interval between tests, and (3) the relatively small sample size. Suggestions for future research are put forth.

The tactile system, subserving incoming information from the skin and subcutaneous tissues of the body, is of primary importance in human activity. For example, the touch system plays a key role in human survival; touch sensations can warn of danger[1] or transmit sexual sensations. In addition, motor activity such as reflexes can be elicited by cutaneous input[2,3] and also, motor planning is highly dependent upon touch sensations.[4,5] Perceptual ability is, in part, dependent upon an adequate amount of tactile experience as well as efficient integration of tactile input.[1,4] Finally, even emotional and social stability is highly dependent upon tactile sensations.[6,7]

Given the variety of human functions subserved by tactile sensations, any disorder concerning tactile processing can severely disrupt the life of a child. One such disorder is tactile defensiveness, which is a disorder of sensory integrative processing. Tactile defensiveness is a syndrome consisting of a collection of adversive reactions to non-noxious tactile stimulation; such input is perceived by the child as noxious. Furthermore, hyperactivity and distractibility may also be associated with the disorder.[1,4]

Tactile defensiveness was first identified and described by Ayres and, subsequently, researchers have continued investigation of the syndrome, delineating its manifestations in learning disabled and developmentally delayed children.[8-10] In tactually defensive children, central nervous system integration centers controlling the sensitivity of incoming afferent signals are probably not functioning optimally. Thus, incoming afferent information is not modulated adequately and aversion to many forms of tactile input results. The integration centers most associated with tactile defensiveness are the dorsal horn of the spinal cord and the reticular formation of the brainstem.[10,11] In order to integrate sensory input optimally, each of these centers

TABLE 1
PSYCHOMETRIC PROPERTIES OF THE TOUCH SCALE

Validity	
Criterion References	The scale differentiates between a sample of tactually defensive and non-tactually defensive children at $p = .0073$ using discriminant analysis with an 85% correct classification rate. (17)
Construct	Domain specification of tactile defensiveness for measurement accomplished by literature review as well as review by A. J. Ayres and a panel of experts. (15)
Reliability	
Internal	Standardized Alpha = .79456 (17)
Interrater	A one hundred percent agreement rate between raters was obtained (Y. Norton, personal communication, February, 1985)

is dependent upon descending influences from supraspinal levels of the central nervous system.[12-14] In cases of tactile defensiveness, descending supraspinal centers cannot effectively modulate incoming sensory input.

Evaluation of tactile defensiveness is part of clinical observations during administration of the tactile discrimination tests of the Southern California Sensory Integration Tests.[4] In order to fulfill the need for psychometric evaluation of tactile defensiveness and to serve as an adjunct to clinical judgement, a touch scale for evaluation of tactile defensiveness in elementary school aged children has been developed.[15-17] The psychometric properties, exclusive of test-retest stability, are presented in Table 1.

The current study was an investigation into test-retest reliability of the newly developed scale.

Method

SUBJECTS

Permission was granted for the research project to be conducted in a large school system in suburban Washington, D.C. A principal willing to allow students from his school to participate in the study was located with the assistance of the school system's Director of Occupational and Physical Therapy Services. Permission to conduct the investigation within the school was granted providing that the principal be allowed to identify parents to whom permission forms could be sent. In addition to regular educational classes, this particular school also had self-contained classrooms for learning disabled children. Subsequently, permission forms were sent to 50 sets of parents whose children were in grades kindergarten to six. Of the 50 sets of parents sent permission forms, 30 returned forms granting permission for their child to participate in the study. Of those 30, two students did not participate since

TABLE 2
DEMOGRAPHIC CHARACTERISTICS OF SUBJECTS

Sex	Male	13
	Female	13
		26 Total
Category	Normal	20
	Learning Disabled	6
		26 Total
Race	Caucasian	19
	Black	2
	Oriental	2
	Spanish	1
	Middle Eastern	1
	Unknown	1
		26 Total

they were younger than six years of age and two students were absent on the days of testing. Thus, 26 children participated in the current study. Tables 2 and 3 present demographic, grade, and age information on those 26 children.

PROCEDURE

The scale, included in the Appendix, was administered in a quiet room by a research assistant. All testing occurred during regular school hours. The reader is referred elsewhere for detailed directions on standardized administration of the scale.[16-17]

DATA ANALYSIS

A Pearson Product Moment Correlation Coefficient was computed on the first and second test scores. A modification of SPSS designed to compensate for the occasional test item not answered by a subject was employed.[18]

Results and Discussion

The correlation between the first testing and second testing was statistically significant (r = .5883, p = .001). The current study indicates that for this sample of children (n = 26) the scale for measuring tactile defensiveness has a correlation coefficient of moderate magnitude. The correlation coefficient (.5883) is close to the value of (.60) specified by Benson and Clark[19] as the minimum acceptable value for test-retest stability. Certain factors need to be considered when evaluating the correlation coefficient. First, the sample size is relatively small. Second, the correlation coefficient is based upon testing employing a two week interval between tests. Most probably the correlation coefficient would be higher if the testing interval was reduced, as length of the time interval between tests is inversely related to the magnitude of the retest correlation.[20] Third, the test instrument is designed such that the three response format ("No," "A Little," "A Lot") is limited in variance. Since calcu-

TABLE 3
SUBJECTS' AGES AND GRADES

Age Category	Number
5.6 – 6.0	3
6.0 – 6.6	0
6.6 – 7.0	3
7.0 – 7.6	1
7.6 – 8.0	1
8.0 – 8.6	0
8.6 – 9.0	2
9.0 – 9.6	2
9.6 – 10.0	3
10.0 – 10.6	1
10.6 – 11.0	4
11.0 – 11.6	1
11.6 – 12.0	4
12.0 – 12.6	1
	26 Total

Grade	Number
Preschool	1
Kindergarten	1
First	2
Second	3
Third	3
Fourth	5
Fifth	5
Sixth	6
	26 Total

lation of correlation coefficients is based upon variance, restricted variance may, as an artifact, have lowered the magnitude of the coefficient.[21]

Considering these three factors and in light of the findings of the investigation, the touch scale appears to have a satisfactory test stability over time. Continued study into the instrument is necessary, however. Investigation into the test-retest reliability over different lengths of time using a random selection of subjects by group (normal and learning disabled) in addition to employing analyses based upon generalizability theory and analysis of variance for evaluation of reliability[22] could further elucidate characteristics of the tests' reliability, in conjunction with replication studies of inter-rater reliability and further study of the concurrent validity of the scale.

A limitation of the study needs to be noted. Since the school system would grant permission to conduct the study contingent upon a principal agreeing to let his or her school participate, and since the principal would participate only if he or she could identify students to whose parents permission forms could be sent, the sample selection may have introduced a systematic bias. Subsequent replication study can address this issue.

Notes

1. Ayres AJ: *Sensory Integration and the Child.* Los Angeles, Western Psychological Services, 1979.
2. Chusid JG: *Correlative Neuroanatomy and Functional Neurology.* Los Altos, CA, Lange Medical Publishers, 1976.
3. Gilfoyle EM, Grady AP, Moore JC: *Children Adapt.* Thorofare, NJ, Charles B. Slack, 1981.

4. Ayres AJ: *Southern California Sensory Integration Test Manual.* Los Angeles, Western Psychological Services, 1973.

5. Lederman SJ: Tactual perception and texture, in Carterette E, Friedman M (eds): *Handbook of Perception.* New York, Alcott Publishers, 1973.

6. Harlow HF: The nature of love. *Am Psychol* 13:673-685, 1958.

7. Montague A: *The Direction of Human Development.* New York, Hawthorn University Press, 1970.

8. Ayres AJ: Tactile functions: Their relation to hyperactive and perceptual motor behavior. *Am J Occup Ther* 18:83-95, 1964.

9. Bauer BA: Tactile sensitivity: Development of a behavioral response checklist. *Am J Occup Ther* 31:357-361, 1977.

10. Larson K. The sensory history of developmentally delayed children with and without tactile defensiveness. *Am J Occup Ther* 36:590-596, 1982.

11. Fisher AG, Dunn WG: Tactile defensiveness: Historical perspective, new research—a theory grows. *Sensory Integration Special Interest Section Newsletter,* American Occupational Therapy Association 6(2):1-2, 1983.

12. Carpenter MB: *Human Neuroanatomy.* Baltimore, William and Wilkins, 1976.

13. Clark RC: *Clinical Neuroanatomy and Neurophysiology.* Philadelphia, FA Davis, 1980.

14. Guyton AC: *Basic Human Neurophysiology.* Philadelphia, Saunders & Sons, 1981.

15. Royeen CB: Domain specifications of the construct tactile defensiveness. *Am J Occup Ther* 5(9): 596-599, 1985.

16. Royeen CB: Adaptation of Likert sealing for use with children. *Occup Ther J Res* 5(1):59-69, 1985.

17. Royeen CB: Development of a touch scale to measure tactile defensiveness in elementary school aged children. *Am J Occup Ther* 40(6):414-419.

18. Royeen CB, Fortune JC: Data modification commands for summated scale reliability analysis. *Occup Ther J Res* 5(4):257-258, 1985.

19. Benson J, Clark F: A guide for instrument development and validation. *Am J Occup Ther* 36:789-800, 1982.

20. Anastasi, A: *Psychological Testing.* New York, MacMillan Press, 1976.

21. Hinkle DE, Wiersma S, Jurs SG: *Applied Statistics for the Behavioral Sciences.* Boston, Houghton Mifflin Co, 1979.

22. Chronbach LJ: *Essentials of Psychological Testing.* New York, Harper and Row, 1970.

Appendix A:
A Scale for Measuring Tactile Defensiveness
by Charlotte Brasic Royeen, PhD, OTR

Date:________________________ Examiner: ______________________________

Subject: ____________________

Response Format: No = 1 A Little = 2 A Lot = 3

(Check One)

1	2	3	No.	Question
[ ]	[ ]	[ ]	1.	Does it bother you to go barefooted?
[ ]	[ ]	[ ]	2.	Do fuzzy shirts bother you?
[ ]	[ ]	[ ]	3.	Do fuzzy socks bother you?
[ ]	[ ]	[ ]	4.	Do turtleneck shirts bother you?
[ ]	[ ]	[ ]	5.	Does it bother you to have your face washed?
[ ]	[ ]	[ ]	6.	Does it bother you to have your nails cut?
[ ]	[ ]	[ ]	7.	Does it bother you to have your hair combed by someone else?
[ ]	[ ]	[ ]	8.	Does it bother you to play on a carpet?
[ ]	[ ]	[ ]	9.	After someone touches you, do you feel like scratching that spot?
[ ]	[ ]	[ ]	10.	After someone touches you, do you feel like rubbing that spot?
[ ]	[ ]	[ ]	11.	Does it bother you to walk barefooted in the grass and sand?
[ ]	[ ]	[ ]	12.	Does getting dirty bother you?
[ ]	[ ]	[ ]	13.	Do you find it hard to pay attention?
[ ]	[ ]	[ ]	14.	Does it bother you if you cannot see who is touching you?
[ ]	[ ]	[ ]	15.	Does fingerpainting bother you?
[ ]	[ ]	[ ]	16.	Do rough bedsheets bother you?
[ ]	[ ]	[ ]	17.	Do you like to touch people, but it bothers you when they touch you back?
[ ]	[ ]	[ ]	18.	Does it bother you when people come from behind you?
[ ]	[ ]	[ ]	19.	Does it bother you to be kissed by someone other than your parents?
[ ]	[ ]	[ ]	20.	Does it bother you to be hugged or held?
[ ]	[ ]	[ ]	21.	Does it bother you to play games with your feet?
[ ]	[ ]	[ ]	22.	Does it bother you to have your face washed?
[ ]	[ ]	[ ]	23.	Does it bother you to have your face touched if you don't expect it?
[ ]	[ ]	[ ]	24.	Do you have difficulty making friends?
[ ]	[ ]	[ ]	25.	Does it bother you to stand in line?

Comments:

Illustrative Example 5–1: Discussion

1. What is the purpose of the research?

The purpose of the research is just that. What does the author suggest is the purpose or reason for the research investigation?

In this example, look at the Abstract. Usually, the abstract of a research article will provide you with a summary statement of the purpose of the investigation. In this case, the Abstract states, "the test-retest reliability of the scale was investigated" (p. 45). One could state, therefore, that the purpose of this research was to investigate the test-retest reliability of an evaluation tool.

2. Does the literature review provide you an understanding of how and why this investigation is important?

Oftentimes in published research there is no heading that labels a section, "Review of the Literature." Usually, it is included in the article's introduction, immediately after the abstract. In this example, there is neither an introduction nor a separate review of the literature. The section in this article containing a review of the literature follows the Abstract and precedes the Methods section.

The Literature section really provides the reader with a background understanding of what is known about the area and why it is important, and then focuses more specifically on why the current research is important as related to the general area. It progresses, therefore, from the general to the specific. In this example, the Literature section is rather sparse. Yet it does provide the reader with a general understanding of the nature of the problem under consideration, why it is important, and how this particular piece of research relates to it.

3. Do you think the investigation is important? Why or why not?

This question can only be answered by you based on your clinical judgement and experience, as well as your understanding of theory. The author of a research article may or may not make an argument for the importance of a piece of research. Many times the importance is merely implied and not explicitly stated. The reader may find reference to the importance of the study in the Introduction and Literature sections, the Discussion, or in the Conclusion or Summary. This varies by article. Whatever the case, however, you are the only one who can really judge the degree of importance related to your interests and practice.

In Test-Retest Reliability, the importance of the study is not explicitly stated. One can infer that it is important for measurement tools to be valid and reliable. And test-retest reliability is an important component of a measurement tool for measuring tactile defensiveness. The reader can conclude, therefore, that the article is important regarding documentation of the test-retest reliability of the touch scale. The article is poorly executed, however, because this conclusion has to be assumed when it should be clearly stated for the reader.

4. What is the theoretical or conceptual basis of the investigation?

This question links the piece of research under study to the larger theory or conceptual framework to which it relates. It is critical to try to understand the link of research to theory development and refinement, so we must consider published research as it relates to theory. If the authors of the research article clearly identify the link between theory and research for the reader, then the research is relatively easy to read for this consideration. If the authors do not clearly present a logical argument of how the research links to theory, the article is usually much more difficult for the reader to understand and appreciate.

In this example, the section that includes a literature review (the section preceding the Methods section) clearly discusses a larger theory—tactile defensiveness related to sensory integration processing and human function. The reader can, therefore, see how this piece of research on test stability of an instrument to measure tactile defensiveness fits into the larger picture of clinical evaluation of the phenomenon.

5. How was the research conducted?

Information about how the research was conducted is usually presented in the Methods section of a research article. Sometimes this section is labeled Procedures or one is a subheading of the other. Rarely, however, can one read only that section and really understand what was done.

Rather, the reader must read through the entire research article and attempt to reconstruct what the investigator actually did. Let us read through "Test-Retest Reliability of a Touch Scale for Tactile Defensiveness" again and identify, step-by-step, how the research was conducted.

6. What type or kind of research is it and why?

Review chapter 2 as you consider what type of research was conducted. Correct identification of the type of research depends on the previous question—only by correctly identifying what was done can you really determine what type of research it is, in spite of what the author of the research may purport. Identifying the type of research really seems to confound students. Yet, if you clearly identify what was done, it is relatively easy to categorize the activities. Look at our example. It is descriptive research, as the purpose of the research, and the data collected, is to identify (i.e., describe) the test-retest stability of the instrument under study.

Did you think it was experimental research? Many beginning-level students think that if subjects are administered an instrument, the research is experimental. Note, however, that in this case all subjects were dealt with in exactly the same manner. Systematic variation in how subjects are administered the test (morning vs. afternoon) could change the research design and transform the type of research into quasiexperimental or experimental. But because it was not done in this case, the study is descriptive.

7. What were the research questions or hypotheses?

This question addresses the very essence of the research. What is the question to be answered? Or were there specific hypotheses tested in the research? Sometimes, the author of a research article clearly states the research questions addressed and even provides hypotheses, usually at the end of the Introduction or the Literature section. Most often, however, they do not. The reader must infer what they are.

It is rarely necessary for a reader to infer what specific hypotheses are being tested. But it is essential for the reader to understand the research question addressed, and whether it is quantitative or qualitative research. In this example, the research question is inferred. Can you guess what it is?

Look at the concluding sentence in the Introduction: "The current study was an investigation into the test-retest reliability of the newly developed scale" (p. 46). This may be rephrased into the following research question: What is the test-retest reliability of the touch scale? This is the question that the research should answer.

8. What are the variables or phenomena under study?

In either quantitative or qualitative research, it is essential, in understanding the research, to know what was studied. Traditionally, this is identification of the variables under investigation. It is less important to be able to identify variables by type (independent, dependent, confounding, extraneous, attribute, etc.) than to have a common sense appreciation of what was studied. Such an understanding requires you to read through a research article and really think about what was done, the purpose, and so on. Refer back to Test-Retest Reliability. Jot down what you think were the topics of study.

Did you guess time? If so, you are correct. If not, reread the article. Stability of the instrument over time is the focus of this study. Thus, it is the characteristic of the instrument over time that is investigated.

9. Who were the subjects or units of study? How many were there?

This may be the easiest, and the hardest, part of understanding research articles. Many articles clearly state who did what to whom. In such cases the reader can easily identify the subjects. But more complex research designs often have multiple groups of subjects who were investigated in different ways. Such research articles can be very complicated, and it can be difficult to ascertain just how many subjects were used. Usually the Methods section of an article includes a subsection or a simple paragraph or two that discusses subjects. Refer to Tables 2 and 3 and the Subjects section in this article. The participating subjects are clearly identified and described. In fact, the reader even knows how the actual subjects were obtained from a larger pool.

10. How were subjects or units of study obtained?

This is often not stated in the research article. The following questions need to be asked:

Were subjects obtained through random selection? Of all subjects who could potentially participate, were certain ones selected using a process of random selection (like pulling names out of a hat!)?

Were subjects selected because they possessed certain characteristics or attributes that are important as related to a certain theory or intervention? This is purposive sampling.

Were subjects selected because they were convenient? This is often the case—such as using college students in psychology experiments. This is convenience sampling. Refer to the article. Read through the Subjects section. It is clear that the subjects were not randomly selected. And parental permission to participate does not constitute an attribute or characteristic warranting the label of purposive sampling. By process of elimination, you can see these subjects were a sample of convenience.

11. What information or data were collected?

Answering this question requires the reader to sift through information presented in a research article to determine just what the data or information was that was collected. In our example, the data collected were students' scores on the touch scale from two testing sessions, 2 weeks apart.

12. If specific evaluation tools were used, what were they? Was information on the reliability and validity of the evaluation tools provided?

Generally speaking, this question addresses psychometric qualities of tests used to measure some aspect of the subjects. Many times, change resulting from treatment is measured using some sort of standardized test. Or subjects may be assigned to different groups or treatment conditions based on certain test scores. In these cases, it is important for the reader to know if the test used is (a) valid, and (b) reliable. It is important, therefore, for the researcher to provide the reader with information about the test. However, this is often neglected in research articles. In this example, determining the reliability of the instrument was the entire purpose of the study. However, Table 1 did provide additional information on validity of the instrument.

13. How was the information or data collected?

Simply stated, Who did what, when, and how? If you can answer these questions, you can identify how the data or information was collected. In the example used here, a research assistant administered the test in a quiet room. Then, 2 weeks later, the research assistant readministered the same test to the same subjects.

14. Will data collected be able to answer or address the research question or problem under study?

This question may appear somewhat stupid. You might well ask, Why would someone go to the trouble of conducting research if it won't answer the research question? In the ideal world, one wouldn't go to all that trouble, but we all know that the world is not ideal. Sometimes a researcher ends up with a plan of research that, for a variety of reasons, does not produce data that answers the question. Let us suppose that the study in Test-Retest Reliability was replicated in a school in Miami, Florida. It could be that the data obtained by subjects in a school in Miami, Florida, really would not give the researcher information about the test-retest reliability of the instrument. Why? In all likelihood the majority of students in a Miami school would be Latino American and may or may not be fluent in English. As this test is English based, the results obtained would not be valid. Thus, the data collected could not provide answers to the research question. You can see, then, how it is possible to collect data that does not answer the research question.

15. How was the information or data analyzed?

This question refers to identifying the procedures used in organizing and analyzing the research data. In qualitative research it may be content analysis. In quantitative research it is usually some sort of statistical procedure. In our example, a clear summary of data analysis is presented. The Pearson Product Moment Correlation Coefficient (r) was computed.

16. What were the criteria for interpreting the data?

Criteria for interpreting the data are usually not stated directly in the research article. Most often, they are implied. Because the research described in this example uses probability values (p values), one can assume the customary .05 level of significance was used. Also, an additional criterion of a minimum correlation of .60 for test-retest reliability was used.

17. What were the findings?

These are usually in the Results section in the article. In this example, the probability value ($p = .001$) far exceeded the customary level of significance ($p = .05$). This means that there is less than 1 chance in 1, 000 that the results were due to chance. One can conclude, therefore, that the effect is due to something other than chance; and in this case, the effect was due to the stability of the instrument.

18. What were the limitations of the study? Was there a critical flaw? What was it?

Many research articles present a Limitations section of the paper. Sometimes limitations are incorporated in the Discussion section. Other research articles may identify a limitation and state it anywhere in the paper. Still others may not identify any limitations. In Test-Retest Reliability, the limitations are embedded in the Results and Discussion sections.

A limitation of the study needs to be noted. Since the school system would grant permission to conduct the study contingent upon a principal agreeing to let his or her school participate, and since "the principal would participate only if he or she could identify students to whose parents permission forms could be sent, the sample selection may have introduced a systematic bias. Subsequent replication study can address this issue."

In this case, the limitation is related to the method of subject selection. Refer to chapter 4 for a review of common critical flaws. Can you find any? None were identified in this article.

19. Are the conclusions of the study warranted?

Given what was done and how, do the findings make sense? Do the authors of the research article appropriately interpret the findings? Sometimes there is a tendency to overinterpret the data and lay claim to more than the results really revealed. In the example used here, the findings are appropriately limited and qualified.

20. How can these research findings be used in occupational and physical therapy?

This is the fun part of reading research. Given everything that was done and your analysis, how could you use the results in your practice or work? The example we used provides information on an evaluation tool that pediatric therapists could be using for screening and in public school settings.

This chapter was designed to accomplish two goals. First, it should have provided you with some of the basic skills necessary to read the foreign language of research. Second, it should have provided you with an "attitude adjustment" about research. Research really isn't boring and hard to understand for those in the know. In the next chapter, we will discuss two types of research—quantitative and qualitative.

References

Adler, A. B., Wright, B. A., & Ulicny, G. R. (1991). Fundraising portrayals of people with disabilities: Donations and attitudes. *Rehabilitation Psychology, 36(4),* 231–240.

Burns, N., & Grove, S. K. (1987). *Nursing research: Conduct, critique and utilization.* Philadelphia: W. B. Saunders.

Campbell, D. T., & Stanley, J. C. (1963). Experimental and quasiexperimental design for research. In N. L. Gage (Ed.), *Handbook of research on teaching* (pp. 171–246). Chicago: Rand McNally.

Cohen, H. (1988). How to read a research paper. *American Journal of Occupational Therapy, 42,* 596–600.

Conover, W. J. (1980). *Practical nonparametric statistics.* New York: Wiley.

Cross, D. L., & Donaldson, D. C. (1992). Abstract: An analysis of the descriptive and demographic characteristics of rehabilitation patients as predictors of their physical versus psychological orientation. *Physical Therapy, 72,* 566.

Frank, R. G., Chaney, J. M., Clay, D. L., & Kay, D. R. (1991). Depression in rheumatoid arthritis: A reevaluation. *Rehabilitation Psychology, 36,* 219–230.

Giannini, M. J., & Protas, E. J. (1992). Exercise response in children with and without juvenile rheumatoid arthritis: A case-comparison study. *Physical Therapy, 72,* 41–48.

Hinkle, D. E. Weirsam, W., & Jurs, S. G. (1979). *Applied statistics for the behavioral sciences.* Boston: Houghton Mifflin.

Hoff, A. L., Riordan, H., O'Donnell, D. W., Morris, L., & DeLisi, L. E. (1992). Neuropsychological functioning of first-episode schizophreniform patients. *American Journal of Psychiatry, 149,* 898–903.

Kerlinger, F. N. (1973). *Foundations of behavioral research* (2nd ed.). New York: Holt, Rinehart and Winston.

PSI International (1989). Evolving methodology in disability research. *Rehab Brief, 12(5),* 1–4.

Royeen, C. B. (1986). *An exploration of parametric versus nonparametric statistics in occupational therapy clinical research.* Dissertation Abstracts International.

Royeen, C. B., & DeGangi, G. (1992). *A synthesis of the literature of neurodevelopmental treatment (NDT) 1980–1990.* Chicago: Neurodevelopmental Treatment Association, Inc.

Royeen, C. B., & Seaver, W. L. (1986). Promise in nonparametrics. *American Journal of Occupational Therapy, 40,* 191–193.

Seaver, W. L. (1979). The right test but the wrong occasion. *Journal of Business Education, 19, 5,* 221–223.

Recommended Readings

Cohen, H. (1988) How to read a research paper. *American Journal of Occupational Therapy, 42,* 596–600.

Conover, W. J. (1980). *Practical nonparametric statistics.* New York: Wiley.

Hinkle, D. E., Weirsma, W., & Jurs, S. G. (1979). *Applied statistics for the behavioral sciences.* Boston: Houghton Mifflin.

Mansfield, E. (1986). *Basic statistics.* New York: Norton.

Ottenbacher, K. J. (1995). The Chi-square test: Its use in rehabilitation research. *Archives of Physical Medicine and Rehabilitation, 76,* 678–681.

Royeen, C. B. (1986). *An exploration of parametric versus nonparametric statistical procedures in the occupational therapy literature.* Dissertation Abstracts International.

Royeen, C. B., & Seaver, W. (1986). Promise in nonparametrics. *American Journal of Occupational Therapy, 40,* 191–193.

Seaver, W. L. (1979). The right test but the wrong occasion. *Journal of Business Education, 19, 5,* 221–223.

Learning Activities

1. Define all key words.
2. Locate three research articles that use a statistical analysis. Interpret the results.
3. Construct a personal diary of research concepts and terms on file cards. Add to this file as you learn new information.
4. Find a basic statistics text. Look up measures of central tendency and measures of dispersion.
5. Interpret each of the following:

   $F = 24.5, df = 1/54, p < .00008$

   $x = 37.4, df = 10, p = .05$

CHAPTER 6

Sampling and Selection

KEY WORDS

Criterion-based selection

Population

Probability sampling

Purposive sampling

Qualitative research

Random sample

Sampling

Selection

Stratified sample

Systematic sample

How do you acquire units of study for quantitative research? How do you acquire units of study for qualitative research? The process of planning for and obtaining units of study in research is called **sampling** (used in quantitative research) and selection (used in qualitative research). This chapter provides the reader with an overview of sampling and selection from both a quantitative and a qualitative research perspective. It presents concepts fundamental to each, and provides illustrative examples from the literature. First, I will discuss sampling and the quantitative perspective.

Quantitative Research and Sampling

Once the investigator has identified the purpose of the research and the type of data needed to answer the research question, he or she must determine who or what (units of study) can provide that data. How the investigator obtains the units that provide the data constitutes the process of sampling or selection. In quantitative research, probability sampling is usually desired because appropriate use of most inferential statistics depends on probability sampling (Burns & Grove, 1987).

Units of study for an investigation in occupational and physical therapy research are most often human subjects. Units of study obtained through sampling, however, may also be other things, such as educational programs, salaries paid to therapists, organizational structure of departments, and so on. What the unit of study is depends on the nature of the research question driving the investigation.

WHAT IS A POPULATION?

A **population** is the entire collection of a defined group of individuals or objects. Populations can vary somewhat depending on how you define them or the criteria you set. Following are theoretical examples of populations pertinent to occupational and physical therapy research:

- all entry-level occupational therapy and physical therapy students in the year 1992
- all males with a diagnosis of head injury in federally funded nursing homes in 1992
- all infants served in neonatal intensive care units during 1991, whose mothers used crack, alcohol, or other drugs during pregnancy.

Clearly, studying the entire population in each of these examples would be difficult, but for different reasons. Thus, one can use a proxy for the population. That is, one can use a subset of the population, obtained in a well defined and clear manner, for study. And it is this subset or a specifically chosen segment of the population that constitutes a sample.

WHAT IS A SAMPLE?

It is difficult to discuss sampling in quantitative research without providing you the larger picture about sampling. Let's assume that you wish to study motor skills in older individuals diagnosed with Alzheimer's disease. The population you wish to study, then, is all older individuals who have been diagnosed with Alzheimer's disease.

Can you do this? Do you have the money, time, and personnel to study all older persons in the United States diagnosed with Alzheimer's disease? Probably not. To study an entire population of interest is usually beyond feasibility. Most investigators cannot afford to study an entire population, even if an entire population could be accessed. Think about other populations of interest to occupational and physical therapists. It may be all students in public schools who have cerebral palsy. Or it may be all persons older than 40 who have heart disease. Clearly, the populations of interest to occupational and physical therapists cannot be studied in their entirety.

The problem, then, is how to study a population of interest without actually studying the entire population. The answer is *sampling*—a collection of units of study drawn from the larger population, but smaller in number and representative of the population overall. Sampling allows us to study populations of interest without the time and expense of studying the entire population. A sample size of less than 30 units would be a small sample (Best & Kahn, 1989). This has implications for data analysis because nonparametric statistical procedures are preferred for small sample sizes (Royeen, 1986).

To illustrate, if we cannot study all geriatric individuals with Alzheimer's disease in the United States, we may be able to study all of them within a small city—say those individuals in Indianapolis, Indiana. Or instead of studying all students with cerebral palsy in public schools across the country, we may study those attending public schools in New Jersey and Ohio. In each case we are taking a smaller number of units from the larger population for investigation.

SAMPLING

There are two broad categories of sampling: probability sampling and nonprobability sampling.

Probability Sampling. Probability sampling refers to selecting your sample based on knowing the likelihood in which each unit of the population will be selected to be included in the sample. Probability sampling, therefore, is based on mathematical probability theory (Hayslett, 1968). Because there is a known probability for inclusion in the sample, the accuracy of the degree to which the sample represents the population can be mathematically calculated. Probability sampling can be simply illustrated using a hat. Put two pieces of paper into a hat. If you were to select one of the two pieces of paper from the hat, each one has a 50% probability of being selected. A 50% chance of being selected refers to the known probability of being used in the sample.

The most common types of probability sampling are simple **random samples**, **systematic samples**, and **stratified samples**. Simple random samples are based on randomly selecting some number of subjects or units from the population overall, wherein all subjects or units have an equal chance of being selected (Mansfield, 1986). The previous example of putting names of all possible subjects into a hat and randomly selecting a sample thereof is a simple random sample.

Let's assume that you are working with all Olympic-caliber gymnasts training for the 1996 Olympics. Let's further suppose that you have a new training technique you wish to study. In such a case you may randomly select one name from the total number of names by selecting one out of a gym bag having all names in it. This would be a simple random sample. You may then conduct a single subject study with this athlete, having randomly selected him or her from the total population.

Systematic samples are often confused with simple random samples, but they are not the same. Systematic sampling may also be called systematic selection with a random start (Fortune & Bender, 1989, chapter 2). For example, you may have access to a list of all patients being served in an outpatient clinic, and wish to give them a survey. You put 10 numbers into a hat and pull out one number. That one number has been randomly selected for your random start. Let us assume it is 6. You then start with patient number 6 on the list and you then survey every 5th patient on the list from and including number 6.

At the clinic or program where you work, ask the records department to pull the names of all clients to whom you provided service in the year 1992. From this total list, randomly pick a number between 1 and 10 as a starting place. Let's assume it is 10. Then, you will select every 10th person from that starting point. This is a systematic sample (choosing subjects at the interval of 10 places) of clients you may wish to follow up for a consumer satisfaction survey.

Stratified samples are samples that are "broken down" or stratified by important variables such as sex, age, diagnosis, socioeconomic status (SES), and so on. The important variables are determined by the research investigator based on previous research literature and "best guesses." Stratified sampling allows for broad representation across varied levels of the variables affecting sample characteristics. Stratified sampling is often used in test development to assure normative data compiled across ages, sex, and social class.

Let's assume that you wish to study the effects of neurodevelopmental treatment (NDT) on victims of stroke. As we know that variables such as age of onset, sex, and location of stroke are very important in outcomes, these are important variables to assure representation in the study. We may therefore wish to stratify our sample by these very variables. We may wish to have 12 subjects for each age category (50s, 60s, and 70s). Furthermore, we may wish to have six males and six females in each age category. Furthermore, we may wish to have three with a left cerebral vascular accident and three with a right cerebral vascular accident within each sex category. This would be an example of a stratified sample, stratified by age, sex, and diagnosis.

Purposive Sampling. The vast majority of quantitative research, however, does not use random samples, the most appropriate and desired type of probability sampling for use with inferential statistics. Instead, most quantitative research uses a form of purposive sampling.

Purposive sampling is not based on probability. Hence, it is often called nonprobability sampling. Purposive sampling is based on what its name implies—a purpose. Generally, the units of study are selected for investigation based on some attribute, trait, or group membership that they possess (Patton, 1980).

There is a prevalent misunderstanding that purposive sampling is, by definition, "bad and inadequate." It is not. It is merely based on different assumptions and principles than probability sampling. It is the selection of subjects or units using a criterion other than probability when conducting a quantitative investigation (Sell, 1968). It is the choice of a sample or sampling unit based on certain characteristics or manifestations.

Purposive sampling is used when random selection does not meet the requirements of what the investigator wishes to study. It is up to the investigator to explicitly state the subject characteristics on which the sampling is based. The primary drawback is that one does not know the degree of error in the sample studied, whereas probability sampling allows for exact determination of the degree of error in a sample. (Recall how surveys report plus or minus certain percentage points when reporting on, for example, political polls. This is based on error calculations.) One must, instead, use logic to determine how representative the purposive sample is to the group under study.

Pull out one of your professional journals and look at the section on subjects in a research article. The odds are that the study will use purposive sampling, but that it will not be identified as such. Whenever random sampling is not used in occupational and physical therapy research, it is likely some sort of purposive sampling is used. Look at the article and see if the investigator presents some sort of rationale or diagnostic criteria for the subjects used. If the article you have uses random sampling, look through the journal and see if another research article has a form of purposive sampling.

An example of subject acquisition that is typical of purposive sampling would be if 30 hospitalized schizophrenics attending an inpatient sheltered workshop were assigned to either work skills training (WST) or a standard treatment control group (Sauter & Nevid, 1991).

Qualitative Research and Selection

Qualitative research, by its very nature, uses nonprobability sampling. But because the very notion of probability infers a statistically based mathematical model, qualitative methodologists call the process of obtaining subjects or units **selection** (Goetz & LeCompte, 1984, chapter 3). The investigator's rationale for who or what is chosen for study constitutes selection.

SELECTION

Selection is to qualitative research as sampling is to quantitative research. The process of selection focuses on who, where, and when units or subjects will be studied in qualitative research. And unlike the strict and predetermined methods of probability sampling in quantitative research, flexibility and adaptability of selection are hallmarks of selection in qualitative research (Goetz & LeCompte, 1984). Selection of initial informants or subjects in qualitative research may lead the investigator to other subjects. This process of going from initial subjects to other subjects as the investigation progresses illustrates the methodological flexibility built into qualitative approaches (Goetz & LeCompte, 1984).

CRITERION-BASED SELECTION

The selection of units for study in qualitative research is criterion based, just as purposive sampling was criterion based in quantitative approaches. Criteria for selection of subjects should address the characteristics of the subjects to be studied. This is a point of commonality between qualitative and quantitative research. Criterion-based selection may be appropriate to function as purposive sampling in quantitatively oriented research when

- the characteristics of the population are unknown
- the groups under study do not have well-defined boundaries
- generalizability of the results is not a primary goal
- the investigator does not have access to the whole population (Goetz & LeCompte, 1984).

Figure 6–1 presents an example of selection in qualitative research.

What Is The Best Sample or Selection?

Realistic considerations enter into the decision about what is the best sample to use in an investigation. The best sample is economical to obtain and representative of the population in which you are interested. And the best sample is one that you really can obtain. Many research proposals include specification of samples that are ideal, and in all likelihood the investigator cannot really access the sample for study. An ideal sample that cannot be accessed is not useful in research. In quantitative research the best sample is a random sample that is large enough to support the data analysis of choice. In qualitative research, the best selection meets the criteria for inclusion in the investigation.

Errors in Sampling and Selection

Having been trained as a quantitative researcher, most of my experience in sampling has been in probability sampling. Let me share with you two experiences illustrating how easy it is to make errors in probability sampling when true random samples are not used.

My first experience was with pilot testing the language of test items. Because it is very difficult to obtain permission to conduct research in public schools, I obtained permission to pilot test questions on developing an instrument in a local private school. What was not apparent at that time was that children attending private school in this region varied systematically from those attending public schools. Only after pilot testing and actually using the instrument in public schools did it become apparent that children in the public schools did not have as high a vocabulary level as those attending the private school. The children attending the private school systematically varied from those attending public school in terms of vocabulary. Thus, the pilot-

FIGURE 6–1. SUBJECT DESCRIPTION IN A QUALITATIVE STUDY

The Eight Study Participants and Their Families

Mother	Family Configuration Summary	Ethnicity	Location and Economic Class	Child's[a] Attributes
Carol	Husband Daughter, adolescent Son, school-aged Daughter[a]	Black	Bronx; Economically depressed	4 years old; spastic diplegic; verbal; uses wheelchair
Donna	Husband Son, school-aged Son[a]	Caucasian	Bronx; Middle-class	3 years old; spastic quadriplegic; does not talk
Fran	Husband Son, 9 years old Daughter, 10 years old Son, 11 years old Son[a]	Black	Manhattan; Public housing	3 years old; right leg impaired; normal IQ
Gail	Husband Sex unknown, married Daughter, married Daughter, college-aged Son, school-aged Son[a]	Black Jamaican	Brooklyn; Renovated area in Flatbush area	3 years old; spastic quadriplegic; blind; totally dependent
Helen	Husband (Photographer) Son, 5 years old Daughter[a] Daughter[a] Daughter, infant	Caucasian English	Manhattan; Middle-class apartment building	4 years old; spastic quadriplegic; both dependent
Irene	Husband (Administrator) Son, 3 years old Son[a]	Black	Manhattan; Public housing	2 years old; spastic hemiplegic; behavior difficulties
Jane	Husband (Art dealer) Daughter[a] Son, 8 months old	Caucasian, English, French	Manhattan; Luxury loft	5 years old; spastic diplegic; crawls; verbal
Kay	Husband (Musician) Son[a] Daughter, 8 months old	Caucasian	Queens; Middle-class	3 years old; spastic quadriplegic; mentally retarded

Note: Children are listed from oldest to youngest.
[a]Preschool child with cerebral palsy.
From J. Hinojosa & J. Anderson (1991). Mother's perceptions of home treatment programs for their preschool children with cerebral palsy. *American Journal of Occupational Therapy, 45(3),* 273–279. Page 275. Reproduced with permission.

testing validity had been compromised because the population on which the pilot testing was conducted was not the same population on which the study itself was to be conducted.

The second example has to do with how random sampling in theory can play out in practice. After much paperwork, I received permission to conduct an investigation in a public school. The permission to conduct such research was pending the approval of the principal. The principal agreed to the research with a provision that no letters of informed consent be sent to certain parents, that is, certain children would be excluded from participating. Thus, a large section of the potential population was deleted as a condition of receiving approval to conduct research in the desired setting. Already, then, my sample was biased before even obtaining a single subject.

Issues of Generalizability in Sampling

In theory, generalizability of quantitative research findings depends on use of random samples. Then the findings of the research study can be generalized to the population. In fact, however, much research that is conducted and published does not use random samples and results are generalized to theory. In fact, most of the research published in psychology is of this model. It may be, therefore, that research using nonrandom samples can generalize findings to theory underlying the investigation, not to populations. There is a growing trend toward using such theory-driven methods of generalizability in research (Chen & Rossi, 1987).

Application

The next part of this chapter contains examples of sampling or selection from published literature in occupational and physical therapy. Ask yourself the following questions for each example:

1. What type of sampling or selection was used?
2. Are criteria stated if nonprobability sampling was used?

Short discussions are provided after each example.

EXAMPLE AND DISCUSSION 6–1

PERSONALITY CHARACTERISTICS OF THE PUBLISHED AND NONPUBLISHED OCCUPATIONAL THERAPIST (RADONSKY, 1980).

Radonsky studied the personality characteristics of therapists who have and have not published. Her "Subjects" section read as follows:

Subjects. A list of 300 therapists was compiled from a random sample of membership of the AOTA, of which half were published authors (publishers). Publishers were defined as those therapists who had published in the American Journal of Occupational Therapy. From this list, 50 publishers and 50 nonpublishers were selected by geographic distribution for this study (p. 10).

What type of sampling or selection was used? This example illustrates stratified random sampling. The variable of publisher was stratified, or divided, two ways: therapists who had published and therapists who had not published. The overall sample was randomly selected, and from that a stratified subsample was obtained.

EXAMPLE AND DISCUSSION 6–2

INTERVENTION APPROACHES WITH STROKE PATIENTS (LOGIGIAN, SAMUELS, FALCONER, & ZAGAR, 1983).

Logigian, Samuels, Falconer, and Zagar (1983) conducted a study of intervention approaches with clients who have experienced strokes.

Intervention strategies consisted of (a) facilitation techniques to promote muscle movements, and (b) traditional forms of occupational and physical therapy. The sample in this study is described as follows:

Subjects. A total of 42 adults (24 men and 18 women) with a mean age of 61.6 years (SD = 21) were admitted to Massachusetts Rehabilitation Hospital from September 1976 through November 1978 with a diagnosis of stroke. Each patient was selected from a larger population of approximately 400 stroke patients admitted with the diagnosis of stroke within the study time period.

Criteria for inclusion within this study group were: (a) stroke documented by CT scan within 7 weeks of onset and prior to initiation of therapy; (b) medically fit to participate in a nonrestrictive program as determined by the attending physician and supported by electrocardiogram, hematology, white blood cell count, electrolytes, blood urea nitrogen, blood sugar, erythrocyte sedimentation rate, and liver function tests; and (c) informed consent.

The patients were separated on three diagnostic CT scan measures: (a) lesion site (middle cerebral artery distribution, lacunar, internal capsule, thalamus, pontine, carotid, corona radiata, temporoparietal, anterior cerebral artery); lesion type (hemorrhage, thrombosis, embolism, lacunar); and (c) right or left hemisphere. There were 16 right middle cerebral artery distribution infarctions; 9 left middle cerebral artery distribution infarctions; and 6 deep lacunar infarctions. The remaining 11 patients had either multiple lacunas, basilar artery distribution infarctions, thalamic hemorrhages, or carotid occlusions. The lesion site, type, and side were thought to be important patient characteristics. The lack of a sufficient number of patients in each group precluded analysis of covariance (ANCOVA) by lesion site, type, and side.

Procedure. The 42 patients who met the study criteria were randomly assigned to one of two different treatment approaches for remediation.

What type of sampling or selection was used? The sample was a purposive sample. That is, patients in this study were selected based on certain criteria having to do with type and location of the stroke, as well as informed consent of the subjects. We have no information about the subjects who did not provide informed consent. Were they systematically different in any way? The random assignment of subjects to treatment is not to be confused with random selection. Random selection would consist of randomly selecting 42 subjects out of the total pool of 400. Instead, 42 out of 400 potential subjects were purposively sampled because they met criteria. Then, these 42 subjects were randomly assigned to one of two treatment conditions. In short, this may be termed criterion-based purposive sampling with which random assignment to treatment conditions is used.

Are criteria stated if nonprobability sampling is used? Criteria are clearly stated. There are many conditions for subjects to meet. This example illustrates a very typical approach to sampling in clinical research. Because random samples are usually very difficult to obtain (primarily because of the informed consent issue), investigators randomly assign subjects to treatments. This then qualifies the investigation as quasiexperimental research. Such selection/assignment is common in what is called clinical trials or efficacy research, that is, research into the effectiveness of one intervention strategy compared to another.

EXAMPLE AND DISCUSSION 6–3

COMPARISON OF SERVICE PROVISION MODELS IN SCHOOL-BASED OCCUPATIONAL THERAPY SERVICES: A PILOT STUDY (DUNN, 1990)

Dunn used the selection assignment approach in studying models of service delivery, that is, direct versus consultation.

Subjects. The subjects for this study included 12 preschoolers and 2 kindergartners (between 35 months and 79 months old) who attended special education programs within their own communities. The communities corresponded to the programs served by the occupational therapists participating in the study. Six subjects were girls and eight were boys. Children were selected for the study based on eligibility and exclusionary criteria that would establish a more homogeneous sample for the study. To be included in the study, children had to display at least a one-year delay in two or more areas of development as measured by the Developmental Programming for Infants and Young Children (DPIYC)...; one of the areas of delay had to be gross motor, fine motor, or self help skills.

Furthermore, the educational team had to have made a recommendation that occupational therapy would be a part of the children's educationally related services within the school program. Deaf and blind children and those who were either nonambulatory or required devices for walking were excluded from consideration, because these factors would affect administration and scoring of many items on the DPIYC.

Children were randomly assigned to one of two conditions, the direct service condition (DS) or the consultation condition (C). Seven children were randomly assigned to each condition at the onset of the study; both groups consisted of four boys and three girls. At the beginning of the study, the DS group had a mean age of 55 months with a range of 39 months to 67 months, while the C group had a mean age of 56 months with a range of 35 months to 79 months. All seven DS children were enrolled in preschool programs; two were classified as educable mentally retarded (one child had Down's syndrome), four were classified as developmentally delayed (one child had a seizure disorder), and one was classified as autistic. Two had received occupational therapy services before this study; six received physical therapy; and five received speech therapy in addition to occupational therapy during the study period. Five of the C children were enrolled in preschool programs and two attended kindergarten. Two of these children were classified as multiply handicapped, one as autistic, one as educable mentally retarded, and three as developmentally delayed (one child had Down's syndrome). Four of these children had received occupational therapy previously, four received physical therapy, and all of them received speech therapy concurrent with occupational therapy services during the study. (p. 203)

What type of sampling or selection was used? Because the author wished to restrict potential confounds of the study, homogeneity of subjects was desired. Thus, subjects were selected based on "eligibility and exclusionary" criteria; therefore, the sample was purposive. Exact criteria are not clear, but are categorically identified.

EXAMPLE AND DISCUSSION 6–4

EFFECTS OF VERY LOW BIRTH WEIGHT AND SUBNORMAL HEAD SIZE ON COGNITIVE ABILITIES AT SCHOOL AGE (HACK ET AL., 1991).

Hack, Breslau, Weissman, Aram, Klein, and Borawski (1991) studied the school-age abilities of low birth weight infants whose head circumferences were smaller than normal at eight months. In this particular publication, the subjects and sampling were described as follows:

Subjects. The population studied at eight years of age included the cohort of 490 children with very low birth weights who were admitted to the neonatal intensive care unit at Rainbow Babies and Children's Hospital in Cleveland from January 1977 through December 1979. Of these children, 316 (64 percent) survived to their second year, and one additional child died of a brain tumor before the age of eight years. Fifty-nine children were not examined at eight years: 22 were lost to follow-up, including 3 who were adopted; 17 families refused further participation; and 20 families moved out of state. Of the remaining 256 children, data were incomplete for 7. Two hundred forty-nine (79 percent) of the surviving birth cohort thus constituted the study population. Maternal demographic data and infant birth data are presented in Table 6–1. The study children differed significantly from the 67 children excluded from the eight-year analyses in only two categories: their mothers were more likely to have been black, and they were less likely to have been transferred from a community hospital. None of the infants had documented major congenital malformations or gestations complicated by interuterine infections. (p. 231)

What type of sampling or selection was used? Again we see in this investigation purposive sam-

TABLE 6–1. MATERNAL DEMOGRAPHIC RISK FACTORS AND PERINATAL DATA FOR THE 249 CHILDREN STUDIED AT EIGHT YEARS OF AGE AND FOR THE 67 CHILDREN EXCLUDED FROM THE STUDY.*

Variable	Study Cohort (N = 249)	Children Not Studied (N = 67)
Maternal risk factor		
Age (yr)	24 ± 2	23 ± 5
Unmarried	91 (37)	23 (34)
< High-school education	61 (24)	20 (30)
Black	140 (56)	27 (40)†
Perinatal data		
Weight (g)	1176.5 ± 218	1198.1 ± 222
Gestational age (wk)	29.7 ± 2	29.7 ± 2
Small for gestational age	51 (20)	12 (18)
Male sex	124 (50)	32 (48)
Multiple birth	42 (17)	8 (12)
Hobel neonatal risk score	55.2 ± 31	57.3 ± 36
Transferred from community hospital	135 (54)	47 (70)

*Reasons for exclusion are given in the Methods section. Unless otherwise stated, values are the numbers of children, with percentages given in parentheses. Plus–minus values are means ± SD.

†P < 0.05 for the comparison with the study cohort.

Hack, M., Breslau, N., Weissman, B., Aram, D., Klein, N. & Borawski, E. (1991). Effect of very low birth weight and subnormal head size in cognitive abilities at school age. *New England Journal of Medicine, 325(4).* 231–237. Page 232.

pling. That is, the subjects were included in this investigation if they met the criteria of (a) being in the original population, (b) being able to be followed for the time period, and (c) having complete data sets. In no way can this sample be interpreted to be a random sample. Yet, this is a typical type of sample seen in longitudinal research, that is, research that follows a set or cohort of subjects over a period of time. Much of the research in development uses this type of sample.

EXAMPLE AND DISCUSSION 6–5

COMPARISON OF TWO METHODS OF DETERMINING CHANGE IN MOTORICALLY HANDICAPPED CHILDREN

Stephens and Haley (1991) investigated the relationship between individual subject goals generated using goal attainment scaling (GAS; Cytrynbaum, Binath, Birdwell, & Brandt, 1979) and the Peabody Development Motor Scales (PDMS; Palisano & Lydic, 1989). Their sampling process was as follows:

Subjects. The subjects for this study were part of a larger sample of children recruited for the program evaluation study, Components of Program Evaluation in Early Intervention: A Model for Practice. Children were recruited from nine early intervention programs in the greater Boston area and ranged from 3 to 32 months at time of entry into the study. Selection of the specific children to participate in the project was made by the staff of each early intervention program. All parents signed a consent form approved by the Human Subjects committees of Boston University and the respective early intervention program. Each of the children was receiving physical therapy as part of early intervention services during the course of the study. The intensity of the services varied from consultation to direct therapy. Some were receiving home-based intervention while others were involved in center-based classrooms.

TABLE 6–2. SAMPLE CHARACTERISTICS

Mean Chronological Age:	19.1 months (7.1)*		
Sex:	34 Males	20 Females	
Race:	69.8% White	18.9% Black	11.3 Other
Mean Peabody Gross Motor Quotient:	0.4	(0.2)*	
Mean Peabody Fine Motor Quotient:	0.5	(0.2)*	
Diagnoses:**	25.9% Down's Syndrome		
	3.7% Spina Bifida		
	9.2% Cerebral Palsy		
	1.9% Autism		
	7.4% Failure to Thrive		
	16.7% Hydrocephalus		
	27.8% Congenital Abnormality		
	5.5% Congenital Infection		
	40.7% < 36 Weeks Gestation		

* Standard Deviation
**Percentages total more than 100% because some children have multiple diagnoses.

From Comparison of two methods for determining change in motorically handicapped children. *POTPeds, 11(1),* 1991. Page 1–17.

A variety of handicapping conditions are included in the sample. Table 6–2 presents the sample characteristics. The early intervention program participants were recruited from both inner city and surrounding towns and cover a broad socioeconomic range. Socioeconomic status is a strong predictor of outcome in high-risk children. In this study, each child's PDMS scores were compared with his or her GAS.

What type of sampling or selection was used? You may be tempted to call this stratified random sampling. One might make this mistake because of the presentation of subject characteristics in Table 6–2. Note, however, that subjects were not selected based on proportions represented by this criteria. Instead, subjects were merely described by these characteristics. This is a big difference. Again, this is a purposive sample. You may be beginning to realize that the majority of the sampling in research is of this type. This is a purposive sample because it is not a random sample, and criteria have been set for subject inclusion.

Are criteria stated if nonprobability sampling is used? Not exactly. The authors state that staff at participating centers selected subjects for participation in the study. The reader does not have a clear understanding of what these criteria were. The only clear criteria is that subjects have a consent form. As you can see, criteria can be extremely varied in purposive sampling. And the investigators can also vary in delineation of just what their criteria was for subject selection. It may also be clear to you that the more specific and detailed an investigator is about a purposive sample, the better you, the reader, are able to understand who were subjects in the study.

Look at the following criteria for sampling specified in a study by Kluzik, Fetters, and Coryell (1990):

Subjects were selected from the Cotting school (Lexington, MA), an academically oriented school for children with physical handicaps. All subjects met the following criteria: (1) have ability to understand and carry out the verbal directions included in the reaching task, (2) have sufficient visual skill to localize an object with both eyes, (3) have sufficient passive range of motion to be able to reach the target, and (4) have a letter of informed consent signed by his or her parent(s).

Compare these subjects with other clients with whom you work. If a sample is not random, the subjects or sampling section should enable you to evaluate how similar or dissimilar the study subjects are to clients with whom you work.

As was previously stated in this chapter, use of a purposive sample is not bad. In fact, most application research in our fields uses it. But use of purposive sampling requires delineation of criteria for subject selection and a detailed description of subjects so that the reader can evaluate the study in terms of applicability to the reader's clients.

This chapter presented an overview of probability sampling and purposive sampling used in quantitative research as well as selection used in qualitative research. Hypothetical and actual examples from the literature were provided for illustration. Finally, important issues related to sampling and selection, such as generalizability, were discussed.

In the next chapter, I will discuss a fundamental aspect of all research, measurement.

References

Best, J. W., & Kahn, J. V. (1989). *Research in education* (6th ed.). Englewood Cliffs, NJ: Prentice-Hall.

Burns, N., & Grove, S. K. (1987). *The practice of nursing research: Conduct, critique and utilization.* Philadelphia: W. B. Saunders.

Chen, H., & Rossi, P. H. (1987). The theory-driven approach to validity. *Evaluation and Program Planning, 10,* 95–103.

Cytrynbaum, S., Binath, Y., Birdwell, J., & Brandt, L. (1979). Goal attainment scaling, a critical review. *Evaluation Quarterly, 3,* 5–40.

Dunn, W. (1990). A comparison of service provision models in school-based occupational therapy services: A pilot study. *Occupational Therapy Journal of Research, 10,* 300–320.

Fortune, J., & Bender, M. (1989). Provisional guidelines for sampling in clinical research. In C. B. Royeen (Ed.), *Clinical research handbook: Analysis for the service professions* (pp. 29–46). Thorofare, NJ: Slack.

Goetz, J. P., & LeCompte, M. D. (1984). *Ethnography and qualitative research design in educational research.* Orlando, FL: Academic Press.

Hack, M., Breslau, N., Weissman, B., Aram, D., Klein, N., & Borawski, E. (1991). Effect of very low birth weight and subnormal head size on cognitive abilities at school age. *New England Journal of Medicine, 325,* 231–237.

Hayslett, H. T. (1968). *Statistics made simple.* Garden City, NJ: Doubleday.

Kluzik, J., Fetters, L., & Coryell, J. (1990). Quantification of control: A preliminary study of effects of neurodevelopmental treatment of reaching in children with spastic cerebral palsy. *Physical Therapy, 70,* 65–76.

Logigian, M. K., Samuels, M. A., Falconer, J., & Zagar, R. (1983). Clinical exercise trial for stroke patients. *Archives of Physical Medicine and Rehabilitation, 64,* 364–367.

Mansfield, E. (1986). *Basic statistics.* New York: W. W. Norton.

Palisano, R. J., & Lydic, J. S. (1984). The Peabody Developmental Motor Scales: An analysis. *Physical and Occupational Therapy in Pediatrics, 4,* 69–75.

Patton, M. Q. (1980). *Qualitative methods.* Beverly Hills, CA: Sage.

Radonsky, V. E. (1980). Personality characteristics of the published and nonpublished occupational therapist. *American Journal of Occupational Therapy, 34,* 208–212.

Royeen, C. B. (1986). *An exploration of parametric versus nonparametric statistics in occupational therapy clinical research.* Dissertation Abstracts International.

Sauter, A. W., & Nevid, J. S. (1991). Work skills training with chronic schizophrenic sheltered workers. *Rehabilitation Psychology, 36,* 255.

Sell, D. L. (ed.). (1968). Nonprobability sampling. In the *International Encyclopedia of Social Science.* New York: MacMillan.

Stephens, T. E., & Haley, S. M. (1991). Comparison of two methods for determining change in motorically handicapped children. *Physical and Occupational Therapy in Pediatrics, 11,* 1–17.

Recommended Readings

Hawkins, G. D., & Cooper, D. H. (1990). Adaptive behavior measures in mental retardation research: Subject description in American Journal of Mental Deficiency Articles (1979–1987). *American Journal of Mental Retardation, 94(6),* 654–660.

Kraemer, H. C., & Thiemann, S. (1987). *How many subjects?* Beverly Hills, CA: Sage.

Learning Activities

1. Define all key words.
2. Find two research articles of interest to you. One should be quantitative research and one should be qualitative research. Delineate the sampling and selection used in each.
3. Generalizability can be to either populations or theory. Explain the difference and rationale.
4. What are characteristics of an "ideal sample" and why?

CHAPTER 7

Measurement

KEY WORDS

Checklists

Construct validity

Content validity

Criterion-referenced tests

Face validity

Instrumentation

Internal consistency

Levels of measurement

Likert scaling

Measurement

Norm-referenced tests

Observations

Protocols

Reliability

Scales

Self-reports

Validity

This chapter presents information about the fundamental tool of research, measurement. The bulk of the chapter addresses measurement and quantitative research, but a later section does discuss comparable issues in qualitative research. I have also included a user's guide for the research consumer to evaluate measurement tools.

Measurement

One of the earliest forms of measurement is described in ancient China when, in 1115 B.C., the first "civil service" exams were administered to potential candidates for public office (DuBois, 1970). In this century, the work of German and

French scientists regarding the assessment of intelligence and biology has contributed to modern-day standards and practice related to measurement.

Measurement is the assignment of numbers to objects, events, or processes according to some rule (Burns & Grove, 1987, p. 748). It allows us to more objectively think about, discuss, and research aspects of behavior or function in a quantifiable manner. Think about the meanings measurement indices convey to you in your professional, as well as your daily, life:

- The consumer inflation index is up 3%
- Mortgage interest rates are at a 30-year low of 8%
- The number of millionaires has increased by 66% in the last decade
- ADL status is independent with assist
- Fair level of resistance is obtained in extensor muscle group
- ATNR is present.

Note that many of these examples did not have numbers associated with them, but the measurement index was a category or descriptor. Thus, measurement includes assignment of not just numbers but categories to objects, performance, events, or people.

Levels of Measurement

There are four levels of measurement that are typically used to determine at what level something is being measured. They are presented in Figure 7–1.

Think about the data you collect on clients in your hospital, clinic, or school. What level of measurement is the data? It is probably a variety of levels of measurement.

It is important to think about the level at which your data are collected in the clinic and in research because certain statistical procedures assume data will be measured at a certain level.

FIGURE 7–1. LEVELS OF MEASUREMENT AND DEFINITIONS

Level of Measurement	Definition	Example
Nominal	This level of measurement is merely categorical. There is no order or numerical meaning.	• Diagnosis • Group membership
Ordinal	Assignment of numbers reflect order effects or increasing or decreasing amounts. Intervals between numbers are not consistent or equal.	• Muscle strength • Grades • Coma levels • ADL status
Interval	Intervals between numbers are consistent. The starting point or zero lacks meaning.	• Motor test scores
Ratio	Intervals between numbers are consistent and zero is meaningful.	• ROM scores • Blood pressure readings

Adapted from Hopkins, Glass, and Hopkins (1987).

For example, most parametric statistics require ratio or interval levels of data. One can always collapse or move data from a higher level to a lower level of measurement (ordinal to categorical) but not vice versa. This has implications for conducting research.

Qualities of Measurement

Generally, when we talk about measurement we also must consider qualities of the measuring process itself, that is, the **validity** and **reliability** of how one is measuring something to obtain the data. These may be called the psychometric qualities of measurement. Traditionally, these psychometric qualities center around validity and reliability.

VALIDITY

Validity refers to the meaningfulness or appropriateness of an inference or interpretation made from a test; it is the ability of a test to really measure what it is supposed to measure (Anastasi, 1989; Dunn, 1989). This concept can be transformed into the question, Does the instrument measure what it purports to measure (Best & Kahn, 1989)?

For example, there is some degree of controversy in the literature that the Southern California Postrotary Nystagmus Test (SCPNT; Ayres, 1975) may not measure discrete vestibular system processing as it was originally envisioned to do (Royeen, Lesinski, Ciani, & Schneider, 1981). Does it measure vestibular system processing or does it measure overall arousal and alertness levels of the central nervous system? The issue of what this test really measures is germane to its construct validity.

Another example of this concept may be illustrated with the development of the Sensory Integration and Praxis Test Competency Exam (SIPT; Royeen, Koomar, Cromack, Fortune, & Domkey, 1991). As the test development team was developing the test questions, the test consultant raised an issue about the length of test questions. He believed that the length of most of the test items had created a test that had more to do with reading ability than with knowledge and skills about the SIPT. Thus, he believed the construct validity of the test being developed would be compromised unless we addressed the issue of length of test items.

There are three general types of validity. **Face validity** is the superficial appearance that an instrument measures the construct it is supposed to measure. Or as a question, Does the instrument appear to measure what it is supposed to measure (Dunn, 1989)?

To illustrate, let's assume that you asked colleagues to review a family-centered interview guide for use with families of stroke victims. You may ask your colleagues to determine if the interview guide appears family centered. And they may say that it does. Yet when the interview guide is really tested with actual families, they find it offensive and intrusive. Appearances and reality are not always the same thing. Face validity, therefore, is the appearance of validity without rigorous testing to determine that it is so.

Construct validity is "the degree to which scores on a test can be accounted for by...the constructs of a sound theory" (Best & Kahn, 1989, p. 171). Reinterpreting the concept as a question, one would ask, Does the instrument measure the construct of interest?

The best example of a measurement tool with strong construct validity is the *Sensory Integration and Praxis Test* (Ayres, 1989). This tool is a collection of tests based on a complex, complicated, and comprehensive theory of sensory integration processing. It is specifically designed to identify patterns of sensory integrative processing in children. The theory is integrally built into the tests, and the tests have further developed the theory.

Content validity is how appropriately or broadly the instrument measures the breadth and scope of what is to be measured. Or one could ask, Does the instrument measure the expected content (Burns & Grove, 1984, p. 275)? Think back to a time when you took a final exam that focused on something that was either not well covered or not emphasized in class. Were you upset and angry? Such instances, where the test material does not match up to class material, illustrate a lack of content validity.

RELIABILITY

[Reliability refers to the degree to which the instrument measures whatever it is measuring consistently (Best & Kahn, 1989).] Consistency of measurement over time reduces testing error. Thus, it is desirable for tests to be reliable. Reliability may be asked as the question, Does it consistently measure the phenomenon? There are three types of reliability to consider when evaluating a measurement tool.

Stability over time refers to test-retest reliability (Best & Kahn, 1989). Test-retest reliability is typically evaluated using a correlation between subjects' scores on a first test correlated with the subjects' scores on a retest at some later interval of time. If a test is stable over time, you would expect there to be a high correlation between the first test and the second test.

Internal consistency reliability refers to the correlation of certain test items with the other test items, that is, the relationship between test items; they should all be measuring the same thing (Dietz, 1989). This may be determined by asking, Do test items correlate? Internal consistency reliability is often obtained by computing a correlation based on the correlation of each single test item with the test overall. This correlation is called coefficient alpha (Crocker & Algina, 1986, p. 119).

Stability of scorers refers to interscorer reliability. Imagine this scenario: Two different people score the same test. If a test has good interscorer reliability, the scores should correlate highly. If the test has poor interscorer reliability, the two scores will not correlate well. This correlation may be called coefficient between scores (Best & Khan, 1989).

An example of determining interscorer reliability would be a research team practicing scoring on a standardized test that requires expert judgments, such as the *Harris Goodenough Draw a Person Test* (Harris, 1963). The scores taken by different members of the team would be compared to see how well they correlate; the correlations would determine if the Goodenough Test has high or low interscorer reliability.

Instrumentation Related to Measurement

Instrumentation is the manifestation of measurement. For example, if you want to measure something, an instrument is a tool for doing so. Instrumentation is the process of using rules to assign numbers to objects or events so that we have a common language, or a common way of looking at something. It is important because it allows us to view human behavior in an objective manner, or at least as objectively as possible.

Why are measurement and instrumentation important in occupational and physical therapy practice? Let me share an event from personal experience: My interest in instrumentation was prompted by frustration. I was having difficulty justifying a diagnosis of tactile defensiveness in parent conferences. It was difficult to explain to a parent the statement, "I think your child is tactually defensive." These are words that parents have never heard before. And I did not have an objective measure from an instrument to support my diagnosis. As a clinician, I wanted face validity behind the diagnosis of tactile defensiveness. My need for credibility drove me to look for instrumentation in tactile defensiveness. I thought that future parent consultations might go better if there was an instrument for measuring tactile defensiveness. The data it would yield could give validity to the occupational therapy diagnosis.

This example illustrates how I became interested in instrumentation for tactile defensiveness (Royeen, 1985, 1986, 1987). We have all been in similar situations where something has been diagnosed based on clinical judgment with no standardized assessment for data-based support. List areas in your practice for which you would like an instrument. Here is my list:

- occupational engagement
- classroom-based sensory motor processes
- sensory integrative disorder processing and the family
- quality of life.

There is a clear need for more and better instrumentation and measurement in occupational and physical therapy. Before discussing measurement in specific terms, let us look further at instrumentation and the role it plays in therapy.

Llorens and Gillette (1985) identified two roles for instrumentation in occupational therapy. One of these is to articulate the domain of concern, that is, to develop a sort of collection of variable specifications pertaining to occupational therapy and physical therapy areas of interest.

Benson and Clark (1982) identified the roles of instrumentation in occupational therapy related to research. They argued that instrumentation in occupational therapy is necessary as a means to measure program effectiveness. This brings us to the question, What is the role of instrumentation in research?

It is easiest to answer this question if we talk about evaluation; not evaluation in terms of evaluating a client, but evaluation in the research sense, that is, how you evaluate a program. There are two levels in evaluation research (Royeen, 1986). First-level evaluation research is where you define roles and functions of your program. In second-level evaluation research you evaluate the effectiveness of your program. In occupational therapy and physical therapy, for example, first-level evaluation research would be to define our roles and functions as an educationally related service in public schools. Only after first-level evaluation research has been accomplished could we then do the second-level evaluation research to measure how effective that program is in the school system. For it is impossible to measure effectiveness (second level) without first knowing what to measure (first level).

Instrumentation and research have a similar relationship. First-level research is having the tools to measure what you want to see change. Second-level research is measuring that change. It is extremely difficult to generate effectiveness studies or documentation of change during treatment until one can adequately measure that change. Thus, instrumentation may be considered the first level of research in occupational therapy and physical therapy. To illustrate, Dr. Lucy Miller wanted to conduct effectiveness studies on treatment with preschoolers. She wanted to do second-level research but discovered she did not have a tool for it, so Dr. Miller developed a nationally standardized instrument for preschoolers, the Miller Assessment for Preschoolers (MAP; Miller, 1982).

Let us now take a look at types of instrumentation or measuring tools, that is, the methods of measurement.

Methods of Measurement

The methods of measurement or types of evaluation tools consist of established procedures or methods for collecting measurement data. There are six main methods of measurement in occupational and physical therapy:

- observations
- interviews
- self-reports and scales
- checklists
- protocols
- standardized tests.

In the following section I define each method and present an example. Validity and reliability concepts apply to each, though perhaps in different ways.

OBSERVATIONS

Observations are a research technique that is "systematic, directed by a specific purpose, carefully focused, and thoroughly recorded" (Best & Kahn, 1989, p. 175). If the researcher does the observation unobtrusively, that is, without the subjects knowing, the likelihood of introducing bias or adversely influencing subject performance is lessened (Kazdin, 1982).

The process of observation is not spontaneous and haphazard. Rather, observations must be based on careful planning and pretesting of data collection guides, methods, and so on (Best & Kahn, 1989). Typically, the investigator "practices" observations many, many times as a sort of pretest, and develops data collection tools based on that practice.

Laver has developed an instrument that provides a standardized format for diagnostic reasoning through observation of performance in simple, daily tasks. Figure 7–2 represents this observation-based data collection tool (Laver, 1990).

SELF-REPORTS AND SCALES

Self-reports and scales are a collection of techniques and strategies commonly used by the social science community (Lodge, 1984). In fact, the techniques date back as far as 150 B.C. when a form of rating scale was used to evaluate the brightness of stars (Lodge, 1984). You are all familiar with Likert-type ratings, but you may not know that they are scales (McIver & Carmines, 1981).

Table 7–1 presents a Likert-type scale by Branholm and Fugl-Meyer (1992). You can evaluate your life in general by using this scale. An additional example is presented in Figure 7–3. Respond to the statements based on how you feel right now; rate the validity of each statement by how much you agree with it.

Figure 7–4 presents a short research plan for developing a rating scale that measures attitudes on the part of parents and professionals regarding the parent-professional partnership in early intervention.

CHECKLISTS

Checklists are rather self-explanatory. They consist of a collection of items that can be checked either as present or absent or as accomplished or not. It is rare indeed for these to appear in the published literature. Rather, they are prevalent in practice with little beyond face value validating them. Do you have any checklists in your paperwork in your current practice?

PROTOCOLS

Protocols consist of step-by-step procedures for executing assessment without having standard-

FIGURE 7–2. EXAMPLE OF AN OBSERVATION-BASED DATA COLLECTION TOOL

Part of an Observational Checklist

Task 1: Eating from a bowl using a spoon

Name: ______________________ Assessor: ______________________

Site of Lesion: ______________________ Deficit: ______________________

Equipment (e.g. glasses, hearing aid): ______________________

Dominant Hand: ______________________ Hand used to hold spoon: ______________________

Action	Able (Yes)	Unable (No)	Further Testing	Comments
*Identifies spoon through touch	R L	R L		
Puts spoon on table on the right of the bowl				
Scans table for objects				
Fixes gaze on objects				
Recognizes objects *names <> points				

From Laver, A. J., & Powell, G. E. (1995). The Structured Observational Test of Function (SOTOF): A standardization of diagnostic reasoning for the assessment of neuropsychological dysfunction through the observation of activities of daily living. Windsor: NFER–NELSON. Reprinted with permission.

ized directions or methods. Many clinics and school systems have their own protocols for initial patient observation. Examples of protocols used in occupational and physical therapy include reflex testing and manual muscle testing. An article published by Ayres and Tickle (1980) reported on a set of clinical procedures that, collectively, constitute a protocol for evaluating modulation of sensory processing.

STANDARDIZED TESTS

Recall your original training as an occupational or physical therapist. Part of your training undoubtedly covered administration and interpretation of one or more standardized tests. Standardized tests are developed according to strict and accepted psychometric principals, and are administered under uniform conditions of directions, setting, and equipment. There are many types of scores and testing terms associated with standardized tests. Figures 7–5 and 7–6 provide reference guides to use with standardized tests. The variety of standardized tests used in occupational and physical therapy are beyond the scope of this text. I refer you to the Recom-

TABLE 7–1. LIKERT SCALE LIFE SATISFACTION CHECKLIST (adapted from Branholm & Fugl-Meyer, 1992)

How satisfactory are these different aspects of your life? Indicate the number that best suits your situation.

1 = Very dissatisfying
2 = Dissatisfying
3 = Rather Dissatisfying
4 = Rather satisfying
5 = Satisfying
6 = Very satisfying

Life as a whole is	1	2	3	4	5	6
My ability to manage my self-care (dressing, hygiene, transfers, etc.)	1	2	3	4	5	6
My leisure situation is	1	2	3	4	5	6
My vocational situation is	1	2	3	4	5	6
My financial situation is	1	2	3	4	5	6
My sexual life is	1	2	3	4	5	6
My partnership relation is	1	2	3	4	5	6
My family life is	1	2	3	4	5	6
My contacts with friends and acquaintances are	1	2	3	4	5	6

mended Readings for more information in this specific area.

Given this overview of types of measurement tools used, how do you know if they are any good? How do you know that they are reliable and valid? You need to go to sources that discuss these key points of measurement tools.

Information on Measurement Tools

There is a wealth of information available on measurement tools and evaluations. A few of the key texts are identified here. These books are the place to go to find out what others think of the test or measurement tool you may be using or thinking of using, or to evaluate tests used in research you read.

- *The Eighth Mental Measurements Yearbook* (Buros, 1980) provides a comprehensive review of over 1,000 tests distributed commercially.
- *Standards for Educational and Psychological Tests* (American Psychological Association, 1974) delineates standards for educational and psychological test developers and test users.
- *Psychological Measurements* (Anastasi, 1976) is a classic text encompassing theory and use of standardized tests.
- *An Annotated Index of Occupational Therapy* (Asher, 1989). Bethesda, MD: American Occupational Therapy Association.
- Linda King Thomas (1987) book.

So far this chapter has addressed measurement related primarily to quantitative research. We will now address measurement in qualitative research.

Measurement Concepts in Qualitative Research

Measurement is a part of qualitative research as well as quantitative research. The exact nature of how things are measured is what differs between

FIGURE 7–3. LIKERT-TYPE RATING SCALE FOR RESEARCH ANXIETY

I feel overwhelmed with research books.

[ ]	strongly agree
[ ]	agree
[ ]	undecided
[ ]	disagree
[ ]	strongly disagree

Research is incredibly stupid!

[ ]	strongly agree
[ ]	agree
[ ]	undecided
[ ]	disagree
[ ]	strongly disagree

Perhaps there is more to research than I used to think.

[ ]	strongly agree
[ ]	agree
[ ]	undecided
[ ]	disagree
[ ]	strongly disagree

Research is really interesting.

[ ]	strongly agree
[ ]	agree
[ ]	undecided
[ ]	disagree
[ ]	strongly disagree

I will use my research knowledge after finishing this book.

[ ]	strongly agree
[ ]	agree
[ ]	undecided
[ ]	disagree
[ ]	strongly disagree

FIGURE 7–4. RESEARCH PLAN FOR SCALE DEVELOPMENT

	Task
Step One	**Domain Specification** Identification of the content to be addressed in the attitude scale, domain specification.
Step Two	**Advisory Board Review** Submission of the content for review by Advisory Board. Revision of content and weighing based upon panel of expert feedback. Discussion of need for one or more versions of the scale.
Step Three	**Specific Objectives** Specifications of content areas to be addressed by objectives.
Step Four	**Table of Specifications** Generation of the Table of Specifications. Define domains.
Step Five	**Panel of Experts** Submission of the Table of Specifications to panel of experts.
Step Six	**Test Item Development and Item Analysis** Generate favorable and unfavorable statements about each attitude to be measured (roughly 60 for each domain). Sources: transcripts of focus groups, existing instruments, and potential subjects. Have Expert Panel review test items and code by Table of Specifications. Have pilot group (n = 50) rate each statement from 1 (strongly agree) to 5 (strongly disagree). Compute each subject's summated score. Identify subjects scoring in the top 25% and bottom 25%. Conduct item analysis with each item based upon high scorers' and low scorers' response patterns. Keep items that discriminate between high and low scorers (n = approximately 20 items). Randomize order of remaining test items.
Step Seven	**Pretest** Pretest of the newly constructed scale including directions, format, etc.
Step Eight	**Revisions** Revise based upon pretesting.
Step Nine	**Pilot Testing** Pilot testing of the attitude scale at select sites. When a large enough sample is obtained for item analysis (n = 100), Step Ten will commence.
Step Ten	**Psychometric Analysis** Calculation of internal consistency of the attitude scale across groups (Coefficient alpha set at a minimum of .80. Items will be deleted or revised to accomplish this.) Investigation of stability of attitude scale with n = 30. (Test-retest reliability set at a minimum of .80.) Generalizability analysis.

FIGURE 7–5. GLOSSARY OF TESTING TERMS (CERMAK, 1989; DIETZ, 1989)

Measurement Error: Any of the factors which can and do influence test scores other than the "true" performance of the subject. It is specifically the difference between a subject's score (observed score) and the subject's score if no measurement error occurred (true score). This difference is, in reality, unknown but can be estimated based upon the Standard Error of Measurement (SEM).

Mean: Arithmetic average of all scores combined.

Median: Score at which 50% of all scores are above and 50% of all scores are below.

Mode: Most frequently occurring score in a distribution.

Norm: The performance on a test of the sample used for standardization.

Norm Referenced: Shows how an individual scored in comparison to the normative group. That is, a test for which interpretation is based on the comparison of the test taker's performance to other people in a specified group, the normative group.

Norm Takers: Data that summarizes the test performance of specified groups, usually by age or grade. This is the sample used for standardization.

Standard Deviation: A measure of the dispersion of all test scores based upon the square root of the overall variance.

Standard Error of Measurement: Arithmetically calculated range of subject's test score when measurement error is considered. It is based upon the standard deviation of the errors of measurement that is associated with the test scores for a specified group of test takers. This may then be used to calculate the probability that the "true score" will fall within a specified range.

Sums: Arithmetically calculated total scores or subscores.

True Score: Refers to the "true" test score of a subject if chance events had not influenced the test performance of the subject. This may be thought of as the average of scores earned by an individual on an unlimited number of parallel or equivalent tests.

Variance: In a set of test scores, the total amount of variability based upon the squared difference between each individual test score and the average score.

FIGURE 7–6. OVERVIEW OF STANDARDIZED TEST SCORES AND THEIR MEANING ADAPTED FROM CERMAK (1989)

Types of Standardized Test Scores	What they mean
Derived Scores	Refers to raw scores which have been transformed into some type of standard score.
Raw Score	Has meaning based upon the scoring system of the test.
Percentile Rank	Some percentage of the raw scores are the same or lesser than this raw score.
Age Equivalent Score	This is based upon the raw score which would be the mean score for a specified age group.
Grade Equivalent Score	This is based upon the raw score which would be the mean score for a specified grade.
Standard Score	Based upon standard deviation, the distance the individual's score is from the average score.
Stanine Score	Based upon the distribution of raw scores into nine parts.
z-Score	Within a given distribution, this reflects the number of standard deviations a score is above or below the average score.

the two. In qualitative research the measurement is usually observational in nature. Structured and unstructured observations are used to study variables of interest (Burns & Grove, 1989). The use of unstructured observation in qualitative research may mean the observation and recording of what is being seen without prior planning or pretesting (Burns & Grove, 1989).

An entire measurement methodology within qualitative research is based on observation as well as participation in the setting in which observation is occurring, and is called participant observation. In this type of observation there are no hypotheses or even identified variables prior to engaging in the observation. The process of measurement in qualitative research has been undergoing methodological refinement in recent years. Burns and Grove (1989) developed 12 qualitative research strategies, based on the work of Miles and Huberman (1984), that assure validity of qualitative measures. Their strategies are presented in Figures 7–7 and 7–8.

Review of all these strategies in Figure 7–7 suggests that there are many, many methods to assure the validity of qualitative research measures.

FIGURE 7–7. STRATEGIES FOR STUDY OF THE VALIDITY OF QUALITATIVE MEASURES (FROM BURNS AND GROVE, 1987, REPRINTED WITH PERMISSION)

1. **Checking for Representativeness.** Qualitative measurement can be biased by either the attention of the researcher or a bias in the people from whom they obtain their measures. To ensure that measures are representative of the entire population, a search should be made for sources of data not easily accessible. The researcher assumes that observed actions are representative of actions that occur when the researcher is not present. However, efforts must be made to determine whether observed activities are representative of events occurring in the absence of the researcher.
2. **Checking for Researcher Effects.** In many cases, the researcher's presence can alter behavior, leading to invalid measures. The researcher must remain on the site long enough to become familiar, use unobtrusive measures and seek input from informants to avoid this effect.
3. **Triangulating.** The qualitative researcher must compare all the measures from different sources to determine the validity of the findings.
4. **Weighting the Evidence.** Qualitative research involves reducing large amounts of data during the process of coming to conclusions. In this process, some evidence is "captured" from this mass of data and is used in reaching those conclusions. The researcher must review the "strength" of the captured data to validate the conclusions. The researcher determines the strength of the evidence from the source, circumstances of data collection and researcher's efforts to validate the evidence. The researcher must actively search for reasons why the evidence should not be trusted.
5. **Making Contrasts/Comparisons.** Contrasts between subjects or events in relation to the study conclusions should be examined. For example, if nursing supervisors consider an action to be very important but staff nurses consider it simply another administrative activity, this is a contrast. The two extreme positions should be examined. Then a decision must be made about whether the difference is a significant one.
6. **Checking the Meaning of Outliers.** Exceptions to findings should be identified and examined. It is these exceptions that are referred to as outliers. The outliers provide a way to test the generality of the findings.
7. **Using Extreme Cases.** Certain types of outliers, referred to as extreme cases, can be useful in confirming conclusions. The researcher can compare the extreme case to the theoretical model that was developed and determine the key factor that causes the model not to fit the case.
8. **Ruling Out Spurious Relations.** This strategy requires the examination of relationships identified in the model in order to consider the possibility of a third variable influencing the situation.
9. **Replicating a Finding.** Documenting the findings from several independent sources increases the dependability of the findings and diminishes the risk of the "holistic fallacy." The findings can be tested with new data collected later in the study or data from another site or data set. The second option is more rigorous.
10. **Checking Out Rival Explanations.** The qualitative researcher is taught to keep several hypotheses in mind and to constantly compare the plausibility of each with the possibility of one of the others being more accurate. However, near the end of data analysis, when the researcher is more emotionally wedded to one idea, it is very useful to get someone not involved in the research to act as a devil's advocate. Questions should be directed toward "what could disprove the hypothesis?" or conversely "what does the present hypothesis disprove?" Evidence that does not fit the hypothesis should be carefully examined.

continued

FIGURE 7–7, CONTINUED

11. **Looking for Negative Evidence.** This action naturally flows from the search for outliers and the search for rival explanations. In this step, there is an active search for disconfirmation of what is believed to be true. The researcher goes back through the data, seeking evidence to disconfirm the conclusions. However, the inability to find disconfirming evidence never decisively confirms the conclusions reached by the researcher.
12. **Obtaining Feedback from Informants.** Conclusions should be given to the informants, and feedback should be sought from them about the accuracy of the casual network developed. Although researchers have been getting feedback from informants throughout the analysis period, feedback after completion of the model will provide a different type of verification of information.

FIGURE 7–8. EVALUATING INSTRUMENTATION

The following guide for evaluating measuring devices or data collection tools used in research is based on the work of Law (1987). It was developed to accommodate qualitative measurement strategies for validity identified by Miles and Huberman (1984) and elaborated on by Burns and Grove (1989). This guide should serve as a starting place when evaluating the measurement strategies used in research.

GUIDE FOR EVALUATION OF MEASUREMENT IN RESEARCH.

1. What type of data collection strategy was used?
   [ ] unstructured observation
   [ ] structured observation
   [ ] checklist
   [ ] protocol
   [ ] standardized test
2. What does the data collection strategy measure?

   ____

   ____
3. Is the measurement strategy clinically useful?

   ____

   ____
4. What type of reliability information is provided?

   ____

   ____
5. What type of validity information is provided?

   ____

   ____
6. What do you think about the measurement strategy used?

   ____

   ____

In this chapter, I presented aspects of measurement related to quantitative and qualitative research. Definitions, descriptions, and examples of specific data collection techniques and measuring devices were given. I also provided a guide for evaluating the usefulness of various measurement tools. In the next chapter, I will address a type or category of research: descriptive research.

References

American Psychological Association (1974). *Standards for educational and psychological tests.* Washington, DC: Author.

Anastasi, A. (1989). *Psychological testing* (6th ed.). New York: MacMillan.

Asher, I. L. (1989). An annotated index of occupational therapy. Bethesda, MD: *American Occupational Therapy Association,* Inc.

Ayres, A. J. (1975). *Southern California postrotary nystagmus test.* Los Angeles: Western Psychological Services.

Ayres, A. J. (1989). *Sensory integration and praxis test.* Los Angeles: Western Psychological Services.

Ayres, A. J., & Tickle, L. S. (1980). Hyper-responsivity to touch and vestibular stimuli as a predictor of positive response to sensory integration procedures by autistic children. *American Journal of Occupational Therapy, 34,* 375–381.

Benson, J., & Clark, F. (1982). A guide for instrument development and validation. *American Journal of Occupational Therapy, 36,* 789–800.

Best, J. W., & Kahn, J. V. (1989). *Research in education* (6th ed.). Englewood Cliffs, NJ: Prentice-Hall.

Branholm, I., & Fugl-Meyer, A. R. (1992). Occupational role preference and life satisfaction. *Occupational Therapy Journal of Research, 12,* 159–165.

Burns, N., & Grove, S. K. (1987). *The practice of nursing research: Conduct, critique and utilization.* Philadelphia: W. B. Saunders.

Buros, O. K. (Ed.). (1980). *The eighth mental measurement yearbook.* Highland Park, NJ: Gryphon Press.

Cermak, S. (1989). *Physical and Occupational Therapy in Pediatrics, 9,* 91–123.

Crocker, L., & Algina, J. (1986). *Introduction to classical and modern test theory.*

Dietz, J. (1989). Reliability. *Physical and Occupational Therapy in Pediatrics, 9,* 125–148.

DuBois, P. H. (1970). *History of psychological testing.* Boston: Allyn & Bacon.

Dunn, W. (1989). Validity. *Physical and Occupational Therapy in Pediatrics, 9,* 149–168.

Harris, D. (1963). *Children's drawings as measures of intellectual maturity.* NY: Harcourt, Brace & Jovanovich.

Hopkins, R., Glass, F., & Hopkins S. (1987). *Basic statistics for the behavioral sciences* (2nd ed.). Englewood Cliffs, NJ: Prentice-Hall.

King-Thomas, L., Hacker, B. (1987). (ed). *A therapist's guide to pediatric assessment.* Boston: Little, Brown.

Laver, A. J. (1990). The structured observational test of function. *Gerontology Special Interest Section Newsletter, 17,* 1–3.

Law, M. (1987). Measurement in occupational therapy: Scientific criteria for evaluation. *Canadian Journal of Occupational Therapy, 54,* 133–138.

Lodge, M. (1984a). *Magnitude scaling: Quantitative measurement of options.* Beverly Hills, CA: Sage.

Lodge, M. (1984b). *Single case research designs.* New York: Oxford University Press.

McIver, J. P., & Carmines, E. G. (1981). *Unidimensional scaling.* Beverly Hills, CA: Sage.

Miles, M. B., & Huberman, A. M. (1984). *Qualitative data analysis: A sourcebook of new methods.* Beverly Hills, CA: Sage.

Miller, L. J. (1982). Miller assessment for preschoolers. Littleton, CO: Foundation for Knowledge in Development.

Royeen, C. B. (1985). Domain specification of the construct tactile defensiveness. *American Journal of Occupational Therapy, 39,* 596–599.

Royeen, C. B. (1986). Development of a scale measuring tactile defensiveness in children. *American Journal of Occupational Therapy, 46,* 414–419.

Royeen, C. B. (1986). Evaluation of school-based occupational therapy programs: Need, strategy and dissemination. *American Journal of Occupational Therapy, 40,* 811–813.

Royeen, C. B. (1987). Test-retest reliability of a touch scale for tactile defensiveness. *Physical and Occupational Therapy in Pediatrics, 7,* 42–45.

Royeen, C. B., Koomar, J., Cromack, T., Fortune, J. C., & Domkey, L. (1991). Evidence for content and discriminant validity of the Southern California sensory integration and praxis test competency exam. *Occupational Therapy Journal of Research, 11,* 1–9.

Royeen, C. B., Lesinski, G., Ciani, S., & Schneider, D. (1981). Relationship of the Southern California sensory integration tests, the Southern California postrotary nystagmus test, and clinical observations accompanying them to evaluations in otolaryngology, ophthalmology, and audiology: Two descriptive case studies. *American Journal of Occupational Therapy, 35,* 443–450.

Thomas, L. K. (1987). Book.

Recommended Readings

Benson, J., & Clark, F. (1982). A guide for instrument development and validation. *American Journal of Occupational Therapy, 36,* 789–800.

Henerson, M. E., Morris, L. L., & Fitz-Gibbon, C. T. (1987). *How to measure attitudes.* London: Sage.

Llorens, L. A., & Gillette, N. P. (1985). The challenge for research in a practice profession. *American Journal of Occupational Therapy, 39,* 143–145.

Learning Activities

1. Earlier in this chapter I suggested looking at the data you collect in your clinic to determine at what level it is measured. Now is the time to really do this! Use the following worksheet section to help your thinking.

Data Level of measurement (n = nominal, o = ordinal, i = interval, or r = ratio)

Write a description of the data here	Circle the level of the data here
1. ________________	n o i r
2. ________________	n o i r
3. ________________	n o i r
4. ________________	n o i r

2. Define all key words.
3. Refer to Figure 7–7. Select two research articles and use the guide to look at measurement in the research.
4. For each of the following tools, write down what you are using:

   Observations

   Self-reports and scales

   Checklists

   Protocols

   Standardized tests.

CHAPTER 8 Descriptive Research

KEY WORDS

Correlational research

Descriptive research

Qualitative descriptive research

Quantitative descriptive research

Survey research

1. There may also be extensive statistical manipulation of the variables of interest in descriptive research.

Descriptive research does what its name implies—it describes variables, events, phenomena, and subjects. Variables are not manipulated by the experimenter in any way, even though extensive testing of subjects may occur to better describe their characteristics.[1] Simply, descriptive research entails the systematic representation of variables of interest to the researcher.

Perhaps the easiest way to learn about just what constitutes descriptive research is to participate in the following learning exercises. Learning by doing may assist you in understanding some of the fundamental concepts behind descriptive research. Take a moment and complete Exercises 8–1 and 8–2.

EXERCISE 8–1. DESCRIPTION OF ROOM USING COUNTS

From where you are sitting, describe the room you are in by counting objects in it, colors of objects in it, number of windows, and so on. Record your observations.

EXERCISE 8–2. DESCRIPTION OF ROOM

Again from where you are sitting, describe the room by how it feels, how it looks, and how it makes you feel. Take 5 minutes and record these observations.

These two simple exercises illustrate two different aspects, qualitative and quantitative, of descriptive research. Exercise 8–1 required counts of objects. This counting, loosely speaking, is counting the variables of interest. This exercise, therefore, is quantitatively based descriptive research.

Contrast the two descriptions. The second description should portray a feeling about the room, a delineation of who was in it, and what happened in it. This noncounting approach is more qualitatively based descriptive research (Miles & Huberman, 1984, pp. 15, 26). Exercise 8–1 illustrates the principals involved in quantitative descriptive research—portrayal of phenomena by counting in some manner. And Exercise 8–2 illustrates the principles involved in qualitative descriptive research—portrayal of phenomena in prose format. Descriptive research is what is common to these two rather different approaches.

Descriptive Research Defined

Let's now look at a broad definition of descriptive research that encompasses both qualitative and quantitative approaches. Look at your responses in Exercises 8–1 and 8–2. Analyze the nature of the different types of information you obtained from the two exercises. Your analysis should provide you with an understanding of the different type of information obtained from qualitative and quantitative descriptive research, respectively.

Taken together, however, the two approaches address the frequency, intensity, or, patterns of objects, events, places, and phenomena (Best & Kahn, 1989, pp. 88-96). Restated another way, descriptive research addresses

- who
- what
- where
- how
- how many
- how much
- any combination of the above.

Descriptive research describes phenomena. Or it gives counts of phenomena. It focuses on indexing some aspect of a phenomenon.

Descriptive research, however, is not just loosely observing something. Rather, it is based on well-defined research questions directing the research and a well-defined method to measure or describe the phenomenon of interest. The description of events, subjects, or variables, therefore, are directed by the clearly defined research questions. Remember that research questions are the guiding force determining what and even how you will research phenomena.

Clinical Application of Descriptive Research

Let's talk about clinical examples that may give you a better idea of what is descriptive research. If you are an occupational therapist, think about the first time you were asked to render a pie chart of your occupations throughout the course of a day. Spenser (1991) conducts descriptive research based on that very concept. She determines the number of occupations (self-care, leisure, work, etc.) and the time period spent on each in groups of elderly individuals across various cultures. She is, therefore, describing their occupational engagement—a form of descriptive research.

If you are a physical therapist, recall the first time you had to analyze the kinesiological components of a body movement. How can this be easily defined and measured in individuals having dysfunction? Fetters and Holt (1990) have investigated movement units in children having cerebral palsy. They found that efficiency of movement in children having cerebral palsy can be portrayed by counting or indexing oxygen use during preferred stride length. Description of such movement patterns in terms of oxygen use is a form of descriptive research.

Both of the previously cited investigations (Fetters & Holt, 1990; Spenser, 1991) used counts of something (occupations, oxygen use) as a way to describe some aspect of an event or phenomenon (occupational patterns, efficiency of muscle movements). Figure 8–1 presents additional examples of descriptive research.

Descriptive research can be thought of as the necessary foundation for almost all other types or categories of research. It is the foundation for almost all other types of research because you must first have a good idea of "What is?" before you can begin to address, "How are things related?" and "What if?" Let us take a further look at this important concept.

Descriptive Research in Occupational and Physical Therapy Research

There is a great effort to demonstrate the effectiveness of occupational and physical therapy services with intervention research (DeGangi & Royeen, 1994). The disciplines of occupational and physical therapy still have considerable need for generating information on phenomena of interest because they are both relatively new. Other disciplines that have a longer research history and that have already defined and described variables and constructs of interest (such as the fields of psychology, education, and medicine) do not have as great a need for descriptive-level research. It is, however, difficult to conduct well-designed intervention studies without a strong descriptive database on pertinent variables. Doing so would be analogous to designing a treatment plan for a client about whom you know nothing.

You cannot design an appropriate treatment plan without knowing about your client. And you cannot design rigorous and appropriate intervention studies without knowing about the pertinent variables. As yet, occupational and physical therapy research has a long way to go toward developing empirical databases about the variables of interest.

For example, answer the question, Who decides the length of your treatment sessions? Were they determined through research suggesting optimal treatment intervals for different client groups? Probably not. Were they deter-

FIGURE 8–1. ILLUSTRATIVE EXAMPLES OF DESCRIPTIVE RESEARCH

Investigator(s)	Descriptive Research Being Conducted
Dyck (1992)	Presents an overview of how an immigrant woman who has rheumatoid arthritis has acquired knowledge of the health care system and how she uses that knowledge.
DeGangi and Royeen (1994)	Present results of a questionnaire examining the variables pertinent to NDT practice.
Kelly, Murphy, Bahr, Brasfield, Davis, Hauth, Morgan, Stevenson, and Eilers (1992)	Identify knowledge of AIDs/HIV risk behavior among the mentally ill.

mined through custom and convenience? You bet! This is one small example of how we operate from something other than a database.

Occupational and physical therapy, therefore, need vast amounts of descriptive research. Only by conducting such foundational research can we effectively move large numbers of investigators into conducting large-scale intervention studies. Descriptive research is something that is relatively easy to carry out and is, consequently, an ideal type of research for clinicians and beginning-level researchers to conduct. The following are examples of the types of research questions that can be addressed using descriptive research:

- What are intervention strategies used by neurodevelopmental treatment-trained therapists?
- What are classroom-based intervention strategies of SI-trained therapists?
- What are the most common mobility problems experienced in the home as individuals age?
- What are the most common functional problems experienced in the home as individuals age?
- How can therapists assist parents bringing home infants from the neonatal intensive care unit?
- What is the incidence rate of sensory integrative dysfunction in "normal" populations?
- How many people display irregular motor patterns during routine exercise?

You could probably add at least ten more questions to this list. In fact, take a moment and identify some of your own research questions for descriptive research. Remember that descriptive research addresses who, what, where, how, how many, how much, or any combination thereof. Keeping this in mind, generate three research questions based on your clinical experience in occupational or physical therapy.

The professional organizations of any field can, and should, do a great deal to address the need for research activity. In the field of occupational and physical therapy, the Neurodevelopmental Treatment Association, Inc., (NDTA) has recognized the great need for more descriptive research on what NDT treatment is, how it is done, and the outcomes. NDTA has funded clinical case studies by clinicians on these topics (DeGangi, 1994a, 1994b). NDTA's commitment to multisite descriptive research conducted by clinicians illustrates how research activity in the field can be increased.

Common Types of Descriptive Research

The previous discussion of qualitative and quantitative descriptive research is but one way to categorize descriptive research. We will discuss three additional types of descriptive research:

- clinical
- correlational
- survey.

CLINICALLY BASED DESCRIPTIVE RESEARCH

Clinical descriptive research serves to describe incidence rates, document the existence of variables and phenomena, and define variables or phenomena of interest in occupational and physical therapy research. Or it may consist of clinical case studies that don't use any type of research design, but that merely describe a client's dysfunction, discuss what was done, and present the outcomes. The previously mentioned NDTA-funded studies are examples of clinical case descriptive research.

The first example in chapter 3 was also of clinical, descriptive research. Please review that example.

CORRELATIONAL RESEARCH

Correlational or associational descriptive research attempts to identify or describe the relationship between two or more variables. Thus, correlational research is quantitatively based and uses some sort of correlational statistical analysis. Examples of this are studying the relationship between motor planning and motor performance, or the relationship between severity of cerebrovascular accidents (CVA) suffered by adults and rehabilitation outcomes.

The second example used in chapter 3 was of correlational research, that is, an investigation of the relationship between variable one (first test administration) and variable two (second test administration). Please review that example. Correlational research is relatively easy to conduct as it can be as simple as scheduling two different testing sessions for a sample of subjects. For this reason, correlational research is a realistic goal for students required to participate in or conduct beginning-level research.

SURVEY RESEARCH

Survey research is a specialized type of quantitatively based descriptive research.[2] Rather than studying single individuals or events, however, survey research is directed toward finding out about the characteristics of a well-defined group of people (population) by investigating a subgroup of that population (sample).

Surveys can use one or more of a variety of techniques for collecting data from the subjects. Such techniques can be personal interviews, questionnaires sent by mail or fax, or telephone interviews. On a large scale, the American Occupational Therapy Association (AOTA) conducts a survey of all their members every few years. You may have participated in an AOTA survey or in one from the American Physical Therapy Association.

The design or plan of survey research is usually based on two main concepts: across time or across subjects. Surveys that collect data across

2. Sometimes, survey research is used for prediction and not just description (Mann, 1985) but that is a specialized case.

FIGURE 8–2. EXAMPLES OF SURVEY RESEARCH FOUND IN OCCUPATIONAL AND PHYSICAL THERAPY LITERATURE

Investigator(s)	Research Topic
Shaw and Taylor (1992)	A questionnaire administered to 200 subjects from six nursing homes in the Memphis, TN, region was designed to find out if the subjects were having wheelchair-related problems and, if so, the nature of the problem.
McMillan (1992)	A questionnaire administered to local education agencies in England, Scotland, and Wales focused on how students in wheelchairs were transported to and from school.
Edwards and Hanley (1992)	A mailed questionnaire addressed interdisciplinary activity between occupational therapists and speech language pathologists working in the public schools.

or over time are called longitudinal surveys (Mann, 1985). This means that the same questionnaire will be administered to the same subjects over set points in time (Year 1, Year 2, Year 3, etc.). Surveys that sample subjects at one point in time, but across the variety of subjects within the defined population are called cross-sectional (Mann, 1985). That is, the survey is administered across a section of the population of interest. A variety of survey research investigations can be found in the literature. Figure 8–2 presents examples of some of that research.

Figure 8–2 reveals that the focus of these surveys is on topics about which relatively little is known. That is when descriptive research is a powerful tool.

Application

The next section of this chapter contains two examples of descriptive research. Read the following examples and answer the interpretation questions for each example. Compare your answers to the answers provided after each interpretation section.

ILLUSTRATIVE EXAMPLE 8–1

Reprinted from *Occupational Therapy Journal of Research,* Number 4, 1984, pp. 237–240. Used with permission.

Incidence Of Hypoactive Nystagmus Among Behaviorally Disordered Children

Charlotte Brasic Royeen

Emotionally disturbed and behaviorally disordered children have displayed a variety of types of irregular responses to vestibular stimulation. Zlotnick et al. (1971) tested the hypothesis that psychotic children show a significant amount of vestibular system dysfunction, and they found that of 61 children, 30 exhibited an abnormal duration of nystagmus. Somewhat similarly, Piggot et al. (1976) conducted a study of the nystagmic response of emotionally disturbed children. They found that the children scoring most poorly on the Lafayette Clinic Cognitive Perceptual Motor Battery (CPM) demonstrated a significantly reduced amplitude and decreased duration of postrotary nystagmus. They concluded that "a vestibular disturbance may be present in many emotionally disturbed children" (p. 724).

Silberzahn (1975) studied sensory integrative dysfunction, which included measures of vestibular system functioning, within a child guidance population. She concluded that "children with behavior disorders should be carefully evaluated for disorders of sensory integrative function, especially those related to the vestibular system" (p. 34).

Support of the concept that the vestibular system has a primary role in emotional development and that vestibular system inefficiency can underlie emotional dysfunction has been provided by an animal model of research. Douglass et al. (1979) investigated spatial orientation and emotionality in mice having genetic defects specific to the static organs, the uticle and saccule, of the vestibular system. Behavioral tests of the mice's performances on different motor and balance tasks were conducted. Compared to a control group of normal mice, the mice with static end organ defects performed significantly poorer during the tests, supporting the hypothesis that the vestibular system is critical for the normal development of spatial orientation, which is crucial for normal ego development. Douglass et al. (1979) also investigated the chemical systems within the nervous system of genetically defective mice. Atypical drug reactions to cholinergic derived drugs were observed, as well as atypical responses to saline injections. The researchers found these results "consistent with the increasingly popular notion that early vestibular defects can lead to emotional deviations or even psychosis" (p. 480).

In light of these findings, as well as the work of Ayres (1978), which indicates that hypoactive postrotary nystagmus underlies certain forms of learning disabilities, duration of nystagmus among behaviorally disturbed children was investigated. Specifically, the incidence of hypoactive postrotary nystagmus in response to spinning was studied.

Methods

SUBJECTS

During one academic year, all children enrolled at the Special Center for Learning in Cincinnati, Ohio, were asked to participate in the study. The Special Center for Learning is a public school servicing behaviorally disordered children in southeastern Ohio. The 43 children were from 6 to 13 years of age, and all but two were male.

EQUIPMENT

The Southern California Postrotary Nystagmus Test (SCPNT) and a switch-back stopwatch were used for measuring postrotary nystagmus.

PROCEDURE

As part of routine testing for children enrolled in the Special Center for Learning, each subject was administered the SCPNT according to standardized procedures by an examiner certified in administration and interpretation of the Southern California Sensory Integration Tests. If a subject displayed 5 seconds or less of postrotary nystagmus after either spinning to the left or right, the response was deemed hypoactive. Postrotary nystagmus greater than 5 seconds after each of the two spins was considered within normal limits.

Results

Twenty-two of the subjects (51%) demonstrated expected or normal responses to vestibular stimulation. Fourteen of the subjects (32.5%) exhibited hypoactive postrotary nystagmus.

Conclusions

Considering that nearly one-third of the subjects displayed hypoactive postrotary nystagmus, this pilot study lends empirical support to the hypothesis that behaviorally disordered children exhibit a greater incidence of hypoactive postrotary nystagmus than would be anticipated in a normal population. Further study is needed to compare the incidence of hypoactive postrotary nystagmus among a sample of normal children as compared to a sample of behaviorally disordered children.

Caution should be exercised in generalizing these results to other clinical populations. However, these results suggest that it may be prudent to include the SCPNT evaluation when working with behaviorally disordered children.

References

Ayres, A. J. (1978). Learning disabilities and the vestibular system. *Journal of Learning Disabilities, 11*, 30–41.

Douglass, R. J., Clark, G. M., Erway, L. C., Hubbard, D. G., & Wright, C. G. (1979). Effects of genetic vestibular defects on behavior related to spatial orientation and emotionality. *Journal of Comparative and Physiological Psychology, 8*, 467–480.

Piggot, L., Purcell, O., Cummings, G., & Cadwell, D. (1976). Vestibular dysfunction in emotionally disturbed children. *Biological Psychiatry, 11*, 719–728.

Silberzahn, M. (1975). Sensory function in a child guidance population. *American Journal of Occupational Therapy, 29*, 29–34.

Zlotnick, G., Iversen, P. B., & Tolstrup, K. (1971). Vestibular function of patients in a child psychiatry department. *Danish Medical Bulletin, 18*, 6.

Illustrative Example 8–1: Questions

1. What is the purpose of the research?
2. Does the literature review provide an understanding of how and why this investigation is important?
3. Do you think the investigation is important? Why or why not?
4. What is the theoretical or conceptual basis of the investigation?
5. How was the research conducted?
6. What type or kind of research is it and why?
7. What were the research questions or hypotheses?
8. What are the variables or phenomena under study?
9. Who were the subjects or units of study? How many were there?
10. How were the subjects or units of study obtained?
11. What information or data were collected?
12. If specific evaluation tools were used, what were they? Was information on the reliability and validity of the evaluation tools provided?
13. How was the information or data collected?
14. Will data collected be able to answer or address the research question or problem under study?
15. How was the information or data analyzed?
16. What were the criteria for interpreting the data?
17. What were the findings?
18. What were the limitations of the study? Was there a critical flaw?
19. Were the conclusions of the study warranted?
20. How can these research findings be used in occupational and physical therapy?

Illustrative Example 8–1: Answers

1. What is the purpose of the research?

The purpose of this research is to determine whether emotionally disturbed children display atypical vestibular system processing evidenced by performance on the Southern California Postrotary Nystagmus Test (SCPNT).

2. Does the literature review provide you an understanding of how and why this investigation is important?

Though brief, the literature cited provides a theoretical and empirical link between irregular vestibular system processing and emotional disturbance.

3. Do you think the investigation is important? Why or why not?

The research appears important as it provides the beginning database linking vestibular deficit and emotional disturbances in school-aged children.

4. What is the theoretical or conceptual basis of the investigation?

The conceptual basis of the investigation is as follows: The vestibular system has an important role in emotional development and, therefore, vestibular system inefficiency or irregularity may underlie some emotional disorders.

5. How was the research conducted?

During the course of a school year, all children enrolled in a special center for students who are emotionally disturbed were used as subjects. They were administered the SCPNT (Ayres, 1975) as part of routine testing.

6. What type or kind of research is it and why?

This research is descriptive because it answers the question, How many? It provides a count of an incidence rate.

7. What were the research questions or hypotheses?

The research question is, What is the incidence of irregular vestibular system processing among students who are emotionally disturbed?

8. *What are the variables or phenomena under study?*

The variables under study are (a) emotional disturbance, and (b) vestibular system processing. The variable emotional disturbance is represented by the subjects diagnosed emotionally disturbed. The variable vestibular system processing is represented by the score on the SCPNT.

9. *Who were the subjects or units of study? How many were there?*

The subjects under study were all students enrolled in the special center for the school year. There were 43 subjects.

10. *How were the subjects or units of study obtained?*

The subjects constituted a sample of convenience. That is, the investigator could access all subjects in this setting.

11. *What information or data were collected?*

Scores on the SCPNT were collected for each subject.

12. *If specific evaluation tools were used, what were they? Was information on the reliability and validity of the evaluation tools provided?*

No psychometric data on the SCPNT was provided.

13. *How was the information or data collected?*

Each subject was administered the SCPNT as part of routine testing.

14. *Will data collected be able to answer or address the research question or problem under study?*

The data collected can address one aspect of the research question under study.

15. *How was the information or data analyzed?*

Logical analysis was used based on a simple descriptive statistic: percentages.

16. *What were the criteria for interpreting the* data?

None stated, logical analysis inferred.

17. *What were the findings?*

One-third of the subjects exhibited hypoactive nystagmus.

18. *What were the limitations of the study? Was there a critical flaw?*

The sample size was limited and poorly defined. The reader really cannot tell who these subjects were. The incidence rate among non-emotionally disturbed subjects is unknown, so a comparison is lacking. The reader does not know who administered the SCPNT. Generalizability is limited because of sample size and method of obtaining sample.

19. *Were the conclusions of the study warranted?*

Given the limitation of the study as noted in the article, the conclusions are warranted.

20. *How can these research findings be used in occupational and physical therapy?*

The article provides data for the need to assess vestibular system processing in those individuals with emotional disturbances. And the article provides a starting point for further research.

Reprinted from
American Journal of Occupational Therapy
Vol. 38, Number 1,
January, 1984,
pp. 44–45.
Used with permission.

ILLUSTRATIVE EXAMPLE 8–2

Initial Profile of Therapists Seeking Certification in Sensory Integrative Testing

Charlotte Brasic Royeen

Specialization into practice areas within occupational therapy has been a controversial issue for the last decade; in fact, it was the theme of the 1978 AOTA Annual Conference. Specialization may well serve as one ingredient in the "professionalization" of occupational therapy (1). However, if specialization will be a significant factor in the continued development of the profession, data are needed on therapists entering the different areas of practice. By developing data bases for each specialty area of practice, the processes contributing to the "professionalization" of occupational therapy via specialization can be better understood. Thus, a pilot study was designed to develop a profile or data base on therapists seeking to specialize in one area of practice—sensory integration—and, specifically, those seeking certification from the Center for the Study of Sensory Integrative Dysfunction (CSSID).

Methods

A questionnaire of 14 items was developed specifically for this study. The items covered topics ranging from age, sex, and years of professional experience, to motivation and reason for seeking specialization. Participants in a 2-day workshop, held in Washington, DC, on administration and interpretation of the Southern California Sensory Integration Tests (SCSIT), were asked to fill out the questionnaire. All 28 therapists who attended the second day of the workshop completed the questionnaire. The subjects' responses were coded for computer analysis and run, using the subprograms frequencies and condescriptive from the Statistical Package for the Social Sciences (2).

Results

Of the 28 subjects, 27 were female and 1 was male; 27 were occupational therapists, and 1 was a physical therapist. Their average age was 33 years, ranging from 23 to 53 years, with a median of 41 years. One therapist was certified in neurodevelopmental treatment (NDT), and all but one were members of the American Occupational Therapy Association (AOTA). In addition, 20 were members of CSSID. Five of the therapists (18%) reported that they had published and 11 that they had conducted research. Other results are presented in tabular form (Table 1).

Discussion

Certain findings are particularly relevant to the "professionalization" of occupational therapy. First, more than half of the therapists seeking certification have advanced degrees, which seems a high proportion. This raises the question about whether or not therapists with advanced degrees are more likely to become practitioners in spe-

TABLE 1

Area of Practice	Frequency	Percentage
Pediatrics	16	57
Psychiatry	1	3
Physical Dysfunction	3	11
Other	3	11
Missing	5	18
	28	100
Area of Work		
Treatment	19	68
Treatment/Administration	5	18
Administration	1	4
Other	3	10
	28	100
Highest Degree Obtained		
B.A./B.S.	14	50
M.A./M.S.	13	46
Ed.D./Ph.D.	1	4
	28	100
Frequency (Per Year) of Attending Continuing Education Presentations		
1/year	1	4
2/year	10	36
3/year	8	28
4/year	3	11
5/year, or more	2	7
Missing	4	14
	28	100
Reason for Seeking CSSID Certification		
Increased Knowledge	12	43
For Private Practice	7	25
Need It for Job	6	21
Other	2	7
Missing	1	4
	28	100
Party/Person Funding Certification		
Self	25	89
Employer (partially)	2	7
Missing	1	4
	28	100

cialty areas than therapists who do not possess advanced degrees. Thus, future consideration might be given to the extent and the nature of the influence of graduate education on specialization within occupational therapy.

Second, most respondents paid for the certification process themselves. This suggests that specialty sections, the AOTA, as well as other organizations should try to obtain private or federal funding to help subsidize therapists' expenses for training in specialty areas of practice. Otherwise, many talented and qualified therapists will be kept from specializing because of the financial burden associated with it.

Third, the finding that nearly one-quarter of the therapists were seeking CSSID certification for use in private practice suggests a changing model of occupational therapy service delivery. The traditional hospital-based delivery of services is being transformed into community-based delivery of services, of which the private practice of occupational therapists might be a significant component.

In summary, the findings of this pilot study indicate that the processes apparently associated with specialization in occupational therapy and, hence, "professionalization" are graduate education, financial resources of the therapists or sponsoring agency, and the mode of the delivery of occupational therapy services.

Delimitations. The results of this pilot study are only preliminary. The sample size was small (N=28) and thus the results cannot be generalized to all therapists seeking specialization in sensory integrative testing or other specialty areas. Furthermore, only those therapists seeking certification were studied; not those who had already received it.

Acknowledgment

Sincere appreciation is extended to Barbara Hanft, M.Ed., OTR, and especially to Dottie Marsh, M.Ed., OTR, for their guidance and support.

References

1. Gillette, N., Keilhofner, G. The impact of specialization on the professionalization and survival of occupational therapy. *Am J Occup Ther* 33:20–28, 1979.
2. Nie, N.H., Steinbrenner, K., Bent, D. *Statistical Package for the Social Sciences* (2nd Edition). New York: McGraw-Hill and Company, 1975.

Illustrative Example 8–2: Questions

1. What is the purpose of the research?
2. Does the literature review provide an understanding of how and why this investigation is important?
3. Do you think the investigation is important? Why or why not?
4. What is the theoretical or conceptual basis of the investigation?
5. How was the research conducted?
6. What type or kind of research is it and why?
7. What were the research questions or hypotheses?
8. What are the variables or phenomena under study?
9. Who were the subjects or units of study? How many were there?
10. How were the subjects or units of study obtained?
11. What information or data were collected?
12. If specific evaluation tools were used, what were they? Was information on the reliability and validity of the evaluation tools provided?
13. How was the information or data collected?
14. Will data collected be able to answer or address the research question or problem under study?
15. How was the information or data analyzed?
16. What were the criteria for interpreting the data?
17. What were the findings?
18. What were the limitations of the study? Was there a critical flaw?
19. Were the conclusions of the study warranted?
20. How can these research findings be used in occupational and physical therapy?

Illustrative Example 8–2: Answers

1. *What is the purpose of the research?*

To better understand specialization of practice in the field of occupational therapy by collecting information on those therapists seeking specialty certification in one area, sensory integration testing.

2. *Does the literature review provide an understanding of how and why this investigation is important?*

No. There is no literature review.

3. *Do you think the investigation is important? Why or why not?*

Because of the emergence of specialization as a trend in occupational and physical therapy, information about who seeks specialization and why is important for educators, clinicians, and policymakers.

4. *What is the theoretical or conceptual basis of the investigation?*

There is none given.

5. *How was the research conducted?*

A 14-item questionnaire was administered on the second day of a two-day workshop for certification in sensory integrative testing and evaluation.

6. *What type or kind of research is it and why?*

This is descriptive survey research.

7. *What were the research questions or hypotheses?*

The research question, though not stated, could be, What are the characteristics of therapists seeking specialty certification in sensory integration testing?

8. *What are the variables or phenomena under study?*

The variables under study are the characteristics of subjects seeking specialty certification in sensory integrative testing.

9. Who were the subjects or units of study? How many were there?

The subjects were the 28 participants in the workshop seeking certification in sensory integration testing.

10. How were subjects or units of study obtained?

The sample was a sample of convenience.

11. What information or data were collected?

The information collected consisted mostly of demographic data and therapist characteristics such as income earned.

12. If specific evaluation tools were used, what were they? Was information on the reliability and validity of the evaluation tools provided?

No information on the development of the questionnaire was provided. The reader has no idea if the questionnaire appropriately covered the scope of what should have been asked, or if it asked the questions in an appropriate manner.

13. How was the information or data collected?

The questionnaire was administered on the second day of the two-day workshop. The reader does not know how it was actually administered or by whom.

14. Will data collected be able to answer or address the research question or problem under study?

Only a small part of the research question can be addressed by the data collected in this investigation.

15. How was the information or data analyzed?

The data was put into a statistical computer package and analyzed using descriptive statistics.

16. What were the criteria for interpreting the data?

None provided.

17. What were the findings?

The findings were that nearly half of those seeking certification had an advanced degree, that they were paying for the training themselves, and that most attended continuing education events two to three times per year.

18. What were the limitations of the study? Was there a critical flaw?

The study can only point to or give preliminary identification of characteristics of those seeking certification, as it was a sample of convenience with limited generalizability. It could be argued that because the reader does not know how the questionnaire was developed, one cannot trust the data obtained from it. It could also be argued, however, that given the straightforward and preliminary nature of the questionnaire, the data could be accepted.

19. Were the conclusions of the study warranted?

Given the limitations identified, the conclusions appear warranted.

20. How can these research findings be used in occupational and physical therapy?

This article provides the professional some preliminary information for a better understanding of the nature of specialization and who obtains it.

This chapter has presented a foundation for understanding descriptive research, and described the types of descriptive research. I defined some of the variety of ways that descriptive research can be categorized (quantitative, qualitative, clinical, associational, and survey), and provided examples of these categories. The next chapter will present you with a foundation in experimental and quasiexperimental research. You will see that compared to the many different ways of categorizing and thinking about descriptive research, experimental and quasiexperimental research are extremely "tightly" defined.

References

Ayres, A. J. (1978). Learning disabilities and the vestibular system. *Journal of Learning Disabilities, 11,* 30–41.

Best, J. W., & Kahn, J. V. (1989). *Research in education* (6th ed.). Englewood Cliffs, NJ: Prentice-Hall.

DeGangi, G. A. (1994a). Examining the efficacy of short-term NDT intervention using a case study design: Part 1. *Physical and Occupational Therapy in Pediatrics, 14,* 71–88.

DeGangi, G. A. (1994b). Examining the efficacy of short-term NDT intervention using a case study design: Part 2. *Physical and Occupational Therapy in Pediatrics, 14,* 21–61.

DeGangi, G., & Royeen, C. B. (1994). Current practice among neurodevelopmental treatment association members. *American Journal of Occupational Therapy, 48,* 803–809.

Dyck, I. (1992). Managing chronic illness: An immigrant woman's acquisition and use of health care knowledge. *American Journal of Occupational Therapy, 46,* 696–705.

Edwards, S., & Hanley, J. (1992). Survey of interdisciplinary activity between occupational therapists and speech-language pathologists in the public schools.

Fetters, L., & Holt, K. (1990). Efficiency of movement: Biomechanical and metabolic aspects. *Pediatric Physical Therapy, 2,* 155–159.

Kelly, J. A., Murphy, D. A., Bahr, G. R., Brasfield, T. L., Davis, D. R., Hauth, A. C., Morgan, M. G., Stevenson, L. Y., & Eilers, M. K. (1992). AIDS/HIV risk behavior among the chronic mentally ill. *American Journal of Psychiatry, 149,* 886–889.

Mann, W. C. (1985). Survey methods. *American Journal of Occupational Therapy, 39,* 640–648.

McMillan, P. H. (1992). A survey of transport for children in wheelchairs. *British Journal of Occupational Therapy, 55,* 179–182.

Miles, M. B., & Huberman, A. M. (1984). *Qualitative data analysis.* Beverly Hills, CA: Sage.

Ottenbacher, K. J., Cusick, A. (1990). Goal attainment scaling as a method of clinical service evaluation. *American Journal of Occupational Therapy, 44(6),* 519–525.

Royeen, C. B. (1984). Incidence of hypoactive nystagmus among behavioral disordered children. *Occupational Therapy Journal of Research, 4,* 127–129.

Royeen, C. B. (1984). Initial profile of therapists seeking certification in sensory integrative testing. *American Journal of Occupational Therapy, 38(1),* 44–45.

Shaw, G., & Taylor, S. J. (1992). A survey of wheelchair seating problems of the institutionalized elderly. *Assistive Technology, 3,* 5–10.

Spenser, S. (1991). A study of time use in the elderly. Conference presentation at the Annual Conference of the American Occupational Therapy Association.

Recommended Readings

Mann, W. C. (1985). Survey methods. *American Journal of Occupational Therapy. 39,* 640–648.

Royeen, C. B. (1988). *Research tradition in occupational therapy.* Thorofare, NJ: Slack.

Learning Activities

1. Define the following:
    a. descriptive research
    b. quantitative descriptive research
    c. qualitative descriptive research
    d. clinical descriptive research
    e. associational descriptive research
    f. survey research
2. Take the research questions you generated early in this chapter. For each research question, think through how you could address it using clinical descriptive research and correlational (associational) descriptive research.
3. Identify a longitudinal survey research that needs to be conducted in occupational or physical therapy. What types of information should be obtained by that survey?
4. Define all key words.

Acknowledgments

Some of the concepts presented in this chapter are acknowledged to originate from R. Forbes and J. Fortune.

CHAPTER 9

Experimental and Quasiexperimental Research

KEY WORDS

Control
Experimental research
Experimenter bias
External validity
Generalizability
History
Instrumentation
Internal validity
Maturation
Measurement error
Mortality
Posttesting
Pretesting
Quasiexperimental research
Random selection
Regression
Research design
Sampling error
Selection
Specification error

Experimental and Quasiexperimental Research Defined

Experimental research is the category of investigations designed to determine the effects of one or more independent variables on one or more dependent variables using one or more groups of subjects for comparisons. Basically, it is specifically designed to look at cause and effect (Kirk, 1982).

Experimental research requires the random assignment of subjects to groups or conditions (Best & Kahn, 1989). Thus, conducting experimental research in clinical settings can be very difficult, and even impossible, because random assignment is usually impossible. As random selection and assignment of subjects is a hallmark of experimental research, experimental research is rarely found in clinical studies. Hence, quasiexperimental research is substituted for true experimentally designed research in many clinic- or field-based investigations.

Quasiexperimental research has many of the same features of experimental research, but it can be carried out in hospital, school, and clinical settings. Quasiexperimental research is similar to experimental designs, but lacks the random selection and assignment of subjects to groups or treatment interventions (Best & Kahn, 1989). Random selection and assignment of subjects to treatment or groups allows for generalizability of the study findings across the entire population of subjects (to apply the findings to other places and people; Gay, 1976). Lack of randomization found in quasiexperimental research limits the generalizability of the research findings.

Origins and Use of Experimental and Quasiexperimental Research

Investigation of cause and effect in experimental and quasiexperimental research evolved out of the study of agriculture (Hayslett, 1968). Originally, many of the research designs that became traditional models of experimental research were based on dividing plots of land into sections and determining the effects of the independent variables (amount of rain, amount of fertilizer) on crop yields (the dependent variable). Remnants of its agricultural beginnings still remain in experimental research, with traditional names for research designs such as the split plot design. The history of this type of research illustrates that research design usually evolves out of a set of needs for research investigation into a particular field or discipline. It may be that the occupational and physical therapy disciplines are in the process of evolving unique configurations of research designs to meet the fields' research needs.

Experimental research designs are used when research into life-and-death decisions is being done. For example, it is critically important to know that a drug is effective if there are serious side effects. Or one must be certain that a particular surgery is really effective before risking anesthesia and the life-threatening complications of surgery. A special type of experimental research is called clinical trials research (Marcus, 1983), and much of the research into drug testing and medical interventions is based on clinical trials.

Figure 9–1 summarizes examples of quasiexperimental research investigations of various interventions. This is typically what is seen in occupational and physical therapy quasiexperimental research. Remember that lack of random selection and lack of random assignment to groups is what differentiates this category of research from experimental research.

Figure 9–2 presents summaries of experimental research investigations. As you can see, the summaries presented in 9–2 are of research in which all subjects were randomly assigned to one of two or more different intervention options. The outcomes of the interventions were then compared. Experimental research, therefore, is designed to reveal cause-and-effect outcomes. Recall that use of random assignment or random selection is the hallmark of experimental research.

FIGURE 9–1. EXAMPLES OF QUASIEXPERIMENTAL RESEARCH

Investigators	Purpose
Dickestein, Hocherman, Pillar, and Shaham, 1986	Two groups were compared. The relative effects of exercise and functional activities were compared to PNF and NDT.
Goodman, Rothberg, Houston-McMillan, Cooper, Cartwright, and Van der Velde, 1985	Low-birth-weight, high-risk infants were divided into two groups. One group received treatment and one group did not.
Logigian, Samuels, Falconer, and Zager, 1983	Compared Rood and Bobath treatment to exercise for victims of stroke.
Watt, Sims, Harcham, Schmidt, McMillan, and Hamilton, 1986	One group study of the effects of inhibitive casting and NDT on motor performance.

PNF=proprioceptive neuromuscular facilitation; NDT=neurodevelopmental treatment.

FIGURE 9–2. EXAMPLES OF EXPERIMENTAL RESEARCH

Investigators	Purpose
Sommerfeld, Fraser, Hensinger, and Beresford, 1981	Compared groups. One received "supervised management" and the other group received physical therapy. Subjects were randomly assigned to groups.
Basmajian, Gowland, Finlayson, Hall, Swanson, Stratford, Trotter, and Brandstater, 1987	A group of victims of stroke receiving NDT were compared to a group of stroke victims receiving behavioral and cognitive training. Subjects were randomly assigned to groups.
Jenkins, Sells, Brady, Down, Moore, Carman, and Horn, 1982	Three group conditions were tested consisting of frequency of treatment. Subjects were randomly assigned to group conditions.

Experimental and Quasiexperimental Research in Occupational and Physical Therapy Research

What is the role of experimental and quasiexperimental research in occupational and physical therapy? Such research is primarily oriented to investigation of the effect of treatment interventions on client performance and status. As discussed in the previous chapter, descriptive research can tell us what and how we work as therapists. Experimental and quasiexperimental research can tell us if our intervention has an effect or changes outcomes. Thus, the call for the efficacy research so needed in our fields is really a call for intervention research in physical and occupational therapy.

Maintaining Control: Experimental and Quasiexperimental Research Designs

The most significant aspect of experimental and quasiexperimental research is that, of all types of research, their research designs can be highly controlled. Maintaining control in research design is an integral part of most research; the degree of control in a research design often determines if the findings of the study will be accepted as valid (I will discuss this situation later in this chapter). **Control** as used here refers to the degree of accuracy or appropriateness of the research design when considering four components:

- how the subjects are sampled
- how the subjects are assessed or measured
- how the data are collected from the subjects
- how the data are used to answer the research questions.

Restated another way, having control in research design means creating a design that allows the investigator to obtain valid data that will appropriately answer the research question.

Good control in research design gives a study internal and external validity, and increases the generalizability of the study's finding. **Internal validity** is the ability of the research to actually study what it is designed to study (Gay, 1976). **External validity** is the generalizability of the research findings to other samples and settings, which is, as previously stated, the ability to apply the findings of the study to other situations. Research design and control are closely linked. The following sections look at the components of a research design and how each component affects control.

Mapping Research: Describing the Research Design

Research designs in experimental and quasiexperimental research are conventionally described by one of two diagramming techniques. Understanding diagramming techniques allows a research consumer to break apart or depict almost any research design. If you can draw, map, or depict a research design, you can usually figure out what the research investigator did. Thus, this is a tool for the research consumer to use in understanding research. The two most common ways to diagram research are matrix and symbol.

MATRIX FORMAT

In the matrix format, groups are crossed by treatments. This means that groups are depicted by row or column, and treatments are then correspondingly depicted by row or column. A matrix display can provide further information if each cell of the matrix specifies the number of subjects or sample units in the cell. This sounds much more complicated than it actually is.

FIGURE 9–3. REPRESENTATIVE RESEARCH DESIGN IN A MATRIX

	*Treatment 1	*Treatment 2	*Treatment 3
Males	30	30	30
Females	30	30	30

* Denotes random assignment to these groups.

Figure 9–3 depicts the following research design: Three treatments are being compared to each other (represented in columns). The nuisance variable of sex is being controlled for by subdividing the sample by sex (depicted in rows) to allow for determination of differential effects of treatment by sex. Cells are the intersecting points of a row by columns. Each cell has 30 subjects (30 subjects receiving Treatment 1, 30 subjects receiving Treatment 2, etc.). If this written explanation of matrix is confusing, try to intuitively grasp what is being portrayed in Figure 9–3.

SYMBOL USE

Research designs can also be graphically represented using symbols. In this technique, shown in Figure 9–4, R is used to indicate random assignment, G is used to indicate a subgroup as the sample, X is used to show treatment, and O is used to indicate the administration of a measurement. Both Xs and Os have subscripts to show different treatments and different assessment periods.

Figure 9–4 basically takes the design from Figure 9–3 and reformats it using a different approach. Line 1 of Figure 9–4 reads:

> random assignment (R) of a group of males (G) to treatment condition 1 and one testing situation.

Line two reads:

> random assignment (R) of a group of males (G) to treatment 2 and one testing situation, and so on.

A classic textbook on quasiexperimental research designs was published by Campbell and Stanley (1966). Their set of research designs uses this symbol format. A few of these "classic" designs using the symbol format are presented here to provide you with a better understanding of how symbol notation can delineate a research design. The designs are presented in a developmental format to give you an idea of how elaboration of research design can allow for more control in the research.

Design 1

$X \quad O_1$

In Design 1, the intervention (X) is provided and then a posttest (O_1) is administered. There is no pretest, and there is no comparison group. You can probably see that this design has little control and that the internal validity of the study is, therefore, questionable.

FIGURE 9–4. SYMBOLIC PORTRAYAL OF RESEARCH

R G (males)	X_1	O_1	R G (females)	X_1	X_2
R G (males)	X_2	O_1	R G (females)	X_2	O_1
R G (males)	X_3	O_1	R G (females)	X_3	O_1

Design 2

$O_1 \quad X \quad O_2$

In Design 2, there is more control. Why? Use of the pretest (O_1) allows for determination of the effect of intervention (X) on the posttest (O_2). Lack of a control group, however, still limits its control provided by the design.

Design 3

$X \quad O_1$

$C \quad O_1$

What is the advantage of Design 3 over the previous designs? If you answered, "Use of a control group," you are correct. In this design, the performance of two groups of subjects is being compared. One group receives the intervention or treatment (X). The other group (C) serves as the control group and receives no treatment. Each group is administered a test to determine group differences. If significant group differences are revealed, can you attribute the difference to the treatment?

Maybe yes, maybe no. What if one group is from the talented and gifted classroom and the other group is from a regular classroom? Could other variables (confounding variables) or predisposing factors such as intelligence affect group performance? Yes, most certainly. So in this case you do not know which cause (treatment or group intelligence) had the effect on the test score. The next research design attempts to control for this issue.

Design 4

$R \quad X \quad O_1$

$R \quad C \quad O_1$

Recall that the R denotes random assignment of subjects to group. By randomly assigning the subjects to group conditions, they are creating equivalent groups. Because the groups are equivalent, any differences in the posttest scores can be attributed to the treatment intervention.

Observe how increasing control in research design increases confidence in the research findings. What about the lack of a pretest before the posttest? Let us now look at one of the most powerful, that is, most controlled, experimental designs.

Design 5

$R \quad O_1 \quad X \quad O_2$

$R \quad O_1 \quad C \quad O_2$

$R \qquad\quad X \quad O_2$

$R \qquad\quad C \quad O_2$

This research design essentially combines Design 3 and Design 4 to allow for consideration of many potentially confounding variables. All groups are randomly assigned. What does this mean? It means that all groups can be assumed to be equivalent, and that the differences on the posttest (O_2) can be attributed to the intervention (X). The presence of control groups (C) allows for determination of the relative effects of treatment to no treatment or control. Finally, pretesting with two groups (O_1) and no pretesting with two groups allows for determination of the effects of pretesting on posttest scores. Perhaps you can see why this design is so much more powerful than the others.

It is beyond the scope of a beginning-level text such as this to elaborate more on research design. Suffice it to say that you get an idea of the relationship between design and control in research.

Threats to the Validity of Research Design

Regardless of how well designed a piece of research may be, it can still have threats to validity. Threats to validity are those that can compromise the accuracy, appropriateness, or validity of the research (Best & Kahn, 1989). There are two general categories of what are commonly referred to as threats to validity: threats to external validity and threats to internal validity.

THREATS TO EXTERNAL VALIDITY

Recall that external validity refers to the generalizability of an investigation's findings to other settings and subjects. Generalizability, therefore, is how applicable the findings are elsewhere. External validity or generalizability of an investigation is not assured, however. There are three common threats to external validity of experimental and quasiexperimental research: sampling error, specification error, and measurement error.

Sampling error refers to a mistake in how the subjects were obtained for the investigation. For example, I can recall a time when I was pilot testing an instrument for language with elementary school-aged children. The pilot testing was conducted in a private school in Alexandria, Virginia. What I did not realize was that the students in this school were all from upper middle-class families. The subjects, therefore, had language skills far superior to the general population. The research's pilot study, therefore, was flawed due to sampling error.

Specification error is an error in the postulated or hypothesized relationship between variables under study in an investigation. It is, in fact, an error or mistake in the fundamental design of the study. For example, it is notoriously difficult to research babies born crack exposed because the researcher is at risk for specification error. That is, one can state that the relationship between crack-exposed babies and developmental milestones would be under study. But crack-exposed babies are usually also victims of exposure to other drugs (alcohol, tobacco), as well as victims of poverty and poor health services. Therefore, the findings of a study that does not consider multiple drug use and poverty as variables would likely have specification error, that is, error in not identifying and considering all relevant variables. Simply stated, this requires creating a research design that includes all of the important variables of interest.

Measurement error, the final threat to external validity, is a very common error. It is due to the lack of or misuse of psychometrically sound measurement tools to collect the pertinent data in an investigation (Burns & Grove, 1987). Using a standardized test with a population for which it was not designed is, in my experience, a common mistake. The results can be compiled into standardized test scores, but they are invalid because they were not developed for that population. Data from such measurement are not data and, when put into a statistical formula for analysis, recalls the maxim, "Garbage in, garbage out"!

THREATS TO INTERNAL VALIDITY

There are other considerations that may be detrimental to the design of the research and may influence the outcome of the research. These considerations are threats to the internal validity of the research, and consist of

- history
- maturation
- pretesting
- regression
- selection
- mortality
- instrumentation
- experimenter bias (Best & Kahn, 1989).

Following is a definition and a theoretical example of each term.

History refers to the differential occurrence of events that influence the dependent variable for one or more values of the independent variables. When my husband conducted his dissertation research, the validity of his data was affected by history. He was studying attitude changes among Taiwanese and Iranian students during their first year of study in the United States. During the year of the investigation, American hostages were taken in Iran. Clearly, this differentially affected the Iranian students compared to the Taiwanese students.

Maturation is the differential growth or change of subjects because of natural causes with the passage of time. Such growth or change may include aging, physical control, growing tired, and practice effects. The effects of treatment may be confounded by prolonged treatment overlapping with maturation. A very common statement about early intervention with infants and toddlers is, The effect was from maturation and not from therapeutic intervention. Investigators typically use control groups to counter this criticism.

Pretesting can affect performance of subjects through learning. If groups that are to be compared are really not equivalent, these effects can be differential. Then learning can be mistaken for treatment effect when it is simply the effect of taking the test on the test scores of the second test administration.

Regression is a statistical phenomenon occurring when a test is administered for a second time. Its effects are most pronounced on the extremes of test score administrations. The effect is due to the lack of perfect reliability in any test with extreme test scores moving toward the mean on retest. Hence, when the researcher elects to single out groups such as students needing remedial studies, the effects of regression confounds the treatment effects, for extreme scores will have a tendency to move toward the average score on retest.

Selection describes the entire process of how subjects are obtained or selected to participate in a study. The process, if not done randomly, can be fraught with unexpected side effects. For example, I conducted research on the touch scale in a private school and pretested test items for language at that school. Later, when normative data were being collected, it was identified that many of the children did not know certain words in the test items. It turns out that where I had pilot tested items was a skewed sample; that is, it was a private school having an unusually large number of students with high vocabularies. Thus, selection of my subjects for pilot testing was compromised, and it adversely influenced later item development.

Mortality refers to losing subjects from the investigation. Loss of subjects can affect the study outcomes. Longitudinal investigations (studies carried out over years) are particularly susceptible to mortality.

Instrumentation refers to how measurement tools used in the investigation can affect subject performance. It may be due to inaccurate or inconsistent tests. It can be due to changes in calibration of a measurement tool. For example, repeated administration of interviews to the same subject can result in the subject being overexposed to the interview and answering haphazardly.

The visual-perceptual tests are administered prior to the tactile tests in the *Sensory Integration and Praxis Tests* (SIPT). If the order were reversed, the spatial test scores could be invalidated because the effects of cumulative touch during the tactile tests might influence the subject's perceptual and attention processing.

Experimenter bias or the researcher's, knowledge of subjects, can subtly influence subject performance. Thus, it is preferred that the investigator be "blind" to subjects' group designation. The threat of experimenter bias is why a therapist should not be the principal investigator as well as the evaluator and treatment provider in a study.

The Superior Research?

Often, when people talk about research, they are really referring to experimental or quasiexperimental research. To many people, this is "real" research and anything else is not as valid. For example, some individuals do not consider single subject research, descriptive research, or qualitative research as valid or "as good" as quasiexperimental and experimental research. This is not true, but it does reflect the attitudes of many professionals. How did such attitudes develop?

The clearest explanation probably has to do with control. As shown in the previous section, of any research design, the designs of experimental and quasiexperimental research have the most control. They are considered the most internally and externally valid of all types of research (Best & Kahn, 1989). Consequently, people tend to be most confident in the findings of such research; they trust that the outcomes are true. This explains why experimental and quasiexperimental research are so valued.

Application

Let's now apply what has been covered about research design as well as experimental and quasiexperimental research. Read the following examples and answer the interpretation sections for each example. Compare your answers with those provided after each interpretation section.

Reprinted from *Perceptual and Motor Skills,* Number 54, 1982, pp. 323–330. Used with permission.

ILLUSTRATIVE EXAMPLE 9–1

Fingertip Textural Perception of Normal Children

Charlotte Brasic Royeen[1,2]

Summary. The current study investigated the influence of masking upon children's fingertip textural perception. While a screen occluded their vision, 52 6- to 10-year-old subjects palpated a pair of equivalent paper-covered sandpaper blocks and judged whether the blocks felt rougher when palpated with or without intermediate paper covering their fingertips. Pressure exerted by the subjects was recorded. It was concluded that children's judgment is independent of pressure exerted; $r = .04$. Masking in children, unlike adults, was related to sandpaper grit, for the children judged the paper condition rougher primarily when the coarser sandpaper was used. Possible explanations are presented.

The concept of haptic masking was investigated by Gordon and Cooper (1975), who noted that, when an intermediate piece of paper was placed under the fingertips while rubbing a surface such as a table top, subtle surface changes became perceptible. That serendipitous finding led them to investigate the effect of using intermediate paper beneath the fingertips on other tactile detection tasks. They found that subjects' perceived orientation of raised strips on a stimulus form was better while using intermediate paper covering their fingertips. Accordingly, they proposed that use of intermediate paper may serve to reduce masking and allow for improved detection of gradual surface changes, hypothesizing that masking is the suppression of information from deeper receptors by a highly sensitive aspect of the tactile system.

Lederman (1978) continued investigations into the phenomenon of masking by measuring subjects' perceptions of roughness while touching paper-covered sandpaper blocks with and without additional loose intermediate paper covering their fingertips. She discovered that the subjects reported an increased perception of roughness when they used an additional piece of loose intermediate paper during palpation. Consequently, Lederman proposed that perception of roughness, primarily mediated via downward forces, was masked by lateral forces interfering with the roughness signal, and that the use of intermediate paper served to reduce the lateral force or masking effect and allowed for an increased perception of roughness transmitted by downward forces.

Since the information on masking is far from complete and limited to adults, it was the purpose of the current study to build on Lederman's investigation of masking to ascertain whether and under what conditions masking influences children's fingertip textural perception of roughness.

Method

The method was developed specifically for the current study. Previous studies were designed for adults and accordingly required subjects to have an understanding of fractions and adequate sequential memory so that they could estimate the relative magnitude of roughness between one stimulus and the next. Since children cannot be expected to do so, the design required subjects to estimate which stimulus form felt rougher, judging between a pair of stimulus forms with sandpaper of equal grit value in a forced-choice format (Anastasi, 1976). During each experimental trial the subject's fingertips alone were used for palpation of one of the pair of equal stimulus forms, and a loose piece of intermediate paper was held under the fingertips while touching the other of a pair of equal forms. Also, the procedure was designed for the most expeditious conduct of the experiment to hold the children's attention and reduce the risk of fatigue.

SUBJECTS

From Saint Boniface School in Cincinnati, Ohio, a sample of normal children was selected. The category of normal children was defined as those attending a regular classroom who were not considered unusual, either emotionally, physically, or academically, by the classroom teacher, and as a result, 76 children were available for this study. When a permission slip was not returned, two or more phone contacts were attempted as necessary. Of all the parents successfully contacted by either letter or phone, only two refused to grant permission for their children to participate in this study. Also, 21 children were not included in the study because no contact was established with their parents. Finally, one child who appeared to have signs of

TABLE 1. AGES OF CHILDREN

Age Category	*N*	M	*SD*
6 yr.	6	6.42	.16
7 yr.	15	7.58	.23
8 yr.	15	8.49	.27
9 yr.	12	9.23	.24
10 yr.	4	10.15	.16

moderate cerebral palsy was dropped from the study. Thus, 13 first graders, 17 second graders, and 22 third graders, a total of 52 children or 69% of the population, participated. The ages of the children in the sample are shown in Table 1. The subjects were almost evenly represented by sex, 25 males and 27 females. Four children were left-handed.

EQUIPMENT

The stimulus forms were constructed to approximate the guidelines specified by Lederman (1978). The current study used sandpaper of 36, 50, 80, 120, 150 and 220 grit.

Sandpaper of 36 grit has the largest particles of sand and is, therefore, the roughest. Sandpaper of 120 grit is approximately mid-range on the roughness continuum. Therefore, two pairs of 15- by 15-cm wooden blocks were covered with sandpaper of 120 grit for use during the practice trials. Next, two sets of six pairs of 15- by 15-cm wooden blocks were made and covered with sandpaper of the full range of grits previously specified. All of the sandpaper-covered wooden blocks also had one layer of Chatwood Bond paper fastened to them, as this was an innovation introduced by Lederman who felt that covering the blocks could maintain the integrity of the sandpaper.[3] The two pairs of practice blocks as well as the two sets of prepared blocks were alternated between subjects to preclude the effects of wear. Finally, the loose intermediate paper used during the experimental trials was also Chatwood Bond, sized 20- by 14-cm.

Besides the stimulus forms, two additional items of equipment were necessary for the study. A 76- by 76-cm wooden frame, hung with a double thickness of black kettle cloth, occluded the vision of the subjects during performance and eliminated visual clues. The cloth in the screen was attached only at the top to allow the subject to pass the preferred hand through the screen near the bottom. Throughout the study a pair of Step-ese Diet Scales were placed on the far side of the screen, to measure the magnitude of the pressure exerted by each subject during palpation of the stimulus forms placed upon it.

3. Paula Bonacci, Chicago sales representative of Weyerhauser Paper Co., verified that this type of paper is the American equivalent of the Canadian paper used by Lederman (1978).

RESEARCH DESIGN

Each subject judged whether the paper or no-paper condition was rougher during 12 experimental trials. There were two independent variables, paper/no-paper condition and six sandpaper grits. Judgments of roughness and finger pressure were the two dependent variables.

In the current study randomization was achieved by first establishing an overall randomized sequence for the 12 trials by drawing the order of the trials out of a box. Each record sheet had the same randomized sequence printed on it, and for any given subject a starting point in the sequence was randomly selected, again by drawing the order out of a box. This starting point was determined just prior to the beginning of each session and was marked on the record sheet.

SCHEDULING

The children were from five different classrooms, and the order of classrooms for testing was randomly selected. Then, since testing occurred during school hours, the children from one classroom were tested in an order which had to be determined at the teacher's discretion. The duration of the experiment for each child was approximately 10 to 15 min., and testing occurred over a 2-wk. period.

PROCEDURE

The hand the child used to write his name at the onset of the session was designated as his preferred hand and used during performance. The investigator then demonstrated proper hand position (10° of flexion at the metacarpal-phalangeal joints of the fingers, full extension of the proximal and distal interphalangeal joints of the fingers, and opposition of the pad of the thumb to the proximal interphalangeal joint of the index finger). The subject was instructed to assume this hand position and, if necessary, was assisted in doing so. The subject had a practice trial, the purpose of which was to teach the procedure for palpating the stimulus forms with additional intermediate paper underneath the fingertips (paper condition) and without intermediate paper underneath the fingertips (no-paper condition).

Once this was accomplished, the entire procedure, with and without intermediate paper, was then done while the screen occluded the subject's vision. Consequently, this necessitated the researcher assisting the subject by holding the dorsum of the subject's wrist and moving him through the procedure: placing her fingers at the subject's medial and lateral epicondyles, she placed the subject's hand in the proper position for each trial, at the point of the block farthest from the subject, to guide the movement of the subject's fingertips along the block toward himself.

The subject practiced until he could perform the task without requiring the researcher to direct the subject's movements actively, except for initial placement of his hand on the stimulus form. However, she continued to hold the subject's wrist at all times during his palpation of the blocks to place his hand easily and quickly on the next block prior to each palpation.

Twelve experimental trials were presented. Each trial consisted of exposure to a pair of interchangeable stimulus forms, for example, two blocks with 36-grit sandpaper. During one exposure to a particular pair of blocks the intermediate paper was employed on the one positioned to the right, and during the other exposure to that set, the intermediate paper was employed on the block positioned to the left.

During each trial the investigator asked, Which one is rougher? This one (the right stimulus form) or this one? (the child is palpating the left stimulus form).

The exposure was repeated twice for a pair of blocks during any one experimental trial unless the subject spontaneously identified which block felt rougher during the first exposure. This procedure decreased the time required to conduct the trial and lessened the risk of losing the child's attention. While the research assistant recorded the maximum pressure exerted by the subject during each palpation of any given trial, the investigator recorded which block the subject reported as feeling rougher. At the end of all experimental trials for each subject, the examiner praised the child for excellent participation.

STATISTICAL PROCEDURE

Confidence intervals were used to assess whether the paper condition was judged rougher. A chi squared test served to determine the relation between the subjects' responses and their sex (Welkowitz, *et al.*, 1976). A Fisher's exact test for small samples was used to assess the relation between the subjects' responses and their ages (Blalock, 1960). A *t* test was used to analyze the differences between the mean pressures exerted by the subjects during the paper and no-paper conditions. Finally, a Pearson product-moment correlation was computed to determine whether the pressure exerted by the subjects was related to their judgments of roughness. A .05 level of significance was selected for these analyses.

Results

For these children, judgments of roughness were related to the use of coarser grit sandpaper. Inspection of Table 2 indicates on Trials 1 and 12, and Trials 9 and 11 (corresponding to sandpaper grits 36 and 50), and for Trial 6 (only one of the two trials corresponding to sandpaper grit 80) was the paper condition judged rougher [sic]. The subjects were not able to discriminate differences in roughness between the paper and no-paper conditions during Trials 3 and 7, Trials 2 and 4, and Trials 8 and 10 (corresponding to the finer sandpaper grits 120, 150, and 220). Only on one trial using rougher sandpaper, Trial 5 (corresponding to sandpaper grit 80), were the subjects unable to discriminate differences in roughness.

Table 3 shows that the subject's choice of conditions was related to sandpaper grit for Trials 1 and 12, and Trials 5 and 6 (corresponding to the rougher sandpaper grits 36 and 80). The subject's choice of conditions during one trial employing a particular sandpaper grit (36 or 80) was related to or statistically dependent upon his choice during the other trial employing that particular sandpaper grit and, therefore, sandpaper grit influenced the subject's choice of conditions for these trials. Furthermore, Table 3 shows that Trials 9 and 11 (corresponding to sandpaper grit 50), even though not statistically significant, appear to group with the other two trials employing rougher sandpaper grits.

TABLE 2

FREQUENCIES AND CONFIDENCE LIMITS OF SUBJECTS' CHOICES REGARDING ROUGHNESS OF PAPER AND NO-PAPER CONDITIONS (*N* = 52)

Grit Value	Trial	Frequency of Choice of Rougher Condition		Confidence Limits		P = 50%
		No-paper	Paper	Lower	Upper	
36	1	13	39	13	37	*
150	2	25	27	34	62	
120	3	24	28	32	60	
150	4	22	30	28	58	
80	5	21	31	26	54	
80	6	19	33	23	49	*
120	7	22	30	28	56	
220	8	20	32	25	51	
50	9	13	39	13	37	*
220	10	25	27	34	62	
50	11	19	33	23	49	*
36	12	15	37	15	42	*
	Total	238	386	25	51	

P = proportion.

*It can be stated with 95% confidence that the interval did not intersect .50.

TABLE 3

CONTINGENCY TABLES OF EQUAL GRIT VALUES BY TRIALS

Sandpaper Grit Value	Trial	Cross Tabulations				*df*	χ^2	*P*
			No-paper %	Paper %	*n*			
Trial 12	1	No-paper	46.7	16.2	13			
36		Paper	53.3	83.3	39			
		n	15	37	52	1	3.78	0.05
Trial 11	9	No-paper	42.1	15.2	13			
50		Paper	57.9	84.8	39			
		n	19	33	52	1	3.34	0.06
Trial 6	5	No-paper	63.2	27.3	13			
80		Paper	36.8	72.7	31			
		n	19	33	52	1	5.04	0.02
Trial 7	3	No-paper	50.0	43.3	24			
120		Paper	50.0	56.7	28			
		n	22	30	52	1	0.03	
Trial 4	2	No-paper	63.3	36.7	25			
150		Paper	36.4	63.3	27			
		n	22	30	52	1	2.70	
Trial 10	8	No-paper	52.0	25.9	20			
220		Paper	28.0	74.1	32			
		n	25	27	52	1	2.70	0.09

Note: On Trials 12 and 1 36-grit sandpaper was used; responses for paper and no-paper were the same for both trials. The same holds for Trials 9 and 11, 6 and 5, 7 and 3, 4 and 2, 10 and 8. For each pair of trials only grit value changes.

Of the 30 possible calculations for age (five age groups for each of six paired trials) four could not be completed due to two or more empty cells within the contingency table. Of the remaining 26 computations, only three were significant. Moreover, considering the unreliability of comparisons based on such small subgroups, it was concluded that the ages of the subjects did not influence their judgments. Also, the subjects' choices were not related to their sex.

For each trial the subjects exerted significantly more pressure during the no-paper condition, exerting approximately 2 oz. of pressure during the paper condition and approximately 3 to 4 oz. of pressure during the no-paper condition. However, no correlation was found between the subjects' choices and the pressure they exerted ($r = .04$, $df = 624$, $p = .14$).

Discussion

The current study indicates that, when palpating a stimulus form with additional loose paper beneath the fingertips, children appear more likely to judge the form as rougher than the form without such intermediate paper if the stimulus form contains rougher or coarser sandpaper (36, 50, or 80 grit). Hence, it may be that, in children, masking is released by use of intermediate paper when coarser sandpaper is used. Further study is necessary to ascertain whether children's judgment of the paper condition as rougher depends upon the use of the coarser sandpaper.

Considering that the children judged the paper condition rougher on five of the trials, it appears that under certain conditions children can make judgments regarding the relative roughness of the paper/no-paper conditions in a manner similar to adults. Also, children's sex and age (6 to 10 yr.) do not appear to affect such judgments. However, children, unlike adults, apparently do not judge the paper condition as rougher primarily when finer sandpaper is used (120, 150, and 220 grit).

For those trials employing finer sandpaper, consider the discrepancy between Lederman's results (the paper condition was judged rougher) and the current study's results (the paper condition was not judged rougher). Lederman employed ratio estimation as a response technique; whereas a forced-choice format was employed in the present study. Thus, the discrepancy regarding the subjects' judgments of roughness for those trials employing finer sandpaper may be due to the use of different methods in the respective studies. Also, Lederman's research controlled for touch-produced sound by the subject's use of earphones but the current study did not attempt to control for such sounds. Hence, during the current study, auditory cues might have influenced the subjects' judgments of roughness. Also, Lederman's research required the subjects to feel the stimulus surfaces for a short time with a light pressure, whereas the present study required the subjects to palpate the stimulus forms in a prescribed manner distally to proximally. Consequently, the manner of the subject's exploration of the stimulus forms could have contributed to the difference in subjects' judgments. It is unlikely that these minor procedural differences account for the respective studies' different results. Rather, three considerations are presented as tentative explanations.

First, based upon normative data derived from a test of tactile localization, it has been suggested that there is an early maturation of this skill (Ayres, 1976).

Similarly, the basic mechanism underlying masking and the release of its effects may also be related to maturation of the nervous system, the mechanism being refined in young adults and underdeveloped in children. Children than may not be able to readily discern differences in texture or roughness when finer distinctions must be made. Children could discern differences in roughness between the paper and no-paper conditions when the stimulus forms contained coarser sandpaper, but children would be less able to discern such differences when finer sandpaper was used.

Second, children's responses to shear force and other mechanical phenomena need to be considered since their fingertips are smaller and shaped differently than adults'. Their skin is not as calloused and so not as thick as adults' skin. It may be conjectured that differences between children's and adults' peripheral mechanical perception of stimuli may occur during palpation of a textured stimulus.

Moreover, if Lederman's explanation of masking, that a decrease in the effect of shear (lateral) force decreases masking and increases the roughness signal, is correct, then the following explanation of the relation between masking and grit value can be proposed. It may be that during palpation, coarser grit sandpaper (having larger particles of sand) elicits disproportionately greater shear or lateral forces in children's fingertips than finer grit sandpaper. Therefore, children's use of intermediate paper with stimulus forms having coarser sandpaper creates a greater effect on perception of roughness than would be found with stimulus forms having finer sandpaper. This greater effect would theoretically result from the intermediate paper decreasing a relatively greater magnitude of shear force or masking.

Third, practice effects and "perceptual learning" may allow for the nervous system with more experience, that is, the adults', to refine perception and, therefore, have greater sensitivity to the roughness signal uncovered by the use of intermediate paper. Further study is needed of the validity of these tentative explanations.

Considering that no correlation was found between the subjects' choices and the amount of pressure exerted, it may be possible to eliminate pressure as affecting normal children's judgment during textural perception tasks, if, as in the current study, the children exercise control over the amount of pressure exerted during the task. Hence, the masking effect appears to be independent of pressure exerted by children, if the pressure is 4 oz. or less.

References

Anastasi, A. J. *Psychological testing.* New York: MacMillan, 1976.

Ayres, A. J. *Interpreting the Southern California Sensory Integration Tests.* Los Angeles, CA: Western Psychological Services, 1976.

Blalock, M. *Social statistics.* New York: McGraw-Hill, 1960.

Gordon, I., & Cooper, C. Improving one's touch. *Nature,* 1975, 256, 203–204.

Lederman, S. J. "Improving one's touch...and more". *Perception and Psychophysics,* 1978, 2, 154–160.

Welkowitz, J., Ewen, R. B., & Cohen, J. *Introductory statistics for the behavioral sciences.* New York: Academic Press, 1976.

Illustrative Example 9–1: Questions

1. What is the purpose of the research?
2. Does the literature review provide you an understanding of how and why this investigation is important?
3. Do you think the investigation is important? Why or why not?
4. What is the theoretical or conceptual basis of the investigation?
5. How was the research conducted?
6. What type or kind of research is it and why?
7. What were the research questions or hypotheses?
8. What are the variables or phenomena under study?
9. Who were the subjects or units of study? How many were there?
10. How were the subjects or units of study obtained?
11. What information or data were collected?
12. If specific evaluation tools were used, what were they? Was information on the reliability and validity of the evaluation tools provided?
13. How was the information or data collected?
14. Will data collected be able to answer or address the research question or problem under study?
15. How was the information or data analyzed?
16. What were the criteria for interpreting the data?
17. What were the findings?
18. What were the limitations of the study? Was there a critical flaw?
19. Are the conclusions of the study warranted?
20. How can these research findings be used in occupational and physical therapy?

Illustrative Example 9–1: Answers

1. What is the purpose of the research?

The purpose of this investigation was to look at the influence of masking on fingertip textural perception in children.

2. Does the literature review provide you an understanding of how and why this investigation is important?

The literature review is limited to presentation of two previous, but key, investigations. But it is clearly identified that the current investigation is built on the investigation of Lederman.

3. Do you think the investigation is important? Why or why not?

This research is basic research into perceptual processing of children. As such, it is not clinically relevant and may not appear to be of real importance to occupational or physical therapy. Rather, the research builds on the body of knowledge about normal perceptual development in children.

4. What is the theoretical or conceptual basis of the investigation?

The phenomenon of masking was first studied by Gordon and Cooper, and then by Lederman. Masking is the phenomenon of improved perception of certain stimuli while the fingertips are "masked" or covered with paper. The work to date had been done with adults, and this study attempted to look at the phenomenon in children.

5. How was the research conducted?

The method was an adaptation of previous methods for appropriate use with children. The treatment (which is what interventions are called in research language) was asking the child to choose one of two conditions (intermediate paper underneath the child's fingertips and no paper) in response to the question, Which one feels rougher?

6. *What type or kind of research is it and why?*

As identified earlier, this is basic research. It is basic research because is does not address a clinically based question. Rather, it seeks to develop more knowledge related to a theory of perceptual processing. I would call this quasiexperimental research because subjects were not randomly selected.

7. *What were the research questions or hypotheses?*

No explicit research question or hypothesis is stated. The general research question may be inferred as, Does masking influence children's fingertip textural perception of roughness? The null hypothesis (remember that this is the statistically based one) would be that there is no difference between conditions (paper and no paper). Many more hypotheses could apply to this study, but that is the main one.

8. *What are the variables or phenomena under study?*

The independent variable was treatment condition (paper and no paper) and the dependent variable was fingertip textural perception (amount of roughness perceived).

9. *Who were the subjects or units of study? How many were there?*

The subjects were children ages 6 to 10 years as presented in Table 1. In total, there were 52 subjects, 25 males and 27 females.

10. *How were the subjects or units of study obtained?*

This was a sample of convenience (not randomly sampled). A private school granted permission for research and subjects' parents were contacted. Of those contacted and permission obtained, all were used in the study.

11. *What information or data were collected?*

The data collected were subjects' (children's) answers to the question, Which one (condition) is rougher?

12. *If specific evaluation tools were used, what were they? Was information on the reliability and validity of the evaluation tools provided?*

Children were asked to write their name at the beginning of the session. This was an informal evaluation tool used to determine handedness. No reliability or validity information was provided on use of this method of determining handedness.

13. *How was the information or data collected?*

Children were administered the protocol of palpating blocks over a two-week period, taking 10 to 15 minutes for each subject. Each child was administered 12 trials once they understood the procedure (the 12 trials consisted of two conditions, paper or no paper, and six levels of sandpaper grit). Sequence of administration of the 12 trials was randomized. And start of the sequence for each subject was also selected randomly.

14. *Will data collected be able to answer or address the research question or problem under study?*

Yes, the data collected regarding which condition is rougher is precise and limited enough to address the question at hand.

15. *How was the information or data analyzed?*

Data were subjected to a variety of statistical procedures consisting of

- confidence intervals for analysis of which condition was judged rougher
- Chi Square for determination of relationship of sex and responses
- Fisher's Exact Test for small samples for analysis of responses and age of subjects

- *t* test for mean pressure exerted during paper and no-paper conditions
- Pearson product moment correlation to look at the correlation between pressure exerted by subjects and judgments of roughness.

16. What were the criteria for interpreting the data?

None was stated a priori. The customary level of p = .05 appears to have been used.

17. What were the findings?

The findings were as follows:

- Confidence intervals for analysis of which condition was judged rougher revealed that for this sample of children, judgments of roughness were related to the degree or coarseness of sandpaper grit
- The Chi Square revealed that sex of subject did not influence responses
- Fisher's Exact Test for small samples for analysis of responses and age of subjects revealed no effects by age
- *t* Test for mean pressure exerted during paper and no-paper conditions revealed that subjects exerted significantly more pressure during the no-paper condition, and
- Pearson product moment correlation to look at the correlation between pressure exerted by subjects and judgements of roughness revealed that there was not a significant correlation between subjects' choices and pressure exerted (r = .04, df = 624, p = .14).

18. What were the limitations of the study? Was there a critical flaw?

None were identified by the author. Sample size is small. The sample is one of convenience, and generalizability is limited.

19. Are the conclusions of the study warranted?

The study conclusions are presented as they apply in general and are not appropriately limited in generalizability.

20. How can these research findings be used in occupational and physical therapy?

Potentially, there may be some application to the theory of tactile defensiveness, but further investigation would be required.

ILLUSTRATIVE EXAMPLE 9–2

Reprinted from *Arch Phys Med Rehabil,* Vol. 68, Number 5, January, 1987, pp. 267–272. Used with permission.

Stroke Treatment: Comparison of Integrated Behavioral-Physical Therapy vs Traditional Physical Therapy Programs

John V. Basmajian, MD, Carolyn A. Gowland, MHSc, M. Alan J. Finlayson, PhD, Anne L. Hall, BS, Laurie R. Swanson, BS, Paul W. Stratford, MS, Judith E. Trotter, MD, Murray E. Brandstater, MD, PhD

Chedoke Rehabilitation Center of Chedoke-McMaster Hospitals, Hamilton, Ontario, Canada L8N 3Z5

In an earlier controlled pilot study,[2] we treated the hemiparetic upper limb in 37 patients with a wide range of severity and duration after stroke. They were randomly assigned to either a five-week, 15-session program of integrated EMG biofeedback (EMGBF) plus physical therapy (PT) or a standard exercise therapy (ET) program with the same time elements and intensity. In both groups, tested independently, some cases showed improved useful function. Patients' conditions were classified as (A) early mild, (B) early severe, (C) late mild and (D) late severe. All in the early-mild group had substantial improvement while those in the late-severe group did not improve. It became imperative to investigate the other two groups: early severe and late mild.

Meanwhile, reports of other independent controlled studies by Wolf and Binder-Macleod[30] and Inglis and associates[15] appeared: EMGBF plus PT had been tested against PT alone. Both studies found that in chronic stroke patients EMGBF, when used as an adjunct to PT, resulted in improvement in upper limb range of movement and muscle strength. Though positive, these authors were more restrained in their enthusiasm for biofeedback for the upper limb than earlier uncontrolled clinical reports.[3,6] Nevertheless they brought new insights into the effects of both standard and biofeedback-behavioral approaches to the hemiparetic upper limb. They also emphasized that EMGBF is an adjunctive and not a total therapy.

At the start of the present study, we were impressed by the apparent importance of the elapsed time before therapy and the severity of the functional loss. In addition, the possible influence of behavioral factors in both groups appeared to require more careful attention. Hence this study was fashioned as a comparison of "integrated behavioral-physical therapy including EMGBF" versus "traditional physical therapy" based on the Bobath "neurodevelopmental" approach, which is well documented elsewhere.[5]

Therapeutic exercise methods, based on the neurologic interpretations of their advocates,[5,7] are widely used and probably often misused: they are rarely studied, usually tolerated, and often scorned by many physicians, who purport to see no clinically useful results directly attributable to the neurologic approaches.[1,25] Each year, therapeutic exercises consume hundreds of thousands of hours of therapy time. Hence our present study also promised to throw more light on the effectiveness of therapeutic exercise with the hemiplegic upper limb.

Our resolve to compare two active therapies and not to use "do-nothing" controls was based on the evidence supporting EMGBF as an effective therapeutic adjunct for the hemiplegic upper limb.[18,29] This resolve was further strengthened by the 1981 report from Smith's group[23] that contradicted the older pessimistic view[13] that any rehabilitation of stroke patients is virtually useless. In a large number of suitable outpatient volunteers randomly assigned to three different courses of therapy, those who received benevolent supervision clearly showed little or no improvement over 12 months, but those who received intensive remedial therapy got clinically useful and statistically significant improvements. The group who received an intermediate level of attention got intermediate results.

Indirect evidence from several inpatient studies[11,12,16,17,24,26,27] strongly suggested that remedial therapies had clinically worthwhile outcomes.

However, one less positive conclusion of the Smith[23] outpatient study warranted attention: only a minority of stroke patients (mostly men) are robust enough for vigorous intensive programs of outpatient rehabilitation; nevertheless for that minority such treatment "is effective and realistic."[23] Since clinical experience supports that conclusion, we modified the patient selection criteria for the present study accordingly.

The present study had four objectives: (1) to determine whether the integrated behavioral therapy program including EMGBF (treatment A) is more effective clinically and statistically than the traditional program (treatment B) in the restoration of useful function in the arm and hand of a recovering stroke patient; (2) to test the hypothesis that there would be a strong correlation between measures of improved physical function and measures of self-control, self-concept, mood and affect; (3) to determine at the nine-month follow-ups whether any differences had occurred between the two groups in physical, social and emotional functioning; (4) to determine the value of all tests and examinations administered in predicting which types of patients are more likely to benefit from the two therapies. This report concentrates on the first three objectives; objective 4 will be addressed in a later report.

Method

Over a three-year span, area outpatients who had suffered a stroke in the previous one to 12 months and fulfilled specific criteria were recruited into the study as volunteers. Extensive and intensive testing in a specially sheltered laboratory were conducted at the start and end of five weeks of therapy and nine months thereafter. Patients were randomly assigned to treatments A and B, and the examiner was never aware of the specific assignments.

Both programs were restricted to five weeks with three sessions of exactly 45 minutes spread through each week on a fairly regular schedule. There were no current or related therapies for the manifestations of hemiplegia during the five weeks, and during the subsequent nine months, patients were not controlled and almost all had no further treatments by others.

ADMISSION CRITERIA AND STUDY POPULATION

The population to be sampled included only patients (a) with no previous history of completed stroke prior to the present illness; (b) 80 years of age or under; (c) with an obstruction involving the territory with distribution centering on the middle cerebral artery (hemorrhagic infarcts were excluded); (d) with impaired motor function of the upper limb but with some ability to extend the wrist or fingers; (e) less than one year poststroke; (f) who, in the estimation of the study physician were able to understand simple commands and the purpose of the treatment; (g) who were well informed, sufficiently motivated and willing to participate; (h) who had the approval of their personal physician; (i) who, in the opinion of the study physician, had a relatively uncomplicated medical history.

Having met the above inclusion criteria, patients also had to have at least one characteristic predisposing to greater recovery as suggested by our pilot study. That is, to be included in the study, a patient had to demonstrate one of the following: mild motor involvement of the hemiplegic hand (a score of 20 or greater on the upper extremity function test (UEFT))[8] if four or more months poststroke—the late mild group; or less than four months poststroke with a score of less than 20 on the UEFT—the early-severe group. Patients falling into the early-mild or late-severe classifications were excluded from the study.

RANDOMIZATION AND STRATIFICATION

Patients who met the entry criteria and had given formal consent were randomly assigned to either the integrated behavioral and physical therapy group or the standard exercise physical therapy group. Within each prognostic stratum, there was a randomization schedule, balanced after every four patients entered. In addition, to prevent a potential final imbalance because of the small sample size, the randomization procedure was also balanced across strata. Patients were subsequently randomly assigned once again to one of the two physical therapists.

PATIENT POPULATION CHARACTERISTICS

Twenty-nine patients, 19 men and 10 women, were included in the study. The mean age was 62 years, range 39 to 79 years. Patients had been treated medically during the early stages of their strokes in community general or rehabilitation hospitals. No systematic, regular treatment had been provided to improve upper limb function. Routine management included the provision of a passive support to prevent subluxation of the shoulder, the teaching of autoassisted exercises to maintain mobility and careful instruction to avoid trauma to the arm.

Conditions of 18 patients were classified as early and severe, 11 as late and mild; mean length of time poststroke for all patients was 16 weeks, range 4 to 44. Sixteen patients had right hemiplegia. Therapist A treated 16 patients; therapist B, 13.

Table 1 describes the patient characteristics of the two study groups at the time of admission to the study.

TABLE 1
PRETEST PATIENT CHARACTERISTICS OF THE TWO THERAPY GROUPS

Characteristic	Biofeedback (n = 13)	Bobath (n = 16)	Type of analysis***
Gender	9 men	10 men	
Age, yr	60.77 (8.50)*	63.77 (13.07)	t
Time poststroke, wk	16.38 (7.60)	16.00 (11.74)	t
Early sev/late mld	7/6	11/5	χ^2
Side of hemiplegia	9 right, 4 left	7 right, 9 left	χ^2
Therapist	9 A, 4 B	6 A, 10 B	χ^2
UEFT[8]	28.85 (27.71)	29.44 (27.69)	t
Trails A	74.92 (60.30)	69.38 (49.28)	t
Trails B	199.46 (99.29)	185.38 (84.66)	t
Finger oscillation[22]	12.15 (15.73)	11.31 (14.22)	t
Beck[4]	4.00 (7.16)(n = 10)**	4.64 (3.32) (n = 11)	t
Health belief[28]	38.80 (6.97)(n = 10)	37.73 (7.11)(n = 11)	t
Token test[10]	4.92 (9.02)	4.06 (6.84)	t
Finger writing	10.08 (8.35)	6.75 (7.51)(n = 15)	t
Finger agnosia	3.46 (6.21)	2.63 (5.86)	t
Word finding[21]	20.46 (14.22)	18.88 (18.43)	t
Category[22]	74.08 (23.79)	69.88 (30.08)	t
Motivation	3.08 (1.85)	3.87 (1.99) (n = 15)	t
Aphasia screening test[20]	1.92 (1.55)	1.75 (1.44)	t
AST-spatial	2.00 (0.82)	2.44 (1.15)	t
16 PF[9]			
A	5.71 (1.70)	4.90 (2.42)	t
B	5.14 (1.46)	5.10 (0.74)	t
C	4.86 (2.12)	5.60 (1.78)	t
E	5.43 (1.90)	4.80 (2.15)	t
F	4.71 (1.38)	4.20 (2.15)	t
G	6.29 (2.29)	6.50 (2.01)	t
H	4.14 (2.27)	5.20 (2.44)	t
I	3.57 (1.72)	4.50 (1.84)	t
L	6.29 (1.79)	6.30 (1.77)	t
M	5.29 (1.60)	4.30 (2.16)	t
N	6.00 (1.73)	6.30 (1.64)	t
O	5.71 (2.14)	5.20 (1.62)	t
Q1	5.57 (2.15)	5.40 (2.72)	t
Q2	7.14 (1.68)	6.30 (2.06)	t
Q3	6.14 (1.22)	6.60 (1.58)	t
Q4	6.43 (1.90)	6.00 (1.94)	t

*Mean (standard deviation).

**Sample size when data missing.

***None of the differences was statistically significant.

COMPLIANCE

To ensure therapist compliance with the maneuvers, a detailed program was prepared and adhered to, with a monitor therapist to act as an observer at random intervals, and to evaluate the treatment according to the set of preestablished criteria. Therapists were evaluated during a treatment session to determine the amount of time spent on goal setting, instructing, and observing the patient in repetitive exercise, hands-on exercises, and delivering selective sensory input. Such a measure helped maintain the motivation of the principal therapists and assured a continuing evaluation of the therapy being administered.

In the pilot study, it was found that experience with EMG feedback caused the treating therapists to change their conventional therapeutic approach. To control for this the protocol was carefully designed to provide the therapists with specific directions and options.

We rejected a study design where one therapist would perform the integrated therapeutic approach while the other performed the exercise approach because of the bias that might have been introduced by each therapist's personality. Clearly the personality of the patient's therapist might affect motivation and, hence, outcome. If one of the approaches is superior to the other, it had to be demonstrated as significantly better for the patients of both therapists.

INTEGRATED BEHAVIORAL AND PHYSICAL THERAPY METHOD—TREATMENT A

Treatment A, developed and refined in our pilot study, was based on cognitive models that employ EMG feedback as an invaluable adjunct to therapy. This approach recognizes the role of the patient's cognitions or thought processes during treatment and how they affect the recovery process. What the patient says to himself and how he appraises his status has a large influence on the responses. The cognitive behavioral model as put forth by Meichenbaum[19] consists of four phases: (1) conceptualization, (2) skill acquisition, (3) skill rehearsal, and (4) skill transfer. During conceptualization, by demonstrations and dialogue the patient is converted as much as possible from a passive recipient to an active participant in treatment. During skill acquisition, EMG feedback goals are learned and the patient is taught how to direct cognitive skills. During repeated skill rehearsal, home practice of the specific rehearsed skills is emphasized and results are carefully monitored and discussed with the patient. The final phase is skill transfer.

EMG biofeedback. Several strategies are used to achieve these skills. EMG feedback is pivotal for precise goal setting, e.g., the EMG output of lights and sounds may be fixed at a specific EMG level or bilaterally symmetric electrodes may be used for the patient to compare and match. The information from the EMG feedback guides the identification of optimal strategies and goals during the skill acquisition phase. Only one or two clear and attainable goals are set for each session.

Using the Cyborg BL900 dual processor, the therapist attaches pairs of standard surface biofeedback electrodes to the patient's skin over muscles that are being targeted for either active recruitment or active inhibition. At different times these may include many of the main muscle groups of the limb.

EXERCISE PHYSICAL THERAPY—TREATMENT B

This approach, based on neurofacilitatory techniques, is in general use for rehabilitation of stroke in the United States and Canada. The physical therapist's technical ability is of major importance in its implementation. Techniques of facilitation and inhibition are used with selected sensory input to bring about automatic, high-quality motor output. The quality of the performance is stressed in all of the techniques. The process is iterative, ie, the therapist is constantly reassessing and retesting the therapeutic strategies based on the patient's response on a moment-to-moment basis. The concept of home practice although verbalized is not specifically emphasized. As a result, a dependency situation may develop in which the patient presents his useless arm for the therapist to "make it better."

The approach used in treatment B strictly adhered to the principles described in detail in Bobath's text.[5] Extensive literature and training in this neurodevelopmental treatment approach are widely available.

TESTING PROCEDURES

A specially trained examiner who was kept unaware of all patient treatment programs performed all tests before randomized assignment, after the course of treatment, and at a nine-month follow-up.

Specific outcome measures for objectives 1, 2, and 3. The primary objective was to demonstrate a clinically and statistically significant difference in upper limb function between the two groups at the end of therapy and at nine-month follow-up. Specifically, the objective was to show that a greater number of patients in treatment group A improved at least 10 points on the upper extremity function test (UEFT).[8] As shown in the pilot study,[2] the UEFT is a valid indicator of upper limb function. It meets essential criteria by correlating well with ADL functions, being quantitative, valid and reliable; providing an indication of the amount of change needed to demonstrate significant clinical improvement or regression; and being useful in predicting functional outcome. A second measure of physical ability, the finger oscillation test,[22] was used to supplement the UEFT by providing information on speed of movement.

Because we expected to see a strong correlation between measures of improved physical function and measures of self-control, self-concept, mood and affect, we looked for secondary changes in the emotional functioning of the patients. The experimental group in treatment A were being exposed to procedures that encouraged greater personal and self-control in the management of their difficulties, but no such expectations occurred in the exercise physical therapy group in treatment B. Consequently, we expected that assessment measures selected would reflect improved self-concept and self-control in the treatment A group. To accomplish this goal the Health Belief Survey,[28] a locus of control scale, was administered to all subjects. It was also expected that improvement in motor functioning would contribute to more positive affect and a better mood state. Thus, mood and affect were measured with the Beck[4] and the 16 PF.[9]

Specific measures for objective 4. Not only were we concerned with therapeutic effectiveness of treatments A and B but we also designed the total study to permit retrospective judgment on the value of our tests in predicting outcomes in the study patients overall and then in the A and B subgroups. That part of the investigation will be reported in detail elsewhere.

DATA ANALYSIS

The statistical analysis for this report is divided into two sections. The first section examines the initial values of all variables considered in the study and determines whether statistically significant differences exist between the two treatment groups. The analysis of the data for this section (Table 1) was that of a *t*-test for independent samples when the data were continuous and a chi-square test when the data were nominal.

The second section determines whether, during the course of the study, significant change in function occurred in the study patients overall and then within the treatment subgroups which could be attributed to differences in the therapeutic interventions. The analysis for functional change included all five outcome measures: the UEFT, finger oscillation test, the Health Belief Survey, the Beck and the 16 PF. The fundamental outcome measure of whether or not the maneuvers were efficacious was based on the proportion of patients in each treatment group who attained a clinically significant 10-point improvement on the UEFT after treatment, and at the nine-month follow-up. A chi-square test of significance was used. In addition, it was of interest to determine if the mean posttest score in group A was 10 points or more greater than the mean posttest score in group B. The data on all outcome variables were analyzed using a repeated measures analysis of variance. A formal stepwise multiple regression analysis was performed to identify predictor variables (objective 4); an analysis of covariance was performed to adjust for differences in the identified predictor variables.

Results

PATIENT CHARACTERISTICS

When the initial data of the two groups were compared for gender, age, time post-stroke, clinical status, and 15 additional characteristics, no statistically significant differences were found for any of the variables. Therefore, randomization was accepted as satisfactory.

TREATMENT OUTCOMES

The repeated measures analysis of variance detected significant differences ($p<0.001$) over time in the study patients overall for the outcome measures UEFT and finger oscillation. No significant change over time was observed in the Beck or the Health Belief Survey (Table 2). Since all the initial findings on the 16 PF were within the expected normal range there was little room for change and no improvement seen in subsequent measures. Values for the 16 PF, although not reported, are available for the interested reader.

TABLE 2: COMPARISONS OF PRETEST, POSTTEST AND FOLLOW-UP SCORES FOR THE FOUR OUTCOME MEASURES (*N* = 29)

Measure	Pretest $\bar{x}$	Pretest (*SD*)	Posttest $\bar{x}$	Posttest (*SD*)	Follow-Up $\bar{x}$	Follow-Up (*SD*)	*p* value
UEFT	29.17	(27.20)	49.96	(30.04)	61.59	(35.36) (*n* = 27)*	< 0.001
Finger oscillation	11.69	(14.65)	16.70	(16.27)	19.77	(16.96) (*n* = 26)	< 0.001
Health belief	38.71	(6.95) (*n* = 21)	38.45	(8.19) (*n* = 20)	39.00	(7.53) (*n* = 17)	NS
Beck	4.33	(5.36) (*n* = 21)	4.25	(3.43) (*n* = 20)	3.69	(3.40) (*n* = 16)	NS

*Sample size when data missing.

The chi-square test of proportions failed to demonstrate that one treatment was more efficacious than another either when comparing pre- and posttest scores (8 of 13 in group A and 9 of 16 in group B demonstrated change scores equal to or greater than 10 points, X^2=0.08, 1 *df*) or when comparing pretest and follow-up scores (10 of 13 in group A and 11 of 16 in group B demonstrated change scores equal to or greater than 10 points, X^2=0.0008, 1 *df*).

The repeated measures analysis of variance failed to detect any significant differences due to group or group-time interaction on the outcome measures: UEFT, finger oscillation, Health Belief Survey, Beck and the 16 PF (Table 3).

The authors' a priori estimations of clinically significant change scores for the UEFT and the finger oscillation test were 10 points and 5 points respectively. Of particular interest is the finding that the 90% confidence interval for the outcome measure UEFT does not include +10, and that the 95% confidence interval for the finger oscillation test does not include +5. Based on these findings, there is at least a 90% chance that the behavioral-biofeedback approach is not clinically better than the exercise approach.

Regression analysis identified the UEFT, the category test and the time poststroke as the most significant independent variables for prognosticating outcome on the UEFT (R^2=0.84) (Table 4). Subjects within the two study groups are similar on all three of these variables.

Discussion

In our controlled pilot study[2] and other independent controlled studies[15,30] EMGBF had been found to be an effective form of therapy for restoration of range of motion (ROM) and strength of the hemiplegic upper limb in select populations of stroke patients. EMGBF compared favorably with traditional exercise therapy based on Bobath techniques given over the same time periods. Our present extended study suggests that the functional recovery following a formal behavioral approach (including biofeedback and cognitive therapy) is probably equal to, but not superior to, a

TABLE 3: BETWEEN GROUP COMPARISONS OF PRETEST, POSTTEST AND FOLLOW-UP SCORES FOR THE FOUR OUTCOME MEASURES (N = 29)

Treatment A (n = 13)

Measure	Pretest $\bar{x}$	(*SD*)	Posttest $\bar{x}$	(*SD*)	Follow-up $\bar{x}$	(*SD*)
UEFT	28.85	(27.71)	47.00	(27.04)	56.25	(34.77)
					(n = 12)*	
Finger oscillation	12.15	(15.73)	16.85	(17.43)	18.00	(19.05)
					(n = 11)	
Health belief	39.80	(6.97)	36.56	(7.21)	39.00	(8.56)
	(n = 10)		(n = 9)		(n = 7)	
Beck	4.00	(7.16)	4.00	(3.43)	4.33	(4.13)
	(n = 10)		(n = 9)		(n = 7)	

Treatment B (n = 16)

Measure	Pretest $\bar{x}$	(*SD*)	Posttest $\bar{x}$	(*SD*)	Follow-up $\bar{x}$	(*SD*)
UEFT	29.44	(27.69)	52.37	(32.94)	65.87	(36.44)
					(n = 15)*	
Finger oscilliation	11.31	(14.22)	16.56	(15.84)	21.06	(15.82)
					(n = 15)	
Health belief	37.73	(7.11)	40.00	(8.94)	39.00	(7.21)
	(n = 11)		(n = 11)		(n = 10)	
Beck	4.64	(3.32)	4.45	(3.59)	3.30	(3.06)
	(n = 11)		(n = 11)		(n = 10)	

*Sample size when data missing.

TABLE 4: PREDICTOR EQUATION FOR THE POST UPPER EXTREMITY FUNCTION TEST SCORE*

Predictor variable	R^2	Multiple R
Square root of pre-UEFT	0.6457	0.80
+		
Category	0.7691	0.88
+		
Weeks poststroke	0.8369	0.91

*Post-UEFT score = 45.98 + (9.6 × sq rt of pre-UEFT score)–(0.357 × category)–(10.92 × wk poststroke)

matched program of Bobath-based PT. This result of "hands-off" versus "hands-on" therapy in this controlled study of a selected population is impressive in that both approaches were clinically effective.

Where does this lead us in clinical practice? Physical therapy is traditionally "hands-on" although subtle behavioral components are often used informally and intuitively by individual therapists. Our results do not tell us to advocate dropping one form of therapy in favor of the other. Instead, they dramatize that in a substantial but still poorly defined proportion of stroke patients with hemiplegic upper limbs, clinically useful improvement is achievable and worth the effort. But the specific patients who would benefit most from one or the other of these two approaches is still not clarified and further study is needed.

Further study is also needed to establish the physiologic basis of the functional changes. "Motivation" enhancement is not the answer. It is obviously needed in both approaches, and in this study, the behavioral approach was no more successful than the PT approach in altering locus of control, mood, affect, etc. Thus we cannot invoke superior psychologic changes as having come from the "psychologic" approach.[14] We lack neurophysiologic correlates of the clinical improvements and these must be sought by the rehabilitation research community.

In conclusion, this controlled study of upper limb hemiplegia in fairly early stroke patients had revealed an optimistic prospect: both a behavioral technique by physical therapists (including EMGBF and cognitive therapy) and traditional neurophysiologic "hands-on" PT may bring about clinically worthwhile and lasting improvement in substantial numbers of patients. The time and costs required are modest and the treatments can be done on an outpatient basis.

References

1. Basmajian JV (ed): Therapeutic Exercise, Ed. 4, Baltimore, Williams & Wilkins, 1984
2. Basmajian JV, Gowland C, Brandstater ME, Swanson L, Trotter J: EMG feedback treatment of upper limb in hemiplegic stroke patients: pilot study. Arch Phys Med Rehabil 63:613-616, 1982
3. Basmajian JV, Regenos EM, Baker MP: Rehabilitating stroke patients with biofeedback. Geriatrics 32:85-88, 1977
4. Beck AT, Beck RW: Screening depressed patients in family practice. Postgrad Med 52:81-85, 1972
5. Bobath B: Adult Hemiplegia: Evaluation and Treatment, Ed 2. London, Heinemann, 1978
6. Brudny J, Korein J, Grynbaum BB, Friedmann LW, Weinstein S, Sachs-Frankel G, Belandres PV: EMG feedback therapy: review of treatment of 114 patients. Arch Phys Med Rehabil 57:55-61, 1976
7. Brunnstrom S: Movement Therapy in Hemiplegia: Neurophysiological Approach. New York, Harper & Row, 1970
8. Carroll D: Quantitative test of upper extremity function. J Chronic Dis 18:479-491, 1965

9. Catell RB, Eber HW, Tatsuoka MM: Handbook for the sixteen personality factor questionnaire. Champaign, IL, Institute for Personality and Ability Testing, 1970

10. De Renzi E, Vignolo LA: Token test: sensitive test to detect receptive disturbances in aphasics. Brain 85:665-678, 1962

11. Garraway WM, Akhtar AJ, Hockey L, Prescott RJ: Management of acute stroke in elderly: follow-up of controlled trial. Br Med J 281:827-829, 1980

12. Garraway WM, Walton MS, Akhtar JA, Prescott RJ: Use of health and social services in management of stroke in community: results from controlled trial. Age Ageing 10:95-104, 1981

13. Gowland C: Predicting sensorimotor recovery following stroke rehabilitation. Physiother Can 36:313-320, 1984

14. Hyman MD: Social psychological determinants of patients' performance in stroke rehabilitation. Arch Phys Med Rehabil 53:217-226, 1972

15. Inglis J, Donald MW, Monga TN, Sproule M, Young MJ: Electromyographic biofeedback and physical therapy of hemiplegic upper limb. Arch Phys Med Rehabil 65:755-759, 1984

16. Lehmann JF, DeLateur BJ, Fowler RS Jr, Warren CG, Arnhold R, Schertzer C, Hurka R, Whitmore JJ, Masock AJ, Chambers KH: Stroke: does rehabilitation affect outcome? Arch Phys Med Rehabil 56:375-382, 1975

17. Logigian MK, Samuels MA, Falconer J, Zagar R: Clinical exercise trial for stroke patients. Arch Phys Med Rehabil 46:364-367, 1983

18. Marzuk PM, Health and Public Policy Committee, American College of Physicians: Biofeedback for neuromuscular disorders. Ann Intern Med 102:854-858, 1985

19. Meichenbaum D: Cognitive-behavior Modification: Integrative Approach. New York, Plenum, 1977

20. Reitan RM: Aphasia and Sensory-perceptual Deficits in Adults. Tucson, Neuropsychology Press, 1984

21. Reitan RM: Verbal problem solving as related to cerebral damage. Percept Mot Skills 34:515-524, 1972

22. Reitan RM, Davison LA (eds): Clinical Neuropsychology: Current Status and Applications. Washington DC, Winston, 1974

23. Smith DS, Goldenberg E, Ashburn A, Kinsella G, Sheikh K, Brennan PJ, Meade TW, Zutshi DW, Perry JD, Reeback JS: Remedial therapy after stroke: randomised controlled trial. Br Med J 282:517-520, 1981

24. Smith ME, Garraway WM, Smith DL, Akhtar AJ: Therapy impact on functional outcome in controlled trial of stroke rehabilitation. Arch Phys Med Rehabil 63:21-24, 1982

25. Stern PH, McDowell F, Miller JM, Robinson M: Effects of facilitation exercise techniques in stroke rehabilitation. Arch Phys Med Rehabil 51:526-531, 1970

26. Stevens RS, Ambler NR, Warren MD: Randomized controlled trial of stroke rehabilitation ward. Age Ageing 13:65-75, 1984

27. Strand T, Asplund K, Eriksson S, Hägg E, Lithner F, Wester PO: Non-intensive stroke unit reduces functional disability and need for long-term hospitalization. Stroke 16:29-34, 1985

28. Wallston BS, Wallston KA, Kaplan GD, Maides SA: Development and validation of health locus of control (HLC) scale. J Consult Clin Psychol 44:580-585, 1976

29. Wolf SL: Electromyographic biofeedback applications to stroke patients: critical review. Phys Ther 63:1448-1459, 1983

30. Wolf SL, Binder-Macleod SA: Electromyographic biofeedback applications to hemiplegic patient: changes in upper extremity neuromuscular and functional status. Phys Ther 63:1393-1403, 1983

This study was supported by grant 6606-2083-44 from the National Research and Development Program of the Department of Health and Welfare, Canada. Submitted for publication April 28, 1986. Accepted in revised form September 2, 1986.

Illustrative Example 9–2: Questions

1. What is the purpose of the research?
2. Does the literature review provide you an understanding of how and why this investigation is important?
3. Do you think the investigation is important? Why or why not?
4. What is the theoretical or conceptual basis of the investigation?
5. How was the research conducted?
6. What type or kind of research is it and why?
7. What were the research questions or hypotheses?
8. What are the variables or phenomena under study?
9. Who were the subjects or units of study? How many were there?
10. How were the subjects or units of study obtained?
11. What information or data were collected?
12. If specific evaluation tools were used, what were they? Was information on the reliability and validity of the evaluation tools provided?
13. How was the information or data collected?
14. Will data collected be able to answer or address the research question or problem under study?
15. How was the information or data analyzed?
16. What were the criteria for interpreting the data?
17. What were the findings?
18. What were the limitations of the study? Was there a critical flaw?
19. Are the conclusions of the study warranted?
20. How can these research findings be used in occupational and physical therapy?

Illustrative Example 9–2: Answers

1. What is the purpose of the research?

The purpose of this investigation was to look at the efficacy of two forms of therapy on the upper limb functions of subjects who had had a stroke.

2. Does the literature review provide you an understanding of how and why this investigation is important?

Yes!

3. Do you think the investigation is important? Why or why not?

It is critically important to, when possible, document the relative effects of different types of interventions with different types of clients. Only in this manner will we know preferred therapeutic interventions for a given client.

4. What is the theoretical or conceptual basis of the investigation?

The theoretical approaches of neurodevelopmental treatment (NDT) compared to EMG biofeedback are the conceptual basis of the study.

5. How was the research conducted?

R O_1 (UEFT) X_1 (EMG) 0_2 (UEFT)

R 0_1 (UEFT) X_2 (NDT) 0_2 (UEFT)

Treatment is well described on page 269 (of the study). Compliance checks are exemplary.

6. What type or kind of research is it and why?

This is experimentally based research because of the random assignment of subjects to treatment conditions (EMG or NDT).

This is, essentially, a clinical trial investigation.

7. What were the research questions or hypotheses?

Research questions addressed could be:

(1) Is there a difference in effect on upper limb function between NDT and EMG biofeedback treatment?

(2) Is there a difference in effect on activities of daily (ADL) status and emotional adjustment between NDT and EMG biofeedback treatment?

Specific hypotheses were not stated.

8. *What are the variables or phenomena under study?*

The independent variable was treatment condition (NDT or EMG). The dependent variable was upper limb function and related issues such as emotional adjustment, ADL, and so on.

9. *Who were the subjects or units of study? How many were there?*

Subject criteria are clearly stated on page 8. Twenty-nine subjects, with an average age of 62, met the criteria. Subjects were further classified by severity and timing of stroke.

10. *How were the subjects or units of study obtained?*

It appears that all subjects who met criteria at this institution were enrolled in the study over a three-year period. It is not clear if others met criteria but could not be recruited, which could have introduced systematic bias into subject selection (theoretically controlled for with the randomization procedures).

11. *What information or data were collected?*

Subject performance data on a variety of tests such as the upper extremity function test (UEFT), and others listed on Table 1, was collected. No reliability or validity data are provided for any of the tests used.

12. *If specific evaluation tools were used, what were they? Was information on the reliability and validity of the evaluation tools provided?*

See answer to question 11.

13. *How was the information or data collected?*

Subjects were tested at the start and end of therapy. See page 269 of the study. An examiner unaware of subject assignment administered all tests.

14. *Will data collected be able to answer or address the research question or problem under study?*

Yes and no. Data will be able to answer the questions. But one cannot evaluate how good the data is without knowing more about the psychometric characteristics of the tests used.

15. *How was the information or data analyzed?*

Many data analysis procedures were used. The basic gist of the report is that "there is a 90% chance that the behavioral-biofeedback approach is not clinically better than the exercise approach" (p. 270 of the study).[1]

16. *What were the criteria for interpreting the data?*

Not stated. We can assume it is $p = .05$.

17. *What were the findings?*

Patients improve with these interventions, but one intervention is not more beneficial than the other.

18. *What were the limitations of the study? Was there a critical flaw?*

Perhaps suffice it to say that there are questions to be discussed and addressed in future investigations. First, tests to measure change need to be assured of a range of scores to show change and not have ceilings that reduce ability to document changes. Second, it may be appropriate to factor out therapist effects from inter-

1. Just a comment—it is interesting that the investigator equates NDT treatment with exercise. This suggests the degree of theoretical understanding possessed by many investigators into OT and PT interventions!

vention technique effects. Third, there is a question of the number of statistical analyses done with a relatively small sample size.

19. *Are the conclusions of the study warranted?*

Discussion appropriately limits conclusions.

20. *How can these research findings be used in occupational and physical therapy?*

It should spur us on to do our own studies, rather than those directed by other disciplines.

You have just completed a difficult chapter on experimental and quasiexperimental research, which also discussed research design. I presented control and the relationship of control to research design. And I stated that these research designs are typically what people think of when they refer to research. Do not expect to master this chapter at all once. Reread it a few times and then, I guarantee, things will begin to click. The next chapter presents more information on a special type of quasiexperimental research: single subject research.

References

Ary, S., Jacobs, L. C., & Razavieh, A. (1979). *Introduction to research in education* (2nd ed.). New York: Holt, Rinehart, & Winston.

Ayres, A. J. (1989). *Sensory integration and praxis tests.* Los Angeles: Western Psychological Services.

Basmajian, J. V., Gowland, C. A., Finlayson, A. J., Hall, A. L., Swanson, L. R., Stratford, M. S., Trotter, J. E., & Brandstater, M. E. (1987). Stroke treatment: Comparison of integrated behavioral-physical therapy versus traditional physical therapy program. *Archives of Physical Medicine and Rehabilitation, 68,* 267–272.

Best, J. W., & Kahn, J. V. (1989). *Research in education* (6th ed.). Englewood Cliffs, NJ: Prentice-Hall.

Burns, N., & Grove, S. K. (1987). *The practice nursing research: Conduct, critique and utilization.* Philadelphia: W. B. Saunders.

Campbell, D. T., & Stanley, J. C. (1966). *Experimental and quasiexperimental designs for research.* Chicago: Rand McNally.

Dickestein, R., Hocherman, S., Pillar, T., & Shaham, R. (1986). Stroke rehabilitation: Three exercise therapy approaches. *Physical Therapy, 66,* 1233–1238.

Gay, L. R. (1976). *Educational research: Competencies for analysis and education.* Columbus, OH: Charles E. Merril.

Goodman, M., Rothberg, A. D., Houston-McMillan, J. E., Cooper, P. A., Cartwright, J. D., & Van der Velde, M. A. (1985). Effect of early neurodevelopmental therapy in normal and at-risk survivors of neonatal intensive care. *The Lancet, 2(8468),* 1327–1332.

Hayslett, H. T. (1968). *Statistics made simple.* Garden City, NY: Doubleday.

Jenkins, J. R., Sells, C. J., Brady, D., Down, J., Moore, B., Carman, P., & Horn, R. (1982). Effects of developmental therapy on motor-impaired children. *Physical and Occupational Therapy in Pediatrics, 2,* 19–28.

Kirk, R. E. (1982). *Experimental design* (2nd ed.) Belmont, CA: Brooks Cole.

Logigian, M. K., Samuels, M. A., Falconer, J., & Zager, R. (1983). Clinical exercise trial for stroke patients. *Archives of Physical Medicine and Rehabilitation, 64,* 364–367.

Marcus, J. (Ed.). (1983). *Clinical research design and statistical analysis of individuals and subgroups.* Chicago: University of Chicago Press.

Sommerfeld, C., Fraser, B., Hensinger, R. N., & Beresford, C. V. (1981). Evaluation of physical therapy service for severely mentally impaired students with cerebral palsy. *Physical Therapy, 61,* 338–444.

Watt, J., Sims, D., Harcham, F., Schmidt, L., McMillan, A., & Hamilton, J. (1986). A prospective study of inhibitive casting as an adjunct to physiotherapy for cerebral-palsied children. *Developmental Medicine and Child Neurology, 28,* 480–488.

Recommended Readings

Ary, S., Jacobs, L. C., & Razavieh, A. (1979). *Introduction to research in education* (2nd ed.). New York: Holt, Rinehart, & Winston.

Best, J. W., & Kahn, J. V. (1989). *Research in education* (6th ed.). Englewood Cliffs, NJ: Prentice-Hall.

Ottenbacher, K. J., & Bonder, B. (1986). *Scientific inquiry: Design and analysis issues in occupational therapy.* Rockville, MD: American Occupational Therapy Association.

Learning Activities

1. Continue to work on your glossary. On file cards, develop a conceptual definition for each of the key words in this chapter.
2. Locate two quasiexperimental or experimental research articles. Read them. Using either symbol or matrix format, map them graphically.
3. Identify an intervention you would like to investigate and design a quasiexperimental study for investigating it. What are the problems you encounter?

CHAPTER 10 Single Subject Research

KEY WORDS

Baseline

Celeration line

C statistic

Ideographic research

Purposive sampling

Time series methodology

In the previous chapter I discussed quasiexperimental and experimental research. We will now look at a special form of quasiexperimental research called single subject research. Single subject research is especially useful when the purpose of the research is to evaluate the effects of an intervention with a particular individual, or when the purpose is to test the effects of a particular intervention with repeated investigations on a variety of subjects having a variety of diagnostic categories. Single subject research has been promoted as a practical method for therapists to use in developing a research database in occupational therapy (Ottenbacher, 1986). (This may apply to physical therapy as well.)

Single Subject Research Defined

Single subject research has many synonyms. By varying authors (Best & Kahn, 1989, chapter 6; Ottenbacher, 1986), it has been called

- "n = 1" research
- applied behavioral analysis
- time series methodology
- ideographic research.

Simply stated, single subject research is research on a single subject using an experimental design of repeated measurement of the dependent variable in response to the independent variable over time. Thus, single subject research is really a specialized type of experimental-quasiexperimental research. And single subject research is usually conducted over some period of time ranging from weeks to months.

Recall that quasiexperimental and experimental research resulted from the need to evaluate crop yields. Similarly, single subject research resulted from a specific need, that is, the need to study the effect of an intervention with a specific organism. The earliest single subject studies may have been conducted by B. F. Skinner and then adapted for use in the 1950s with individuals who were mentally retarded or autistic (Skinner, 1953).

Single subject research encompasses a variety of types of designs. (Such designs will be discussed later in this chapter.) Because there are specific and planned research designs for single subject research, it is distinctly different from clinical case study research or case study methodology (neither of which really have research designs per se). Single subject research is a special form of experimental research and, therefore, does address cause and effect. Let us analyze how it is different.

Single Subject Research Versus Clinical Case Study and Case Study Research

Clinical case study research and case study research are different from single subject research, yet many people confuse them. Clinical case study research consists of systematically reporting on a single case or cases. No baseline data prior to intervention, however, is usually associated with case study research. Moreover, case study research lacks rigor, that is, there is usually uncontrolled variation in the study. And case study research is difficult to replicate because there is no real research design. As mentioned in chapter 3, the work of Piaget (1926) was based on clinical case study.

The methodology of the case study as developed by Yin (1984) focuses on in-depth analysis of programs or projects. It is a specialized form of evaluation research used to determine worth or value of what is studied, and may be associated with policy analysis of social programs (Yin, 1984).

Case study reports are in sharp contrast to single subject research. Single subject research uses variations of experimental designs. (Recall some of the basic research designs presented in chapter 9.) Single subject research usually has some sort of baseline measurement of the variable of interest. These variables of interest (also called the *dependent variable*) may be motor performance, activities of daily living level, amount of drooling, level of sensory integration, occupational performance, and gait. Using strict and well-defined conditions of measurement, the dependent variable is repeatedly measured to determine change because of the intervention (or independent variable).

Design of Single Subject Research

There are classic designs used in single subject research, and they are modifications of the experimental designs presented in chapter 9. Following are two of the more common designs for single subject research that can serve as illustrative examples for any other designs you may encounter. These are the ABA design and the ABAB design.

ABA design consists of the

- A phase (taking a baseline measurement on the dependent variable)
- B phase (administering the intervention—the independent variable)

- A phase (taking another measurement on the dependent variable to determine the effects of the intervention).

You can see why repeated measurement on the variable of interest is a hallmark of single subject research.

ABAB design is similar to the previous design, but there are two measurements during the absence of intervention (two A phases). The first A phase is baseline and the second captures the nature of the dependent variable after removing the intervention. This design would read

- A phase (baseline measurement of dependent variable)
- B phase (delivery of the intervention or independent variable and measurement of its effects)
- A phase (measurement of the dependent variable after removal of the intervention)
- B phase (second administration of the intervention with measurement of its effects).

Single subject research has an entire collection of statistically based data analysis procedures that are clear and well defined. Such statistically based data analysis techniques do not exist for case study research.

Control in Single Subject Research

Recall that in the quasiexperiemtal and experimental research presented in chapter 9, control was established by the use of control groups of subjects. In single subject research an analogous form of control is achieved not by using comparison groups but by using the subject under study as his or her own control. That is, improvement is compared to baseline measures on the subject. Basically, by repeatedly presenting and removing the intervention in elaborations of the ABA or ABAB designs, the investigator attempts to determine the effect of the intervention on the subject.

Data Analysis in Single Subject Research

As a major point of contrast to clinical case study research, single subject research has an entire methodology of data analysis underlying its use. There are two broad categories of data analysis in single subject research:

- visual interpretation of the data
- statistical analyses.

These data analytic approaches can be used together for a design used with a single subject. In the past, visual interpretation of the data was sufficient for data analysis. More recently, however, statistically based data analysis procedures are required in single subject research if, for example, the study is for submission to a peer reviewed journal for possible publication.

VISUAL INTERPRETATION OF THE DATA

In visual interpretation of the data, one looks for patterns and trends in the graphic portrayal of the measurements taken during conduct of the study. An investigator would look at how the dependent variable changes over time in response to the independent variable. This is a common form of data analysis in single subject research.

Figure 10–1 presents typical examples of visually displayed data from single subject research.

Review of Figure 10–1 shows the dependent variable (range of motion) plotted by weeks after surgery. The A phase would be time until Week 32, when the splint was applied (B phase).

FIGURE 10–1. TYPICAL EXAMPLES OF VISUALLY DISPLAYED DATA FROM SINGLE SUBJECT RESEARCH

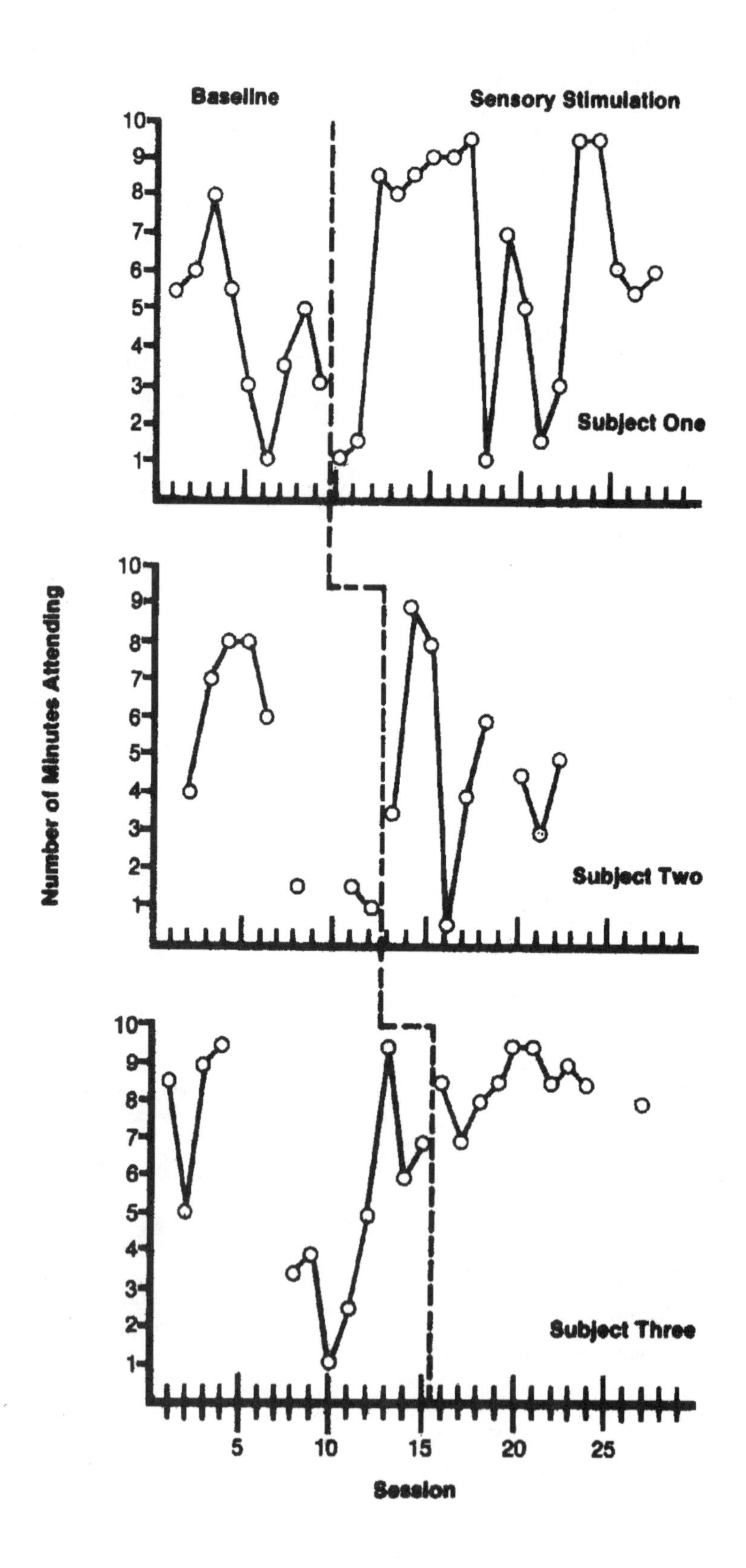

ANALYSIS OF THE DATA

Procedures developed to assist in the analysis of data from single subject research include the **celeration line** and the **C statistic** (Ottenbacher, 1986). The celeration line represents a series of data in a transformed state, with half of the observations represented below the line and half of the observations represented above the line (Ottenbacher, 1986, pp. 137–166). The c statistic is based on an estimate of the stability of variance of one data point to another (Ottenbacher, 1986).

Who Are Subjects in Single Subject Research?

Recall that random sampling and random assignment to group conditions is the hallmark of experimental research. Such random selection of subjects is not relevant in single subject research. Rather, subjects are selected, obtained, or recruited based on their unique problems, needs, or characteristics that are of interest to the research investigator. Single subject research, therefore, uses a form of purposive sampling, that is, the subjects are selected according to some purposive criteria other than random sampling.

It is critically important that subjects be well described in single subject research, for it is only by thorough description of the subjects that the research consumer can determine whether the research results have meaning or application to the individuals that he or she is serving. And many of the published studies using single subject research do not have adequate subject description for this purpose. Better subject description in published single subject research is a goal for investigators to strive to achieve.

Figure 10–2 presents a sample of subject description in single subject research in occupational and physical therapy literature.

This description of the subject provides the reader with a general understanding of the subject characteristics. It is up to you, the reader, to determine whether enough information is presented to give a sufficient understanding of who the subjects were.

FIGURE 10–2. SUBJECT DESCRIPTION IN SINGLE SUBJECT RESEARCH

Subjects. Three male subjects, two aged 11 and one aged 13 years, were chosen from students enrolled in a therapeutic and educational day program for children with behavior problems and mixed psychiatric diagnoses. Selection of the subjects was made in conjunction with the staff occupational therapist.

It was based on criteria routinely used at the agency to determine appropriateness for treatment by sensory stimulation, that is, significantly low postrotary nystagmus, and difficulty assuming or maintaining the prone extension posture. All subjects were enrolled in the same classroom where they were involved in an ongoing academic program. During portions of this program, children were exposed to simple mathematical computations. No subject had received specific treatment by sensory stimulation before.

Taken from Madsen, P. S. & Conte, J. R. (1980). Single subject research in occupational therapy: A case example. *American Journal of Occupational Therapy, 34(4),* 263–267.

FIGURE 10–3. SAMPLES OF SINGLE SUBJECT RESEARCH IN OCCUPATIONAL AND PHYSICAL THERAPY

Investigation	Purpose	Independent Variable	Dependent Variable
DeGangi, Hurley, and Linscheid, (1983)	Develop method to measure short-term effects of NDT treatment	NDT treatment	Individualized subject goals on quality of movement
Laskas, Mullen, and Willson-Brayles, (1985)	Assess NDT treatment effects using EMG and behavioral observations	NDT treatment	EMG recording and observations of equilibrium

NDT = Neurodevelopmental treatment; EMG = electromyograph

Single Subject Research in Occupational and Physical Therapy Research

Single subject research allows for the in-depth study of therapeutic interventions when it may not yet be possible to appropriately design large-scale intervention studies (Ottenbacher, 1986, chapter 3). And it allows for the study of rare or unusual cases. Figure 10–3 presents some of the ways single subject research has been used in occupational and physical therapy research.

The material in Figure 10–3 reveals different applications for single subject research in the therapy fields. Pay particular attention to the dependent variables as depicted in the Figure. I cannot overemphasize the importance of how the dependent or outcome variable is measured in single subject research, and all other types of research. Because there is usually repeated measurement of the dependent variable over time, it is critically important that the measurement be objective and reliable.

Application

Let us now apply these concepts by reading actual articles that use case study and single subject methods. Read the following examples and answer the interpretation questions for each example. Compare your answers with the answers provided after each interpretation section.

Reprinted from *American Journal of Occupational Therapy*, Vol. 44, Number 5, May, 1990, pp. 454–458. Used with permission.

ILLUSTRATIVE EXAMPLE 10–1

An Intervention Program for a Fraternal Twin With Down Syndrome

Sandra J. Edwards, Hon Keung Yuen

Key Words: developmental therapy • neurodevelopmental therapy • patient care team • physical stimulation

Two of the current therapeutic intervention modalities that have been widely used for the treatment of persons with developmental disabilities are neurodevelopmental treatment and sensory stimulation (Harris, 1987; Pothier & Cheek, 1984). The effects of these treatments on the sensorimotor performance of infants and children with Down syndrome have been inconsistent (Harris, 1981; Kantner, Clark, Allen, & Chase, 1976; Lydic, Windsor, Short, & Ellis, 1985; MacLean & Baumeister, 1982). For example, Harris (1981) and Lydic et al. (1985) were unable to demonstrate significant improvement in the motor performance of children with Down syndrome after administering either neurodevelopmental treatment or vestibular stimulation. Vestibular stimulation is regarded as an essential component in sensory stimulation due to its hypothesized positive effect on hypotonicity, which is so commonly observed in children with Down syndrome. Additionally, children with Down syndrome have been observed to have increased alertness after receiving calibrated rotary vestibular stimulation (Lydic et al., 1985).

We incorporated both neurodevelopmental treatment techniques (Bobath & Bobath, 1976) and vestibular and tactile stimulation techniques (Ayres, 1979) into an intervention program for a girl with Down syndrome who was the second born of fraternal twins. "If a child is generally hypotonic, considerable amounts of excitatory tactile and vestibular stimuli are in order and few precautions are necessary" (Ayres, 1979, p. 118). Our objective was to facilitate her motor, reflex, prelinguistic, and cognitive development. We also used a transdisciplinary approach, as advocated by McCormick and Goldman (1979). This approach required a collaborative treatment planning effort across disciplines and left the implementation of the treatment to a single team member.

Case History

This female twin weighed 2,954 g at birth and was born breech. Two days after birth, she was admitted to the hospital because of weak sucking and swallowing reflexes, and tube feeding was required. During this hospitalization, examinations revealed that the child had group B streptococcic sepsis and questionable seizure disorder; however, no abnormality showed in an electroencephalogram. When the child was 2 months old, an atrial septal defect was detected and treated with digoxin until she received a cardiac catheter. A history of recurring bilateral otitis media and upper respiratory tract infections since birth were reported by the nurse practitioner.

FAMILY BACKGROUND

The twin brother weighed 3,210 g at birth, had no difficulty during birth, and was confirmed by a genetic examination to be chromosomally normal. When the twins were born, the mother was 35 years old and in the 37th week of gestation. During her pregnancy, the mother had been on medications to control seizures and a thyroid malfunction.

The physical and medical problems of the twin with Down syndrome and the responsibilities involved in raising twins were a challenge for this single mother. In addition, she had limited social and financial resources, which could have a negative effect on her parenting skills.

PREINTERVENTION EVALUATION

The female twin was evaluated at 11 months 6 days of age with the Bayley Scales of Infant Development (Bayley, 1969), reflex testing (Bleck, 1975), the oral and feeding assessment (Coley, 1978), the Receptive Expressive Emergent Language Scale (Bzoch & League, 1970), the Sequenced Inventory of Communication Development (Hedrich, Prather, & Tobin, 1984), clinical observation, and neuromuscular examinations. All evaluations were administered in the child's home to obtain a natural sampling of her behavior. They were completed by the first author, who is certified in sensory integration testing, and by a speech–language pathologist.

To establish the interrater reliability of the Bayley Scales of Infant Development, a registered occupational therapist with extensive pediatric experience, who was unaware of the purpose of the study, sat next to the first author and rated the Bayley scales independently as the child was evaluated. A 100% agreement in scoring was achieved in all areas of the Bayley scales evaluations. The percentage of agreement for interobserver reliability was calculated as follows:

$$\frac{\text{no. of agreed items}}{\text{no. of agreed items} + \text{no. of disagreed items}} \times 100$$

The results of the Bayley scales are shown in Tables 1 and 2.

Reflex testing indicated the presence of several primitive reflexes and the absence of sitting equilibrium and optical righting reactions in tilting (see Table 3). The combined motor and reflex delays warranted the use of neurodevelopmental treatment. The correlation of the low score on the Bayley Motor Scale (5.5 months) and the poor postural reactions of the child was consistent with Haley's (1986) findings.

On the basis of clinical observation, we found that the child demonstrated tactile defensiveness by withdrawing from being touched and resisting toys hidden in rice. She also demonstrated signs of vestibular dysfunction, as evidenced by her poor sitting balance and her withdrawing or crying when engaged in such vestibular stimulation as slow spinning, rocking, and rolling. These signs indicate a need for vestibular stimulation (Montgomery, 1985).

An oral-motor assessment showed poor sucking and swallowing responses, strong bite reflex, tongue protrusion, and other oral-motor dysfunctions (see Table 3).

Neuromuscular examinations revealed low muscle tone, as demonstrated by hyperextension of the finger and wrist joints, excessive dorsiflexion of the ankles,

TABLE 1

A COMPARISON OF SCORES ON THE BAYLEY SCALES OF INFANT DEVELOPMENT[a] FOR THE TWIN WITH DOWN SYNDROME

Scale	Preintervention	Postintervention
Mental		
Raw score	78	93
Mental Development Index	52	<50
Age equivalent (months)	4.5	10.0
Developmental quotient	40.90	47.62
Motor		
Raw score	25	38
Psychomotor Development Index	<50	<50
Age equivalent (months)	5.5	9.0
Developmental quotient	50.00	42.86

Note: Developmental quotient = (age equivalent/chronological age) x 100. The child's chronological age before intervention was 11 months; after intervention, 21 months.
a. (Bayley, 1969).

TABLE 2

A COMPARISON OF THE INFANT BEHAVIOR RECORD[a] BEFORE AND AFTER INTERVENTION FOR THE TWIN WITH DOWN SYNDROME

Preintervention	Postintervention
Displays little body motion	Displays active body motion
Is accepting	Is friendly
Watches warily	Smiles, vocalizes
Bangs toys infrequently	Bangs toys frequently
Does not mouth toys	Actively mouths toys

a. From the Bayley Scales of Infant Development (Bayley, 1969).

hyperabduction and flexion of the hip joints, and noticeable lordosis of the back. Extreme hypotonia has been correlated with the absence or persistence of some of the pathological reflexes in children with Down syndrome (Cowie, 1970).

The child scored 3 months behind her age level in both receptive and expressive language on the Receptive Expressive Emergent Language Scale and the Sequenced Inventory of Communication Development.

INTERVENTION

On the basis of these evaluation results, we designed an intervention that focused on facilitating fine and gross motor developmental milestones; reflex and equilibrium reactions; and oral-motor, prelinguistic, and cognitive skills. The first author and a speech–language pathologist designed and selected activities to meet both disci-

TABLE 3
A COMPARISON OF THE REFLEX AND FEEDING EVALUATIONS FOR THE TWIN WITH DOWN SYNDROME BEFORE AND AFTER INTERVENTION

Evaluation	Preintervention	Postintervention
Reflex		
Moro	–	–
Parachute	+	+
Neck Righting	–	–
Asymmetrical tonic neck reflex	–	±
Extensor thrust	–	–
Foot placement	–	±
Symmetrical tonic neck reflex	–	–
Landau	+	–[a]
Optical righting	±	+
Feeding		
Rooting reflex	±	±
Sucking reflex	+	–[a]
Swallowing	+	+
Bite reflex	+	–[a]
Tongue protrusion	+	–[a]

Note: – = absent; + = present; ± = beginning or fading.
a. Indicates a maturation in development.

plines' goals and objectives (see Table 4) and to efficiently use the child's limited attention span and energy. We adapted programming resources from Developmental Programming for Infants and Young Children (Schafer & Moersch, 1981) and Time to Begin: Early Education for Children With Down Syndrome (Dmitriev, 1982). Preparation time for the programming (after the initial assessment) took approximately 2 weeks.

A home-based program was selected to promote the parent's participation. A home interventionist implemented the treatment under the supervision of the first author and the speech–language pathologist. The home interventionist had strong parenting skills: She had raised four healthy children of her own and had adopted two children with Down syndrome. She was also a student in an occupational therapy program at the time and was under the supervision of the first author and of a faculty member in the speech–language pathology department.

Treatment consisted of weekly 30-min sessions for a 9 1/2-month period. The parent observed and participated in treatment, and the rationales for each intervention were discussed and explained to her.

To facilitate gross motor skills, the home interventionist stimulated the child's sitting equilibrium and optical righting reactions in tilting. The child was positioned in a cross-legged sitting style and gently pushed on either side at shoulder level to challenge her sitting equilibrium. To strengthen the trunk muscles, stimulation such as tapping and vibrating were applied to the extensor muscles on either side of the spinal column. In addition, techniques described by Bobath (1969) were used to place the child in prone and 4-point kneeling positions in order to facilitate righting and equilibrium reactions in the quadruped and sitting positions.

Because the child was resistant to vestibular and tactile stimulation, both were introduced slowly and carefully. The home interventionist began vestibular stimulation by holding the child in her lap and rocking her side to side and back and forth. Gradually, the child was seated in a snow dish and spun slowly for 2 to 2 1/2 revolutions while her nystagmus responses were observed. After 4 months of holding and gentle spinning, the home interventionist introduced a rubber rocking horse for vestibular stimulation.

Tactile stimulation was implemented through a search for objects of various sizes hidden in rice. At first, the child was resistant to this type of tactile experience but, through a gradual introduction, she became more responsive to it. The child also accepted firm pressure on her hands and demonstrated less defensiveness to it than she did to light stroking.

The development of eye–hand coordination was facilitated by the use of an enlarged pegboard with pegs 2 cm in diameter to foster success in placing pegs on the board. To encourage eye tracking, the home interventionist blew soap bubbles in specific directions.

To facilitate oral-motor function, the home interventionist placed peanut butter on the lateral side of the child's tongue to facilitate tongue movement and lip

TABLE 4
SAMPLE OF INTERVENTION ACTIVITIES

Net Activity

Materials: Low-hanging vestibular net, objects.

Position: Prone, supine, side-lying, or sitting.

Procedure: Encourage child to push with hands to swing self in net; child may reach for objects.

Place different textures on ground to increase tactile stimulation. Alternatively, simply swing or twirl the child.

Goals: *Occupational therapy.* Improve neck cocontraction, facilitate back extension, facilitate labyrinth righting and sitting equilibrium reaction, stimulate tactile sense, stimulate utricle and saccule of the vestibular system, facilitate weight bearing and shifting.
Speech therapy. Gesture and vocal imitation; associated bubbling for imitation.

Bubble Activity

Materials: Soap bubbles.

Position: Child placed in sitting position, supported at hips; therapist positioned to side of child.

Procedure: Blow bubbles and produce the word *more*; prompt child to approximate the word *more*; when approximation is made, present bubbles at the child's side and encourage the child to pop bubbles with opposite hand.

Goals: *Occupational therapy.* Improve sitting equilibrium and labyrinth righting reactions, increase trunk rotation, upgrade weight shift for mobility.
Speech therapy. Word or gesture approximation.

closure. Crackers were introduced on either side of her mouth to encourage chewing. Different shapes of cups were introduced to encourage mouth closure that allowed her to swallow liquid.

The home interventionist used language to encourage vocalization and to imitate the child's and the brother's sounds. A mirror was placed in front of the child to augment visual feedback so she could see the formation of the adult's lips when the adult made sounds. The adult was seated on the floor behind the child to augment positioning of the lower extremities and trunk and to simultaneously talk to the child. Using the mirror, the child could see the adult's lips and be kept in a desirable developmental position for sitting. The mother was encouraged to facilitate language by asking the child to make a sound instead of a gesture for an object.

Besides providing therapy for the child, the home interventionist demonstrated to the mother how to stimulate and facilitate the child's motor, cognitive, and prelinguistic development as a carryover of the same program. Strategies to deal with the child's behavioral problems and to discipline the brother were discussed and implemented. For instance, after discovering that the mother sometimes punished the children by sending them to bed with no supper (the children were underweight), the home interventionist recommended an alternative disciplinary action of time out in the bedroom for shorter periods of time to accomplish the necessary discipline without sacrificing the loss of a healthy meal. The mother used this suggestion.

The child also attended an hour each of special education and physical therapy twice a week in a public school. Over the 9 1/2-month period of the intervention, neither occupational therapy nor speech–language therapy was provided in the school program. Objectives from the special education teacher and the physical therapist were incorporated in treatment planning. The intervention and school program began within 2 weeks of each other.

POSTINTERVENTION EVALUATION

The child was reevaluated at the age of 21 months 5 days after 9 1/2 months of intervention. An analysis of the developmental quotient from the Bayley Scales of Infant Development in preintervention and postintervention evaluations showed a gain in the Mental Scale of .72 points (see Table 1).

A comparison of the child's behaviors before and after intervention showed that some improvement had occurred (see Table 2). The child appeared more relaxed, attentive, confident, and interested in the activities, and she responded more readily to the examiner during the reevaluation (e.g., she was smiling and interacting, moving a lot more, and acting more sociable). The child's attention span for playing with and manipulating toys increased from seconds at the beginning of therapy to 5–7 min at the end of therapy. She also played more purposefully. For example, before the initiation of therapy, the child would throw blocks without interest or attention; with therapy, she developed more interest in banging them, stacking them, and watching where they landed when she threw them.

Improvement was observed in the foot placement response and in the optical righting reaction. The feeding evaluation showed an inhibition of the biting reflex, less tongue protrusion, and an improvement in sucking reflex (see Table 3). The mother and home interventionist reported that the child was generally easier to feed.

The results of the language development evaluation, as reported by the speech–language pathologist, indicated that the child demonstrated a gain of 3 months in her expressive language score but made no gain in her receptive language score.

Discussion

Prior studies with standardized developmental tests have shown that children with Down syndrome exhibit a pattern of a decreasing rate of development throughout infancy and early childhood in both the mental and motor domains (Carr, 1970; Dicks-Mireaux, 1966, 1972). Hanson (1981) reported a gradual decline in scores on the Bayley Scales of Infant Development over the first 2 years, particularly in the area of motor development. This was true even for Down syndrome children who had participated in an intervention program.

The present study suggests that occupational therapy through home intervention and the incorporation of neurodevelopmental treatments and vestibular and tactile stimulation techniques have successfully decreased the decline in the development of a child with Down syndrome, as determined by the age equivalent scores on the Bayley Scales of Infant Development and on reflex testing. We cannot, however, eliminate the possibility of maturation or the effects of physical therapy and special education as alternative explanations.

The home-based program gave the parent a better understanding of the abilities of the twin with Down syndrome, thus facilitating more realistic expectations and a more positive attitude toward the twin. Parental participation in intervention has been identified as an essential component in sustaining the gains from therapeutic intervention once the formal programming has ended (Hanson, 1977). After the intervention period, the parent in the present study reported that she gained more confidence and competence in her daily management of the child by using the emotional support provided by the home interventionist.

The transdisciplinary approach allows team members to share their professional expertise (Wolery & Dyk, 1984), thus avoiding the role conflicts and time clashes that result when team members feel they must defend their professional territories. Additionally, the possibility of overstimulating the child may be reduced.

The success of this intervention can be attributed to (a) the combining of the theoretical principles of neurodevelopmental treatment and vestibular and tactile stimulation, (b) the strategic planning and implementation of treatment through the team members' collaboration (transdisciplinary approach), and (c) the inclusion of parental skills training as part of home-based treatment.

Acknowledgments

We thank Shirley Sparks, CCC-SP, for testing the twins, and Sarah Austin, MOTS, Mary Rambosck, MOTR, and Dolores Harley-Gleason, MOTR, for their suggestions. We also thank Noreen Jolliffe for her work with the parent and child, the multiclinic staff for their contributions, Al Garcia for his help with the editing and the statistics, and Dr. Lela Llorens for consultation.

References

Ayres, A. J. (1979). *Sensory integration and learning disorders.* Los Angeles: Western Psychological Services.

Bayley, N. (1969). *Bayley Scales of Infant Development.* New York: Psychological Corporation.

Bleck, E. E. (1975). Locomotor prognosis in cerebral palsy. *Developmental Medicine and Child Neurology,* 17, 18–25.

Bobath, B. (1969). The treatment of neuromuscular disorders by improving patterns of co-ordination. *Physiotherapy,* 55, 18–22.

Bobath, B., & Bobath, K. (1976). Cerebral palsy. In P. H. Pearson & C. E. Williams (Eds.), *Physical therapy services in the developmental disabilities* (3rd ed., pp. 31–185). Springfield, IL: Charles C Thomas.

Bzoch, K., & League, R. (1970). *Receptive Expressive Emergent Language Assessment Scale.* Tallahassee, FL: Anhinga Press.

Carr, J. (1970). Mental and motor development in young mongol children. *Journal of Mental Deficiency Research,* 14, 205–220.

Coley, I. L. (1978). *Pediatric assessment of self-care activities.* St. Louis: Mosby.

Cowie, V. A. (1970). *A study of the early development of mongols.* New York: Pergamon.

Dicks-Mireaux, M. J. (1966). Development of intelligence of children with Down's syndrome: Preliminary report. *Journal of Mental Deficiency Research,* 10, 89–93.

Dicks-Mireaux, M. J. (1972). Mental development of infants with Down's syndrome. *American Journal of Mental Deficiency,* 77, 26–32.

Dmitriev, V. (1982). *Time to begin: Early education for children with Down syndrome.* Milton, WA: Caring.

Haley, S. M. (1986). Postural reactions in infants with Down syndrome: Relationship to motor milestone development and age. *Physical Therapy, 66,* 17–22.

Hanson, M. J. (1977). *Teaching your Down's syndrome infant: A guide for parents.* Baltimore: University Park Press.

Hanson, M. J. (1981). Down's syndrome children: Characteristics and intervention research. In M. Lewis & L. A. Rosenblum (Eds.), *The uncommon child* (pp. 83–114). New York: Plenum.

Harris, S. R. (1981). Effects of neurodevelopmental therapy on improving motor performance in Down's syndrome infants. *Developmental Medicine and Child Neurology,* 23, 477–483.

Harris, S. R. (1987). Early intervention for children with motor handicaps. In M. J. Guralnick & F. C. Bennett (Eds.), *The effectiveness of early intervention for at-risk and handicapped children* (pp. 115–173). New York: Academic Press.

Hedrich, D., Prather, E., & Tobin, A. (1984). *Sequenced Inventory of Communication Development.* Seattle: University of Washington Press.

Kantner, R. M., Clark, D. L., Allen, L. C., & Chase, M. F. (1976). Effects of vestibular stimulation on nystagmus responses and motor performances in the developmentally delayed infant. *Physical Therapy, 56,* 414–421.

Lydic, J. S., Windsor, M. M., Short, M. A., & Ellis, T. A. (1985). Effects of controlled rotary vestibular stimulation on the motor performance of infants with Down syndrome. *Physical and Occupational Therapy in Pediatrics, 5*(2/3), 93–144.

MacLean, W. E., & Baumeister, A. A. (1982). Effects of vestibular stimulation on motor development and stereotyped behavior of developmentally delayed children. *Journal of Abnormal Child Psychology, 10,* 229–245.

McCormick, L., & Goldman, R. (1979). The transdisciplinary model: Implications for service delivery and personnel preparation for the severely and profoundly handicapped. *American Association for the Education of the Severely/Profoundly Handicapped Review, 4*(2), 152–161.

Montgomery, P. (1985). Assessment of vestibular function in children. *Physical and Occupational Therapy in Pediatrics, 5*(2/3), 33–55.

Pothier, P. C., & Cheek, K. (1984). Current practices in sensory motor programming with developmentally delayed infants and young children. *Child: Care, Health and Development, 10,* 341–348.

Schafer, D. S., & Moersch, M. S. (Eds.). (1981). *Developmental programming for infants and young children.* Ann Arbor, MI: University of Michigan Press.

Wolery, M., & Dyk, L. (1984). Arena assessment: Description and preliminary social validity data. *Journal of the Association for the Severely Handicapped, 9,* 231–235.

Illustrative Example 10–1: Questions

1. What is the purpose of the research?
2. Does the literature review provide you an understanding of how and why this investigation is important?
3. Do you think the investigation is important? Why or why not?
4. What is the theoretical or conceptual basis of the investigation?
5. How was the research conducted?
6. What type or kind of research is it and why?
7. What were the research questions or hypotheses?
8. What are the variables or phenomena under study?
9. Who were the subjects or units of study? How many were there?
10. How were subjects or units of study obtained?
11. What information or data were collected?
12. If specific evaluation tools were used, what were they? Was information on the reliability and validity of the evaluation tools provided?
13. How was the information or data collected?
14. Will data collected be able to answer or address the research question or problem under study?
15. How was the information or data analyzed?
16. What were the criteria for interpreting the data?
17. What were the findings?
18. What were the limitations of the study? Was there a critical flaw?
19. Are the conclusions of the study warranted?
20. How can these research findings be used in occupational and physical therapy?

Illustrative Example 10–1: Answers

1. *What is the purpose of the research?*

The authors state, "Our objective was to facilitate her motor, reflex, prelinguistic, and cognitive development" (p. 454). They are referring to the development of a girl with Down's syndrome who was a fraternal twin. In fact, they wanted to look at the intervention strategy using, as the authors claim, neurodevelopmental treatment (NDT) and sensory stimulation techniques.

2. *Does the literature review provide you an understanding of how and why this investigation is important?*

In a scant two paragraphs, the authors set the stage nicely, and the reader gets an idea of the literature related to this case report.

3. *Do you think the investigation is important? Why or why not?*

It is important because it is immediately clinically relevant and related to intervention services typically provided by therapists.

4. *What is the theoretical or conceptual basis of the investigation?*

NDT and sensory stimulation are cited as the therapeutic frame of reference.

5. *How was the research conducted?*

This is not research per se. Rather, the authors are reporting on a clinically based intervention.

6. *What type or kind of research is it and why?*

One may consider this report to be a clinical case study report that can be argued by different experts to be research or not to be research, depending on their definition (remember the earlier discussion of how different people view research). If deemed to be research, it would be a very simple form of descriptive research.

You might argue that this is a form of quasiexperimental research with no control because there is a pretest, posttest, and intervention. Or you could argue that it is a single subject investigation with little control. In a sense, all of these answers are correct. What is important is for you to see what was done and understand why the study can be considered to be descriptive, quasiexperimental, or single subject research.

7. *What were the research questions or hypotheses?*

The question may be inferred to be, What are the effects of NDT and sensory stimulation on a girl with Down's syndrome?

8. *What are the variables or phenomena under study?*

Because this study is a clinical report and not a true single subject or quasiexperimental design, the use of the terms dependent and independent variables are somewhat inappropriate. But they will be used, nonetheless, as they allow for clear communication about intervention and outcome.

The independent variable was the intervention, a home-based program consisting of weekly, 30-minute sessions over a 9 1/2-month period. The dependent variable was motor and mental functioning of the subject as measured by the Bayley Scales of Infant Development reflex testing, oral motor assessment, neuromotor assessment, and clinical observations of touch.

9. *Who were the subjects or units of study? How many were there?*

A girl with Down's syndrome, aged 11 months 6 days was the subject.

10. *How were the subjects or units of study obtained?*

No information provided.

11. *What information or data were collected?*

The section on preintervention evaluation provides this. The testing was done in the subject's home.

12. *If specific evaluation tools were used, what were they? Was information on the reliability and validity of the evaluation tools provided?*

The Bayley Scales of Infant Development was used. Because this is a standardized assessment, however, it was confusing that interrater reliability of the Bayley was computed and reported. No attempts at interrater reliability was attempted for the other measurement procedures.

13. *How was the information or data collected?*

By testing the subject in her home setting.

14. *Will data collected be able to answer or address the research question or problem under study?*

Yes and no. Because this is fundamentally a descriptive study with a lack of control, the lack of reliable and valid methods of subject assessment are typical.

15. *How was the information or data analyzed?*

To the authors' credit, they made no attempt at statistically based data analysis. Doing so would have been inconsistent with a clinical case study. Instead, logical and descriptive analysis of the data was provided (see p. 457). The authors' merely described the behavioral changes seen in the child, as well as reported changes in the Bayley Scales scores.

16. *What were the criteria for interpreting the data?*

Clinical judgment.

17. *What were the findings?*

Some improvement occurred. "The child appears more relaxed, attentive, confident, and interested in the activities, and she responded more readily to the examiner during the reevaluation" (p. 457). Expressive language improved.

18. What were the limitations of the study? Was there a critical flaw?

It really is not appropriate to critique this like a research study because it is a clinical case report. The reader, however, should have an intuitive feel, based on reading through this analysis, of what some of the problems would be if one were to consider this like a research investigation.

19. Are the conclusions of the study warranted?

I find them acceptable. What do you think?

20. How can these research findings be used in occupational and physical therapy?

Primarily in replication of the findings. If a clinical report like this one was similarly reported from other sites and therapists across the country, it would provide the database needed to then design a series of single subject investigations or quasiexperimental intervention studies with similar subjects.

ILLUSTRATIVE EXAMPLE 10–2

Reprinted from *American Journal of Occupational Therapy*, Vol. 44, Number 2, February, 1990, pp. 139–145. Used with permission.

Measuring the Effects of Neurodevelopmental Treatment on the Daily Living Skills of 2 Children With Cerebral Palsy

Lee Ann Lilly, Nancy J. Powell

Key Words: cerebral palsy • neurodevelopmental therapy • sensorimotor therapy

Neurodevelopmental treatment (NDT), the neurophysiological treatment approach for central nervous system dysfunction developed by the Bobaths (Bobath & Bobath, 1964), is widely used in the allied health professions to treat young children with cerebral palsy. Occupational therapists in particular describe one goal of NDT as providing foundational patterns for the learning of such self-care skills as feeding, dressing, and washing. Studies attempting to document NDT's effects, however, have been unable to validate this treatment approach. Little research has been conducted on the carryover effects of NDT to functional abilities.

Literature Review

Traditionally, studies attempting to substantiate the use of neurophysiologically based treatment approaches such as NDT have examined their long-term effects. Research designs can be descriptive designs, contrast designs, or control group designs. Researchers using descriptive designs to examine the efficacy of therapeutic intervention have usually demonstrated positive change as a result of intervention (Kong, 1966; Norton, 1975). Similarly, the few researchers using contrast designs to compare the effects of neurophysiologically based treatment with the effects of more traditional programs such as functional treatments or passive range of motion have supported NDT (Carlsen, 1975; Sherzer, Mike, & Ilson, 1976).

Most researchers employing the more rigorous control group designs, however, have usually not demonstrated favorable outcomes in children as a result of NDT. Wright and Nicholson (1973) randomly assigned 47 children with spastic cerebral palsy, aged birth to 6 years, to treatment and no-treatment groups. After up to 12 months of therapy, experimental and control groups had made similar gains in passive ankle dorsiflexion, hip abduction, and loss of primary automatic reflexes. Sommerfeld, Fraser, Hensinger, and Beresford (1981) supported Wright and Nicholson's (1973) findings in their study of 29 severely mentally retarded children with cerebral palsy. Harris (1981) examined the performance of 20 infants with Down syndrome on the Peabody (Folio & DuBose, 1974) and Bayley (1969) tests before and after either receiving NDT or participating in an infant learning program. She found no statistically significant difference in favor of NDT except in the attainment of individual treatment goals. Likewise, d'Avignon, Noren, and Arman (1981) found no statistically significant differences in preventing uncomplicated cerebral palsy in 30 infants randomly assigned to experimental (physical therapy based on Vojta's [1976] or Bobaths' [1967] methods) and control groups. Finally, Palmer et al. (1988) randomly assigned 48 infants to groups receiving either 12 months of physical therapy based on NDT or 6 months of physical therapy based on NDT preceded by 6 months of infant stimulation. Using standardized measures of motor and mental quotients, they found a significant difference in favor of the group receiving infant stimulation before NDT.

In response to the mixed results of earlier studies, DeGangi, Hurley, and Linscheid (1983) addressed the development of a reliable method of measuring the short-term effects of NDT in children with cerebral palsy. They said that this type of measurement may permit researchers to control for some methodological difficulties that plagued previous studies examining the long-term effects of NDT. DeGangi et al. stated that "if there is no carryover immediately following a treatment session, the positive effects of NDT are debatable" (p. 483). Furthermore, this approach reflected Harris's research (1981), which suggested that NDT treatment effectiveness may be better assessed with individualized measures associated with therapy goals than with standardized motor assessments.

DeGangi et al. (1983) replicated a single-subject design with 4 subjects receiving NDT and nonspecific play over a 5-week period. Pretest and posttest items designed to reflect qualitative changes in movement, postural tone, and reflex activity were administered during each treatment session and videotaped for later scoring by trained psychology students. Interrater reliability was high. No significant improvements, however, were consistently observed with either NDT or play for any subject. Although the results of the study did not validate NDT, the examination of the short-term (as opposed to the long-term) effects of NDT via a single-subject design emerged as a promising approach to the evaluation of the efficacy of NDT techniques.

In the present study, we employed methods similar to those used by DeGangi et al. (1983). Our objectives were to (a) improve the methodology used to measure the short-term effectiveness of NDT, including the use of individualized therapy goals as the dependent measures, and (b) measure the immediate carryover effects of NDT and play intervention on dressing skills. We sought to address problems identified in previous research by such authors as Erhardt (1983) and Magrun, deBenabib, and Nelson (1983). These problems were insensitivity of test measures, brief length of study, and use of unskilled raters to observe videotapes of children with cerebral palsy. First, we chose to measure the changes in the quality of dressing skills in children with cerebral palsy. This evaluation was designed to reflect individualized treatment goals and to upgrade data from a nominal to an ordinal level of measurement. Whereas the raters in DeGangi et al.'s study had to identify specific categories of behaviors as present or absent (nominal scale) or had to time behaviors, the raters in the present study described behaviors on 3- to 5-point scales (ordinal scale) or counted the number of behaviors. Second, treatment and measurement in the present study occurred for 12 weeks instead of 5 weeks. Third, we used raters with experience in observing children with cerebral palsy.

Methods

SUBJECTS

A single-subject design was repeated with 2 female subjects selected from the patient population of an experienced NDT-certified occupational therapist. These subjects demonstrated appropriateness for treatment by the NDT approach and normal or near-normal intelligence with no secondary disabilities. The subjects, aged 27 and 32 months, had spastic diplegic cerebral palsy. Subject 1 had limited shoulder girdle mobility and trunk rotation; poor sitting balance; increased extensor tone in the lower extremities; and increased flexion, pronation, and ulnar deviation in the upper extremities. Subject 2 had limited trunk rotation, neglect of the right side with limited weight shift over the right side, dyspraxia, and ataxia.

PROCEDURE

Subject 1 received NDT once a week and Subject 2, twice a week, for 12 weeks. For six of these treatment sessions, each subject received 20–25 min of NDT and 20–25 min of play intervention and completed pretesting and posttesting. For all other sessions, each subject received NDT for 45 min. Subject 1 received a total of 390 min of NDT and Subject 2, 885 min, for 12 weeks. The order of the NDT and play treatments was alternated over the course of the study (see Table 1). Although we intended to administer NDT and play conditions alternately on Weeks 1–4, 6, 8, 10, and 12, we had to change our plans due to the subjects' illness and uncooperative behavior.

NDT for both subjects was administered by the same NDT-certified occupational therapist; play intervention was administered by the first author, an occupational therapy student. NDT involved specific therapeutic handling and positioning based on Bobath methods. General components of the NDT intervention included activities to normalize muscle tone and controlled movement in and out of developmental positions. A rigid program of activities for each subject was not used over the study period; rather, NDT handling, which incorporated play tasks, was used according to the child's response to therapy.

Play intervention involved spontaneous touch, encouragement to move, and interaction with the researcher. The child was encouraged to play with toys similar to those used by the NDT therapist, but the play situation was kept as child-directed as possible. The play condition did not require controlled handling in and out of developmental positions or specialized therapeutic equipment (e.g., bolsters or therapy balls) except as objects for play. Play activities included stringing beads, throwing and catching a ball, drawing on a blackboard while kneeling, and dressing a doll.

The services of the NDT-certified physical therapist offered by the center in which the study was conducted were available to both subjects during this study. In addition, the subjects' parents were allowed to continue any home treatment activities begun before the start of the study. These activities consisted largely of fine motor play and some range of motion exercises and did not involve the practice of the dressing skills used as test measures in this study. The treating therapist indicated that home treatment was not a large portion of the total treatment provided by the center, except as particular positioning eased the parents' ability to care for the child.

Data Collection

Each subject was given a pretest before each therapy session, a posttest immediately after the initial 20-min therapy session, and a posttest immediately after the second 20-min therapy session (see Table 1). For each subject, the tests encouraged

TABLE 1
TREATMENT SCHEDULE

	Subject 1		Subject 2	
Week No.	1st Treatment	2nd Treatment	1st Treatment	2nd Treatment
1	NDT	Play	—	—
2	Play	NDT	—	—
3	NDT	Play	NDT	Play
4	—	—	NDT	Play
5	—	—	—	—
6	Play	NDT	Play	NDT
7	—	—	—	—
8	NDT	Play	NDT	Play
9	—	—	—	—
10	—	—	Play	NDT
11	—	—	—	—
12	NDT	Play	NDT	Play

Note: NDT = neurodevelopmental treatment.

the performance of specific dressing skills consistent with each child's level of dressing performance and the attainment of goals set by the treating occupational therapist. For Subject 1, appropriate test items, as determined by parental interview and clinical assessment, were (a) removal of a T-shirt with one arm free of one sleeve and (b) removal of a sock. For Subject 2, appropriate test items were (a) removal of a jacket and (b) removal of a sock.

All test items were administered by the occupational therapist providing NDT in the study. The sessions were videotaped for later scoring. For all tests, the subject was placed in a cube chair (a square, plastic chair with a back and armrests) facing the camera and given 60 sec from the start of cooperative behavior to complete each task. The methods of clothing removal were identical for all tests and were appropriate for each child on the basis of that child's current motor problems. The test administrator began each task using the same verbal and physical prompts for all pretests and posttests. As needed, the test administrator offered specific physical and verbal aids to minimize the child's frustration and maximize cooperation.

TABLE 2
SAMPLE MEASUREMENT CRITERIA FOR PRETESTS AND POSTTESTS

Criterion	Procedure
Separation of lower extremity	Indicate the maximum height to which the foot wearing the sock is lifted to reach hand during removal of sock. Score 0 if foot wearing sock is not lifted from near floor. Score 1 if foot is lifted to between floor and half the height of chair seat. Score 2 if foot is lifted to between half the height of seat and level of seat. Score 3 if foot is lifted to above level of seat.
Associated reaction of lower extremity	Indicate the presence of the greatest associated reaction in the opposite lower extremity while foot wearing sock is lifted to reach hand during sock removal. Score 0 if lower extremity extension results in loss of sitting balance and falling backward. Score 1 if tonal changes result in lower extremity extension lifting foot to half the height of chair seat. Score 2 if tonal changes result in lower extremity extension lifting foot 1–2 in. off floor. Score 3 if tonal changes result in toe and foot movements (e.g. toes curl, hallux extends, foot dorsiflexes). Score 4 if lower extremity is relaxed with foot on floor.
Functional shoulder mobility	Score 0 if shirt is not removed over the head. Score 1 if shirt is removed over the head with difficulty following assistance of shirt to over face. Score 2 if shirt is removed over the head smoothly and easily following assistance of shirt to over face. Score 3 if shirt is removed over the head with difficulty without assistance. Score 4 if shirt is removed over the head smoothly and easily without assistance.
Bilateral use of upper extremity	Describe the best use of each upper extremity during sock removal. Score 0 if left upper extremity alone removes sock while right upper extremity rests in lap or is otherwise not functionally used. Score 1 if left upper extremity alone removes sock while right upper extremity performs a stabilizing function (e.g., holds onto chair). Score 2 if both upper extremities remove sock by pushing down together using same functional movement. Score 3 if both upper extremities remove sock by pushing down in alternating movements.
Hand-to-foot coordination	Indicate the number of trials to remove sock from foot. One trial is one push or pull on sock that ends with the arrest of pushing or pulling movement, the release of grasp on sock, or both.

Four sets of measurement criteria were established for each dressing skill for each subject. Measurement criteria were intended to be objective measures of expected outcomes of NDT, as expressed in functional activity. Most measurement criteria were on a 3-, 4-, or 5-point scale that yielded ordinal data. Three criteria, however, required the raters to count the number of behaviors, thus generating interval-level data. See Table 2 for examples of the main types of ordinal scales and behavior counts used. Other criteria with the same kinds of measurement procedures included measures of shoulder girdle mobility, trunk rotation and sitting balance, spontaneous use of the upper extremity, extraneous body movement, and task initiation.

Occupational therapists experienced at observing children with cerebral palsy served as the raters. The raters first received verbal and demonstrated instruction in the measurement criteria. Individual raters were requested to score at least one test item on one measurement criterion and assign a rating independently. When viewing test items on videotape, the raters did not know whether the particular test session that they were viewing was pre- or posttest, or whether the test session occurred in the earlier or later weeks. Eleven therapists participated as raters, yielding 12 sets of matched scores (pretest, post-NDT, and postplay) from each measurement criterion for each test item. The 12 sets of matched scores resulted from 6 sets of pretest, post-NDT, and postplay scores from one rater plus 6 sets of pretest, post-NDT, and postplay scores from another rater for each measurement criterion. Each rater did not score all of the measurement criteria used in this study, but rather, only a few criteria according to his or her available time. The result was that the scores from two different raters were obtained for all of the measurement criteria.

Results

Scores from two criteria were eliminated from the analysis because the videotape did not permit full viewing of the subject, which was needed to score a sufficient number of pretests and posttests. For each remaining measurement criterion, the G index of agreement was used to determine interrater reliability (Holley & Guilford, 1964). The G index yields an overall proportion of agreement based on the number of perfect matches among scores assigned by two raters. The reliability scores ranged from 0.50 to 1.00, with a mean proportion of agreement of 0.77 (see Table 3).

A comparison of improvement after NDT and after play was made for ordinal data with the Friedman analysis of variance by ranks (see Table 3). The Friedman test (Siegel, 1956) used the test statistic Fr to test the null hypothesis, which stated that median ranks of matched samples (pretest, post-NDT, and postplay) were the same. A modified Friedman test formula was used to correct for the effects of tied ranks among matched sets. Also, an analysis of variance (ANOVA) was used to compare the improvement after NDT and after play for the three measurement criteria yielding interval-level data. The ANOVA used the test statistic F to test the null hypothesis, which stated that the means of the pretest, post-NDT, and postplay groups were the same. As shown in Table 3, these analyses revealed no statistically significant differences among effects due to NDT and play for any criterion.

TABLE 3
RELIABILITY OF MEASUREMENT CRITERIA AND COMPARISON OF IMPROVEMENTS AFTER NEURODEVELOPMENTAL AND PLAY TREATMENTS*

Test Item	Measurement Criterion	G Index	Fr[a] Value	F^b Value
	Subject 1			
T-shirt	Functional shoulder mobility	0.60	0.00	—
	Shoulder abduction	0.60	1.23	—
	Sitting balance	0.70	—	0.13
	Associated reaction of lower extremity	0.90	0.18	—
Sock	Separation of lower extremity	0.90	0.20	—
	Trunk rotation	0.70	0.20	—
	Use of both upper extremities; sitting balance	0.90	2.60	—
	Associated reaction of lower extremity	1.00	0.44	—
	Subject 2			
Jacket	Task initiation	0.58	2.42	—
	Spontaneous use of right upper extremity	0.50	0.63	—
	Extraneous body movement	0.92	4.89	—
	Bilateral coordination of upper extremity	0.76	—	2.29
Sock	Bilateral use of upper extremity	0.92	1.42	—
	Hand-to-foot coordination	0.94	—	0.61

a. Fr = Friedman test (Siegel, 1956) (critical value = 6.20).
b. Critical value ($\alpha = .05$; *df* between = 2; *df* within = 30) = 3.32.
* p = not significant.

Ordinal and interval data were also analyzed for the effects of treatment order. We used a Wilcoxon rank sum test (Siegel, 1956) to compare interval scores from two periods, one in which NDT was the initial treatment condition and one in which play was the initial treatment condition. This test showed no significant differences ($p < .05$). Visual inspection of a graph of pretest and posttest scores from each measure over time was used to assess the effects of order for ordinal data. This visual inspection suggested no differences due to treatment order and revealed an increase in scores over time for measures of shoulder mobility (for Subject 1's T-shirt test) only.

Discussion

This study has expanded the existing single-system methodology for the measurement of the effect of NDT on children with cerebral palsy. Using individualized therapy objectives as outcome measures, we found that we could reliably measure qualitative changes in the dressing skills of children with cerebral palsy. We believe that the measurement of the effects of NDT on daily living skills is particularly relevant to the field of occupational therapy. Occupational therapists should be concerned that gains made in therapy are reflected in a child's increased ability to perform daily living tasks.

The overall results of this study agree with the findings of DeGangi et al. (1983). Neither study showed significant differences between the effects of NDT and play on functional activity. In consideration of the limitations of the present study, however, these results must be interpreted cautiously; they neither support nor discredit NDT as a treatment approach.

The measurement criteria used in earlier research were not sensitive enough to detect small changes occurring due to NDT. Thus, one purpose of the present study was to improve the methodology used to measure the effects of NDT. We enhanced test sensitivity by increasing the level of measurement from a nominal to an ordinal scale and by using individual treatment goals instead of standardized tests or developmental milestones. Perhaps, as recommended by DeGangi et al. (1983), future studies will use more sensitive computerized videotape analyses to measure small changes in angles of movement. Computerized analysis would enhance the level of measurement to a ratio scale, although it would require the researcher to relate resultant angles of movement to functional abilities.

A comparison of raw data from the present study with the DeGangi et al. (1983) study shows that in our study, post-NDT scores were frequently better than postplay scores, and fewer tied scores occurred. Although the number of tied scores remaining in the present study indicates that some rating scales failed to distinguish small differences between tied observations, the data suggest that an ordinal level of measurement may be more useful than categorical data for detecting changes due to NDT. Compared with the DeGangi et al. study, however, our study showed a decrease in overall reliability of measures with some ordinal scales.

Diminished interrater reliability of some measurement criteria is probably a function of insufficient rater training combined with the difficulties of making observations in small increments of ranges from videotape. Although the data analysis methods partially compensated for the raters' limited training by comparing their pretest and posttest scores individually, the differences between the raters may have obscured small effects due to NDT. Additional research is needed to determine whether human observers can detect from videotapes many of the subtle physical changes that occur due to NDT.

Another possible explanation for a lack of significant findings may relate to methods of statistical analysis. In reviewing the research on the effectiveness of NDT with pediatric clients, Ottenbacher et al. (1986) identified a small effect size of 0.31 due to NDT. This finding suggests that analysis may require many scored observations to detect statistically significant changes. Thus, we recommend replication of the present study with a larger sample or over a longer period of time.

Certainly, in view of the small effect size of NDT, an increase in the amount of NDT from the 390 or 885 min provided seems warranted. Perhaps if we had completed testing after the 45-min NDT sessions instead of after the 20–25 min sessions, we would have found differential treatment effects. Clinicians debate the length of treatment required to effect measurable changes in subjects with cerebral palsy. Treatment lengths is therefore a significant variable for future study.

A third consideration is that no significant differences were found between NDT and play because play was more like an additional treatment than like a control condition. Magrun et al. (1983) pointed out that "movement experiences in NDT and play are not mutually exclusive" (p. 848). Another limitation of the present study is that practical considerations demanded that the first author administer play intervention to both subjects. The first author may have unintentionally modeled techniques used by the NDT therapist, thus introducing bias in the play condition. Perhaps the contrast condition should involve developmental play or stimulation as provided by a non-NDT-trained discipline as well as a videotape of both play and NDT conditions for a closer comparison of experiences provided in each treatment.

Finally, like many previous studies, the present study is limited by its inability to withdraw NDT from its subjects. This study design was in part selected to eliminate a baseline or treatment withdrawal condition, thus enabling subjects to continue to receive occupational therapy through NDT. Furthermore, NDT-oriented physical therapy and home programming offered by the study center were not denied to the subjects. In this study, however, we question whether the minimal home treatment could sufficiently mask the gains observed on study measures. Additionally, the effects of physical therapy and home treatment as well as maturation were constant across all tests for each session. That is, posttests for each session were compared with regard to improvement to a pretest for that same session.

Summary

As a result of the present study, we recommend that researchers do the following:

- Continue to refine ordinal test measures, including pilot tests, to eliminate unreliable and nondiscriminating criteria.
- Use computerized videotape analysis to measure small changes in movement, as suggested by DeGangi et al. (1983).
- Train raters thoroughly in test criteria and use three ratings (versus two) for each observation to improve the analysis of reliability.
- Procure a large number of scored observations by increasing the length of the study, the number of treatments given, or both, to detect statistically significant changes.
- Provide longer NDT sessions.
- Use non-NDT-trained special educators to provide the play condition based on their own play and stimulation programs.
- Videotape both NDT and play conditions for closer comparison of treatments.
- Withhold NDT treatment provided in the home and by other members of the treatment team.

This study adds to a growing number of studies that have failed to demonstrate the efficacy of NDT. Perhaps the results of this study demonstrate the influence of the confounding factors to which this type of study is susceptible, such as an inability to withdraw NDT. More controlled research is needed to substantiate NDT as a method for the increased attainment of individual treatment goals. Future studies need to explore the relationship of these short-term outcomes and the long-term attainment of motor skills, functional gains, and deformity prevention. This study may also serve to remind occupational therapy practitioners of the value of play in the treatment of children with cerebral palsy as well as to reemphasize that treatment's primary goal is to increase functional ability.

Acknowledgments

We thank Nancy Gluek, OTR/L, and the Easter Seals Rehabilitation Center, Columbus, Ohio; the many therapists who served as raters; and Biomedical Communications Television Services, the Ohio State University, Columbus, Ohio.

References

Bayley, N. (1969). *Bayley Scales of Infant Development.* New York: Psychological Corp.

Bobath, K., & Bobath, B. (1964). The facilitation of normal postural reactions and movements in the treatment of cerebral palsy. *Physiotherapy, 50,* 3–19.

Bobath, K., & Bobath, B. (1967). The very early treatment of cerebral palsy. *Developmental Medicine and Child Neurology, 9,* 373–390.

Carlsen, P. N. (1975). Comparison of two occupational therapy approaches for treating the young cerebral-palsied child. *American Journal of Occupational Therapy, 29,* 267–272.

d'Avignon, M., Noren, L., & Arman, T. (1981). Early physiotherapy and modum Vojta or Bobath in infants with suspected neuromotor disturbance. *Neuropediatrics, 12,* 232–241.

DeGangi, G. A., Hurley, L., & Linscheid, T. R. (1983). Toward a methodology of the short-term effects of neurodevelopmental treatment. *American Journal of Occupational Therapy, 37,* 479–484.

Erhardt, R. P. (1983). Letters to the Editor—NDT study raises concerns. *American Journal of Occupational Therapy, 37,* 769.

Folio, R., & DuBose, R. F. (1974). *Peabody Developmental Motor Scales. IMRID Behavioral Sciences Monograph, 25,* Nashville, TN: George Peabody College.

Harris, S. R. (1981). Effects of neurodevelopmental therapy on motor performance of infants with Down's syndrome. *Developmental Medicine and Child Neurology, 23,* 477–483.

Holley, J. W., & Guilford, J. P. (1964). A note on the G index of agreement. *Educational and Psychological Measurement, 32,* 281–288.

Kong, E. (1966). Very early treatment of cerebral palsy. *Developmental Medicine and Child Neurology, 8* 198–202.

Magrun, W. M., deBenabib, R. M., & Nelson, C. (1983). Letters to the Editor—More criticism—Article on neurodevelopmental treatment. *American Journal of Occupational Therapy, 37,* 846–848.

Norton, Y. (1975). Neurodevelopment and sensory integration for the profoundly retarded multiply handicapped child. *American Journal of Occupational Therapy, 29,* 93–100.

Ottenbacher, K. J., Biocca, Z., DeCremer, G., Gevelinger, M., Jedlovec, K. B., & Johnson, M. B. (1986). Quantitative analysis of the effectiveness of pediatric therapy. *Physical Therapy, 66,* 1095–1101.

Palmer, F. B., Shapiro, B. K. Wachtel, R. C., Allen, M. C., Hiller, J. E., Harryman, S. E., Mosher, B. S., Meinert, C. L., & Capute, A. J. (1988). The effects of physical therapy on cerebral palsy. *New England Journal of Medicine, 318,* 803–808.

Scherzer, A. L., Mike, V., & Ilson, J. (1976). Physical therapy as a determinant of change in the cerebral palsied infant. *Pediatrics, 58,* 47–52.

Siegel, S. (1956). *Nonparametric statistics for the behavioral sciences.* New York: McGraw-Hill.

Sommerfeld, D., Fraser, B. A., Hensinger, R. N., & Beresford, C. V. (1981). Evaluation of physical therapy service for severely mentally impaired students with cerebral palsy. *Physical Therapy, 61,* 338–344.

Vojta, V. (1976). *Die cerebralen bewegungstorungen im sauglingsalter.* Stuttgart, Germany: Ferdinand Enke.

Wright, T., & Nicholson, J. (1973). Physiotherapy for the spastic child: An evaluation. *Developmental Medicine and Child Neurology, 15,* 146–163.

Illustrative Example 10–2: Questions

1. What is the purpose of the research?
2. Does the literature review provide you an understanding of how and why this investigation is important?
3. Do you think the investigation is important? Why or why not?
4. What is the theoretical or conceptual basis of the investigation?
5. How was the research conducted?
6. What type or kind of research is it and why?
7. What were the research questions or hypotheses?
8. What are the variables or phenomena under study?
9. Who were the subjects or units of study? How many were there?
10. How were the subjects or units of study obtained?
11. What information or data were collected?
12. If specific evaluation tools were used, what were they? Was information on the reliability and validity of the evaluation tools provided?
13. How was the information or data collected?
14. Will data collected be able to answer or address the research question or problem under study?
15. How was the information or data analyzed?
16. What were the criteria for interpreting the data?
17. What were the findings?
18. What were the limitations of the study? Was there a critical flaw?
19. Are the conclusions of the study warranted?
20. How can these research findings be used in occupational and physical therapy?

Illustrative Example 10–2: Answers

1. What is the purpose of the research?

The purpose of this study is to explore the effects of neurodevelopmental treatment (NDT) intervention.

2. Does the literature review provide you an understanding of how and why this investigation is important?

A rather nice literature review is provided. It clearly builds on previous research by appropriately replicating, yet adapting, previous work done by other researchers.

3. Do you think the investigation is important? Why or why not?

Again, because of the immediate clinical relevance of what was studied, this type of research is very important.

4. What is the theoretical or conceptual basis of the investigation?

The authors discussed, in the literature review, that control group investigations, that is, quasiexperimental studies, have not demonstrated the effects of NDT treatment. As an alternative research strategy to address this problem, the authors are conducting a single subject investigation.

5. How was the research conducted?

Two single subject research designs were used with two subjects. Subject 1 had NDT treatment one time per week for 12 weeks. Subject 2 had NDT treatment two times per week for 12 weeks. For 6 of the 12 sessions, subjects had approximately 25 minutes of NDT and approximately 25 minutes of play, and had testing before and after the session. For the other sessions, each subject had NDT for 45 minutes.

6. What type or kind of research is it and why?

The authors report this be to single subject research. The repeated use of measurement over time to assess the effects of intervention is a hallmark of single subject research and is what is used in this investigation.

7. *What were the research questions or hypotheses?*

What is the effect of NDT and play on functional performance in subjects diagnosed with cerebral palsy?

8. *What were the variables or phenomenon under study?*

The independent variables were play intervention or NDT intervention. The dependent variable was dressing skills measured by a protocol developed for use in this investigation.

9. *Who were the subjects or units of study? How many were there?*

Two female subjects, aged 27 and 32 months, were selected from a population of subjects treated by an NDT-trained therapist. There were some criteria for inclusion in the study, that is, normal intelligence. These subjects were obtained by purposive sampling.

10. *How were subjects or units of study obtained?*

Selected from treatment load of a therapist.

11. *What information or data were collected?*

Scores on the before-and-after measurements.

12. *If specific evaluation tools were used, what were they? Was information on the reliability and validity of the evaluation tools provided?*

A rather complex procedure for measurement of dressing was developed for each subject (p. 142). Subjects were videotaped and then analyzed. Agreement among therapists was determined.

13. *How was the information or data collected?*

Subjects were tested before and after every treatment session. These data were analyzed.

14. *Will data collected be able to answer or address the research question or problem under study?*

Yes, except for measurement error inherent in the measurement protocol.

15. *How was the information or data analyzed?*

A variety of statistical analyses were done. Subjects data were aggregated or analyzed together.

16. *What were the criteria for interpreting the data?*

We can assume that the $p = .05$ level was used.

17. *What were the findings?*

$p < .05$ is reported for the comparison of NDT versus play order effects. Authors suggest that no significant differences were found. In fact, $p < .05$ is a significant finding because it is less than chance. Thus, either the article has a typographical error or the authors were in error. NDT was not found to be any more or any less effective than play intervention.

18. *What were the limitations of the study? Was there a critical flaw?*

Potential examiner bias (threat to internal validity) was present as the test administrator was the treatment provider. But this was an unfunded study—so, what choices did the investigator have? The authors suggest that measurement limitations influenced the results (that measurement error contributed to lack of significant findings; see discussion of measurement error in chapter 7).

19. *Are the conclusions of the study warranted?*

With recognition of the limitation of the study, yes.

20. *How can these research findings be used in occupational and physical therapy?*

The authors suggest future research to: (a) refine testing procedures, (b) establish better interrater reliability with measurement protocol, and (c) provide longer duration NDT treatment. Thus, this research can be used as a foundation for replication of the study.

Criticism of Single Subject Research

Take a moment and try to recall the threats to internal and external validity that were discussed in chapter 9. Then think about how such threats to validity might affect single subject research. For each of the following, think about how the research findings could be compromised:

- repeated measures on a subject using the same method of measurement
- Hawthorne effect
- history
- maturation
- generalizability.

Let us discuss each finding.

Repeated measures can produce testing effects where the subject reacts to the testing itself—perhaps by getting so familiar with the testing as to render it invalid. Such testing effects can improve or decrease performance. These effects are lessened by using unobtrusive measures for the dependent variable.

The Hawthorne effect suggests that by simply studying something one changes its very nature. The effects caused by treatment in single subject research, therefore, may be due to the Hawthorne effect. This threat to validity is minimized by repeated baseline and intervention measures, particularly with baseline measures after removal of the intervention.

History and maturation are two additional threats to validity that are common criticisms of single subject research. Again, however, the effects of history and maturation can be minimized by repeated data collection during baseline and intervention phases.

Probably the largest criticism of single subject research centers on its generalizability (Hacker, 1980). Recall that generalizability refers to the ability to apply the study findings to the total population. In single subject research the findings can be applied to theory or to other subjects like the one in the study. The findings cannot be broadly applied across populations.

The strongest counterargument to criticisms of single subject research, however, is that by replication of single subject studies one achieves "truth." That is, by repeatedly demonstrating the desired effect again and again with different subjects, one is demonstrating the effect is replicable over time and conditions. This is very powerful information that cannot easily be refuted. Thus, the goal of single subject research is to repeat studies, and by virtue of replication of findings, establish the effects of the intervention.

This chapter presented you with some of the fundamental concepts of single subject research. In the next chapter, I will discuss research that is not experimentally based, qualitative research.

References

Best, J. W., & Kahn, J. V. (1989). *Research in education.* Englewood Cliffs, NJ: Prentice-Hall.

DeGangi, G. A., Hurley, L., & Linscheid, T. R. (1983). Toward a methodology of the short-term effects of neurodevelopmental treatment. *American Journal of Occupational Therapy, 37,* 479–484.

Edwards, S. J., & Yuen, H. K. (1989). Case report: An intervention program for a fraternal twin with Down's syndrome. *American Journal of Occupational Therapy, 44,* 454–458.

Gillete, N. P. (1982). A database for occupational therapy: Documentation through research. *American Journal of Occupational Therapy, 36,* 499–501.

Hacker, B. (1980). Single subject research in occupational therapy. Part One. *American Journal of Occupational Therapy, 34,* 103–108.

Kazdin, A. E. (1982). *Single subject research design: Methods for clinical and applied settings.* New York: Oxford University Press.

Levin, J. R., Marascuilo, L. A., & Hubert, L. J. (1978). Nonparametric randomization tests. In T. R. Kratochwill (Ed.), *Single subject research: Strategies for evaluating change* (pp. 167–196). New York: Academic Press.

Lilly, L. A., & Powell, N. J. (1990). Measuring the effects of neurodevelopmental treatment on the daily living skills of 2 children with cerebral palsy. *American Journal of Occupational Therapy, 44,* 139–145.

Madsen, P. S., & Conte, J. R. (1980). Single subject research in occupational therapy: A case illustration. *American Journal of Occupational Therapy, 34,* 263–267.

McClure, P. W., & Flowers, K. R. (1992). Case Report: Treatment of limited shoulder motion using an elevation splint. *Physical Therapy, 72(1),* 57–62.

Ottenbacher, K. J. (1986). *Evaluating clinical change: Strategies for evaluating change.* New York: Academic Press.

Ottenbacher, K. J. (1986). *Evaluating clinical change: Strategies for occupational and physical therapists.* Baltimore: Williams & Wilkins.

Piaget, J. (1926). *The language and thought of the child.* London: Kegan Paul.

Skinner, B. F. (1953). *Science and human behavior.* New York: MacMillan.

Yin, R. K. (1984). *Case study research: Design and methods.* Newbury Park, CA: Sage.

Recommended Readings

Kazdin, A. E. (1982). *Single subject research designs: Methods for clinical and applied settings.* New York: Oxford University Press.

Kratochwill, T. R. (1978). *Single subject research: Strategies for evaluating change.* New York: Academic Press.

Ottenbacher, K. J. (1986). *Evaluating clinical change: Strategies for occupational and physical therapy.* Baltimore: Williams & Wilkins.

Tracey, T. J. (1983). Single case research: An added tool for counselors and supervisors. *Counselor Education and Supervision, 22 (3),* 185–197.

Learning Activities

1. Think of a particular client with whom you have worked. Consider ways to write up a clinical case study based on your experiences.
2. Think of another client. How would you plan for a single subject research investigation with that client? What would be the independent variable? What would be the dependent variable, and how would it be measured?
3. Contrast quasiexperimental research and single subject research.
4. Contrast clinical case study with single subject research.

CHAPTER 11

Qualitative Research

KEY WORDS

Aggregating
Comparing
Contrasting
Data verification
Ethnographic research
History
Interpretive research
Maturation
Mortality
Observer effects
Ordering
Participant observation
Perceiving
Phenomenological research
Qualitative research
Regression
Reliability
Research Strategies
Rigor
Selection
Speculating
Spurious Conclusions
Validity

Have you ever read a piece of research that you felt was lacking in its portrayal of a client's experience? Have you ever felt that a research article was so reductionistic, that is, limited in scope, that it missed the big picture regarding how the client felt and was challenged?

If so, you are like many current researchers in occupational and physical therapy, as well as other fields, who feel that the quantitative emphasis in research prevents capturing the true meaning of what our clients feel, do, and think. In fact, qualitative research may be termed

interpretative research (Smith, 1988). There is considerable ongoing debate in occupational therapy as well as education and other fields regarding the usefulness of traditional, quantitatively oriented research to address research needs as we go into the future (Short-Debroff, 1994). At its worst, this argument is a battle between the number crunchers and the storytellers (Smith, 1988). There is even a growing recognition of fundamental differences in thought processes underpinning quantitative and qualitative approaches that can be applied beyond research to learning and teaching (Stiley, 1988).

Qualitative Research Defined

Qualitative research "seeks to gain insight through discovering meanings attached to phenomenon" (Burns & Grove, 1987, p. 75). Unlike quantitative research, which is directed toward understanding by determining cause and effect, qualitative research attempts to enhance understanding by comprehending a phenomenon as a whole in its natural setting (Burns & Grove, 1987). The hallmark of qualitative research is the use of words instead of numbers as units of analysis. This may sound simplistic, but the implications of this difference are truly astounding. Qualitative research consists of many approaches that, as methodologies, are established, yet still evolving. The most common of these are phenomenological and ethnographic.

PHENOMENOLOGICAL QUALITATIVE RESEARCH

Phenomenological research captures and describes subjects' experiences "as they are lived" (Burns & Grove, 1987, p. 81). In this type of research the investigator makes the assumption that there is no single reality, but there are multiple realities depending on whose viewpoint is being illustrated. For example, a plan of research for phenomenological research could address

1. what is to be explored
2. the sources or subjects
3. collecting data from the subjects
4. analyzing and interpreting the data.

Data could be collected using observation or interview of subjects. Data analysis could consist of classification and rank ordering, using panels of experts to confirm such categorizations.

ETHNOGRAPHIC QUALITATIVE RESEARCH

Ethnographic research is "analytic descriptions of intact cultural scenes or groups" (Goetz & LeCompte, 1985, p. 2.) Ethnographic research is based on solid research design and methods. Typically, the investigator will immerse him or herself in the culture for extended periods of time. **Participant observation** is a term associated with this research strategy: it implies that the investigator becomes a *participant* in the cultural group under *observation*—hence participant (one who participates) observation (one who observes).

This methodology has been developed primarily in anthropology and has been adopted in other disciplines such as education. A typical ethnographic research design will present

1. research questions and focus of the investigation
2. how the steps of the investigation will be conducted
3. who will be participants for observations, and the context or setting of the observations
4. researcher's experience conducting such a study
5. methods of data collection
6. methods of data analysis and data interpretation
7. presentation of findings.

What typically happens in qualitative research is that the steps of data collection, data analysis, and data interpretation are not distinct. Rather, data interpretation is ongoing and occurs during data collection and data analysis. This blending is in marked contrast to quantitative research, which has distinct steps in data collection, data analysis, and data interpretation.

OTHER QUALITATIVE RESEARCH STRATEGIES

Two other forms of qualitative research strategies are focus groups and interviewing. Focus groups are discussion groups of five to seven people with common backgrounds who are led by a facilitator to explore feelings, attitudes, and beliefs about a topic presented by the group leader (Krueger, 1988). Focus groups are based on a carefully planned and pilot-tested approach to the discussion and are not informal, ad hoc meetings. Typical questions posed in focus groups are (Krueger, 1988)

- What did you think about...?
- How did you feel about...?
- What did you like?

In-depth interviewing is fairly self-explanatory. It is a means to obtain in-depth data about feelings, beliefs, and attitudes about a topic of interest from designated individuals. The most effective interview procedure, like that of focus groups, evolves from pilot-tested protocols, not "quick and dirty" questionnaires.

Data Analysis and Interpretation in Qualitative Research

Quantitative research has many statistical techniques for data analysis. Because words cannot be subjected to statistical analysis like numbers, alternative methods of analyzing the data are used in qualitative research. The key method of analysis in qualitative research is theorizing, a "generic mode of thinking" (Goetz & LeCompte, 1985, p. 165). Theorizing consists of the following intellectual functions:

1. **Perceiving** is identifying the units of analysis for study that are embedded within the bulk of the data obtained. It is the process of perceiving naturally occurring events or segmentation of data in some meaningful or orderly manner.
2. **Comparing** is done after the units of analysis have been identified. It is determining what is similar across units.
3. **Contrasting** occurs after units of analysis have been identified; the researcher contrasts to determine what is different across units.
4. **Aggregating** is the process of grouping units of analysis into categories or groups, with accompanying delineation of what is central within and what is different from other groups or categories.
5. **Ordering** establishes relationship.
6. In **speculating** or hypothesizing, the researcher(s) makes inferences, hunches, or guesses about variables of interest, which are generated from and tested within data collected.

The functions described here are analogous to the statistical procedures used for data analysis in quantitative research; these qualitative data analysis techniques are, however, conducted throughout the research process, not just at the end of the investigation. The definitions just given are based on the work of Goetz and LeCompte (1985) as used in ethnographic research, but the processes for all other types of qualitative research are the same.

Figure 11–1 contains a data analysis process used in qualitative research; it is based, in part, on the work of Miles and Huberman (1984) and LeCompte and Goetz.

FIGURE 11–1. DATA ANALYSIS, INTERPRETATION, AND VERIFICATION IN QUALITATIVE RESEARCH

Data Analysis

- Data reduction using summary forms (perceiving)
- Identification of patterns and themes (comparing and contrasting)
- Counts of patterns and themes (as appropriate)
- Matrix rating of importance of identified patterns and themes
- Matrix of clustering by group of patterns and themes

Data Interpretation

- Inductive reasoning from the particular to the general
- Reflective remarks
- Developing propositions or theoretical coherence
- Matrix of explanatory effects

Data Verification

- Estimate representativeness
- Triangulation
- Check meaning of outlier
- Replication
- Getting feedback from informants
- Validity check

Data Interpretation (repeat)

Don't worry if you do not understand every part of Figure 11–1. What is important is that you realize that qualitative research is not just a bunch of loose observations. In fact, there is a rigorous research strategy with proven techniques underpinning the conducting of any such research.

Rigor, Reliability, and Validity in Qualitative Research

Just as we are concerned with issues of rigor or control over research design in quantitative research, we are concerned about **rigor** in qualitative research. Related concepts of **reliability** and **validity** of the research are also important in qualitative research.

Rigor is beginning to be actively addressed in the qualitative research literature. In my mind, however, rigor is the intensity, quality, and honesty with which the qualitative research investigator confronts his or her own feelings, attitudes, and perceptions. For only by exploring one's own feelings can a researcher identify if and how they differ from the subjects. And it is the subject's reality that is of interest in the study. Rigor may also refer to the quality and integrity with which the research is implemented.

Reliability[1] addresses the ability of others to replicate the same findings under the same con-

1. Many of the concepts on reliability and validity presented here are based on the work of Goetz and LeCompte (1985).

ditions of study, or, consistency (Kreftig, 1991). In qualitative approaches generally, and ethnography specifically, the methods of data analysis and interpretation should be presented in such a manner that others could replicate them. This, in fact, is no different from the goal of quantitatively oriented research. Another technique to build reliability into an investigation is the use of peer examination. Basically, this is using one's colleagues or peers either on the site or elsewhere to affirm descriptions or consultations based on fieldwork observation, with an eye to discrepancies and differences to be resolved.

Validity concerns the truth or accuracy of a study's findings. One way to look at internal validity in this type of research is to consider whether the concepts presented by the research investigator have the same or similar meaning to the subjects as they do to the investigator. It is the ability of the investigator to truly understand the phenomenon under study (Kreftig, 1991, p. 215). Some of the threats to internal validity identified by Campbell and Stanley (1979)—history and maturation, observer effects, selection and regression, mortality, and spurious conclusions—also apply here.

1. **History** and **maturation**. The qualitative researcher simply assumes that these processes will affect the subjects. And the qualitative researcher must ascertain which processes or events are thereby affected and how.
2. **Observer effects**. Sufficient time in the field is thought to mitigate against this threat to internal validity of qualitative research. The difficult question is, how much time is enough?
3. **Selection** and **regression**. Who and what are observed is critical for the findings in qualitative research. This dilemma is not so difficult when the phenomenon under investigation is not too large. But when large groups of subjects or complex situations are to be observed, problems of selection and regression arise. It is then necessary to delineate an "adequate inventory of subgroups, factions, events and social scenes in the field" (Goetz & LeCompte, 1985, p. 226), and to logically ascertain the representativeness of what was observed to the master overall inventory.
4. **Mortality**. Loss of subjects in the studied phenomenon is part of the study. That is why it is important to have an adequate understanding of the situation at the start, that is, the baseline of the study, to look at mortality as the qualitative study unfolds.
5. **Spurious conclusions**. Logically eliminating rival explanations of the results as part of the interpretative process, in part, prevents spurious conclusions.

The most common mechanism of overall validity considerations is triangulation. *Triangulation* is the strategy of using multiple data sources to study the same phenomenon. If the data from the sources agree, the validity of the findings is enhanced (Mathison, 1988). For example, say that after the next continuing education event you attend, the workshop review forms are compared with comments recorded during a break and with perceptions of the workshop presenters; three data sources would be triangulated. If all three sources revealed fabulous reviews on the workshop, the confidence in the findings, or their validity, would be great.

Qualitative Research Versus Quantitative Research

There are three main criteria for determining qualitative research compared to quantitative research. Know, however, that some research may be combinations thereof. The three questions to use in determining the nature of the research are presented in Figure 11–2 (PSI, 1989). This easy-to-use checklist can be used for preliminary determination of the approach of a research investigation—quantitative or qualitative.

FIGURE 11–2. QUESTIONS TO DETERMINE RESEARCH APPROACH

1. What is the nature of the data?

Is it objective, that is, measured in a way to reduce bias of the examiner? (quantitative) [ ]

Is it subjective, that is, does it reveal the experience of the observer? (qualitative) [ ]

2. What is the sample?

Is it based on groups of subjects used to determine general principles or laws? (*nomothetic*—quantitative) [ ]

Is it based on single cases purposefully chosen to increase understanding of individuals or events? (*ideographic*—qualitative) [ ]

3. What is the data analysis technique?

Is it based on counts and numbers? (quantitative) [ ]

Is it based on a word description of the event, process, or individual? (qualitative) [ ]

4. What is the objective?

Truth? (quantitative) [ ]

Understanding? (qualitative) [ ]

Note: Terms in parentheses define type of research.

Qualitative Research in Occupational and Physical Therapy

There is an increasing focus on and use of qualitative research methodology in occupational and physical therapy research. The work of Kielhofner (1982a, 1982b) is predicated on this approach. Similarly, the work of the faculty at the University of Southern California, and the move toward occupation science is, in part, based on increased use of qualitative strategies (Carlson & Clark, 1991). Currently, less focus on quantitative approaches is apparent in the physical therapy literature. Let us now look at some of the qualitatively oriented research found in the literature.

Application

Let's try to apply our ability to recognize the qualitative approach to research. Read the following example and answer the interpretation questions provided. Compare your answers with the answers provided after the interpretation section.

Reprinted from *Occupational Therapy Journal of Research,* Vol. 11, Number 4, July/August, 1991, pp. 195–211. Used with permission.

ILLUSTRATIVE EXAMPLE 11–1

Making a Difference: Occupational Therapy in the Public Schools

Anita N. Niehues, Anita C. Bundy,
Cheryl F. Mattingly, Mary C. Lawlor

Key words: pediatrics • school system practice • qualitative research methods

Occupational therapists (OTs) have been practicing in the public school system for many years and their numbers continue to increase (American Occupational Therapy Association, 1985). Although their services have been well accepted by educational personnel and parents, they have not been well understood (Bundy, Lawlor, Kielhofner, & Knecht, 1989; Royeen, 1986).

Public Law 94–142 (Education for All Handicapped Children Act of 1975), "while rejecting a medical model of disability, recognized that...some students needed more than educational services alone to be successful in school" (Gartner & Lipsky, 1987, p. 370). Since this law designated occupational therapy as a service related to the education of handicapped children, OTs have faced the need to develop educationally related services and strategies and interventions that enable students to be successful in school (American Occupational Therapy Association, 1989). Until recently, however, these same OTs had been trained primarily within theoretical and practical frameworks that embraced the medical model of disability (Hopkins, 1988; Kielhofner & Miyake, 1983), which emphasizes the application of direct treatment techniques to alleviate specific symptoms or problems of individual patients. As they have endeavored to meet the needs of students and team members in the practice environment of the public schools, OTs often have faced the "uncertainty, uniqueness, and value conflict" of an "indeterminant zone" of professional practice (Schon, 1987, p. 6).

It takes time to become situated (Benner & Wrubel, 1989) in a new practice setting, that is, to come to know the cultural values, needs, and expectations of unfamiliar social systems, and also to become known within those systems. As OTs have struggled to find their places on special educational teams, they have necessarily begun to adjust their own habits, skills, and practices to fit into this relatively new practice setting of the public schools.

Although OTs have practiced in schools for more than 15 years, only two major studies have explored the roles of OTs and the services they provide (Bundy et al., 1989; Gilfoyle & Hays, 1979). Thus, little actually is known about the ways in which therapists provide services in schools. In the two major national studies that have been conducted, researchers have explored occupational therapy practice in public schools through mailed surveys using primarily close-ended questions with predetermined response choices. Both groups of investigators found that the most important services OTs provided in schools are directed toward improving students' motor skills and skills in performing activities of daily living.

As Royeen (1986) observed, the results of the Gilfoyle and Hays study in 1979 suggested that the services of OTs in schools differ very little from those provided by therapists who practice in medical settings. Results from the Bundy et al. (1989) study also support this observation. While Ottenbacher (1982) stated that therapists are "striving to develop alternatives to the traditional medical model" of practice (p. 82), the OT literature has not clearly depicted these alternative models. The need to clearly describe our services in public schools is crucial; Royeen cautioned that, unless OTs define our services in more educationally related terms, there may be a decrease in the demand for occupational therapy services in school settings.

Respondents to the surveys by Bundy et al. (1989) and Gilfoyle and Hays (1979) were constrained in their answers by the format used in the surveys. That is, in these written surveys, respondents were required to answer the questions asked by choosing from a limited set of predetermined responses, and many of these responses were phrased in what Coles (1989) described as "medical shorthand." This medical shorthand, which allows therapists to communicate quickly with one another, may have limited the way in which respondents were able to describe their practice in school settings.

Replies to the open-ended questions included in the Bundy et al. (1989) study support this suggestion. When OTs working in schools were allowed to use their *own* words to provide opinions about therapy, the nature of their responses changed considerably. In response to the open-ended questions included in the study, therapists described their practice in ways readily applicable to the educational system as they shared their opinions about the successes, as well as the problems, associated with their practice in schools. It appears, then, that there may be knowledge to be gained about the practice of occupational therapy in public schools that cannot be elicited easily through close-ended survey questions.

Benner (1984) believed that much knowledge could be gained by interviewing expert clinicians and analyzing their narrative accounts of their practice. Mattingly (1989) also focused on the narratives of skilled practitioners. She found that these stories provided access to more than just a description of *what* therapists did; they also allowed therapists to explain *how* an event in their practice related to their own actions in that situation. In the language of story, practitioners described their clinical reasoning process. Both Benner and Mattingly used qualitative research methodology (Bogdan & Taylor, 1984; Glaser & Strauss, 1967; Mattingly, in press; Patton, 1990; Rowles, 1988; Schatzman & Strauss, 1973) to explore the nature of practice of skilled health care professionals. Their data were rich in description. As Kielhofner (1982) noted:

> The qualitative research tradition appreciates that the social behavior of persons depends on their practical everyday experiences within the social system. Data collection and analytic procedures of this tradition aim to explore and discover that world as experienced by others.

> Qualitative research seeks to understand and portray the social life of a particular group within its own physical, social and cultural context (pp. 68-69).

Therefore, in the study described here, in which we set out to discover how occupational therapists practicing in schools viewed their roles and services, we chose to employ qualitative methodology. In open-ended and in-depth interviews, a small sample of experienced school therapists reflected on their own practices and shared accounts of particular situations in which they believed they had been particularly successful. Mattingly (in press) suggested the value of narratives in research when she said:

> Stories not only give meaningful form to experiences we have already lived through. They also provide us a forward glance, helping us anticipate meaningful shapes for situations even before we enter them, allowing us to envision endings from the very beginning (p. 3).

The purpose of this study was to explore the professional knowledge that has accrued over time within the actual practice of expert school system occupational therapists. Two questions have guided this exploratory study: (1) How do expert occupational therapists practicing in public schools describe successful practice in this setting? and (2) What can be learned about educationally related occupational therapy services through experts' reflections on situations when they felt particularly successful with students in public schools?

Methodology

SUBJECTS

The subjects for this study included five OTs who had practiced for more than 5 years in public schools. All had been identified as expert practitioners by two or more peers, and agreed voluntarily to participate in the study. Although these therapists shared the common experience of practice in school settings, their previous professional experiences and personal characteristics varied significantly in several ways. The therapists ranged in age from 35 to almost 50 years. Their previous clinical experiences included working in acute care and rehabilitation hospitals; private, non-profit, outpatient centers; specialized units in large university hospitals; and large state institutions for the developmentally disabled. In addition, the diagnostic categories, age groups, and educational placement of the students with whom they worked and whose stories they shared varied considerably. They varied from severely handicapped preschool students to older, more mildly involved learning disabled students placed in self-contained special education programs, and also included students who attended regular education classes and received only resource assistance from special education personnel.

PROCEDURES

Each of the five expert OTs participated in an open-ended interview 1 to 2 hours long and conducted by the principal investigator at a location convenient to and selected by the participant. Before the interviews, the principal investigator reviewed methods of face-to-face interviewing (Glaser & Strauss, 1967; Patton, 1990; Schatzman & Strauss, 1973) and received feedback regarding her interviewing technique and her use and monitoring of probes, to reduce the risk of bias during data collection. The following verbal instructions were given to each participant about 1 week before the interviews:

> Please think of a time when you have been practicing in the school system and you felt that your intervention made a difference in student outcomes—a time when you felt that your interventions as an occupational therapist really made a difference for a student. Please tell me the story of this incident. Include a detailed description of the incident, the context of the incident, your concerns, thoughts, and feelings about the situation, and why you think this incident stood out in your memory as critical in your practice.

When an interview was conducted, the above instructions were reiterated. Information regarding issues of confidentiality and use of the data collected also was shared. All interviews were audiotaped in their entirety and were transcribed for narrative review. One interview was not completed in one session; a follow-up interview was scheduled and completed at the convenience of the therapist.

DATA ANALYSIS METHODS

The rigor, or trustworthiness, of this qualitative study was addressed by employing practical strategies to ensure the credibility and dependability of the data collected, analyzed, and reported. Two types of triangulation were employed: (a) triangulation of investigators, including the use of two expert occupational therapists who independently analyzed the narratives for thematic content and also shared in the process of developing the key themes, and (b) theoretical triangulation, including the use of ideas from diverse theoretical perspectives to contribute to the conceptual interpretation of the phenomenon under study (Guba, 1981; Knafl & Breitmayer, 1989; Krefting, in press; Lincoln & Guba, 1985).

The principal investigator acknowledged and assessed the influence of her own background as a therapist who had practiced in public schools on the gathering and analysis of the narrative data. This process of reflexive analysis included acknowledging the fact that the principal investigator was part of the research process (Miles & Huberman, 1984; Ruby, 1980). Constant comparative analysis (Glaser & Strauss, 1967) was used to analyze thematic content of the data, and data were analyzed in a three-stage process.

Initially, narratives were analyzed individually to identify the central themes within each narrative; generally, between five and eight themes emerged from each. Themes were developed in three ways: (a) narratively, by titling the stories, dividing them into chapters, and identifying the main players in each story; (b) thematically, by identifying the important meanings each therapist attached to various aspects of her practice story; and (c) symbolically, by identifying phrases and terms that seemed to be emotionally laden or were expressed repeatedly by the therapist, suggesting their importance to the narrator.

After each narrative was analyzed individually, they were compared with one another, successively, until basic commonalities and discrepancies across all five narratives were identified and categorized. Patterns began to emerge as themes were sorted, compiled, reorganized, and recategorized.

The final step of analysis included interpretation of these data in light of (a) theoretical perspectives gathered from review of literature in the following areas: qualitative methodology, clinical reasoning, medical anthropology, and occupational therapy school practice, and (b) the practical perspectives researchers had gained during practice in public school systems.

Results and Discussion

Although these expert therapists were requested to share one story from their practice, they often shared several stories. They accentuated their stories of success by sharing threads of other stories from their practice. These served as background and contrast for the stories of the times when the OTs felt they had made a difference for particular students. Additionally, each therapist spontaneously shared some of her own perspectives on the provision of educationally related occupational therapy services in public schools.

While these therapists had very different experiences with a wide variety of special students, and although many more than five stories actually were shared, three pervasive common themes emerged from the analysis of the narrative data. One theme illustrated the prelude to a unique, collaborative intervention process that became visible within the therapists' actions and resulted in an enhanced fit between difficult or puzzling students and their educational environments. We titled this theme "reframing" because a key element of each of these therapists' stories was a description of helping other team members to view a student in a new or different way; these new frames enabled team members to develop more effective strategies for teaching or parenting the student.

A second theme that emerged from the data analysis described therapists' need to become situated (Benner & Wrubel, 1989) within particular special education programs and with particular team members, students, and families to develop the most effective interventions. Interestingly, therapists often described their need for situatedness by offering glimpses of untold stories. That is, within the context of their success stories, they also made brief references to other times in their practice when situations had been different, when they had felt uncomfortable in some way and, therefore, had not been able to intervene as successfully as they would have liked. Because the therapists expressed the need for situatedness by contrasting their success stories with other times when their intervention had not been as successful, we titled this theme "situatedness and untold stories."

A third powerful theme concerned the ambivalence and paradox that therapists have felt as they have entered practice in this setting and attempted both explicitly, and more often implicitly, to determine for themselves what counts as real therapy in this setting. This theme appeared in the data in a somewhat different fashion than did the other themes; it was constructed by noticing the feelings therapists expressed, the questions they asked themselves, and the qualifiers they used, as they reflected on both successful and discouraging times in practice. Accordingly, we have titled this theme "ambivalence and paradox."

REFRAMING

"Reframing" (Schon, 1979, 1987) emerged as a service that expert OTs have learned to provide in their practice in public schools. As these OTs used their professional experience to (a) understand the reasons that led to the discrepancies between students' performances in school and the expectations held for those students by others, and (b) interpret these students' behaviors for other members of the team in new or different ways, they essentially reframed the students' behaviors and the problems they were having in school. Mattingly (in press) discussed reframing as a process of coming to see a person or a situation in a new way because one has changed the framework, or lens, through which one views that person or situation. By reframing students' behaviors, the OTs enabled team members to view the students in more positive ways and gave them a basis for developing new and more effective strategies for teaching or parenting the students.

Therapists did not necessarily approach situations intending to frame students' problems differently for team members nor were they consciously aware of using such a process. As therapists developed, and carried out, individualized interventions with challenging students and collaborated with parents and other team members, their actions provided the structure through which this implicit process of reframing became visible.

The process of reframing, although clearly visible within therapists' practice stories, did not follow a sequential and orderly pattern that was employed predictably in every school practice situation. That is, reframing was sometimes a part of evaluation and sometimes a result of intervention.

In one story, a process of reframing was initiated when a therapist shared her assessment information about a student with team members. When Sharon, an occupational therapist, intervened with Mike, a student placed in a self-contained learning disabilities classroom, she listened first to what the teachers had to say about him and then supplemented that information with other assessments to get a sense for what Mike might need from occupational therapy. Sharon included functional and standardized assessments as well as an assessment of Mike's learning environment (both the physical layout and human expectations and interactions).

Sharon described Mike's teachers as "just totally frustrated" with him because "nothing they had tried with him worked." She described Mike as a student who was so motorically involved that he would easily have fit in a program for the physically handicapped. She thought that the teachers knew that Mike's problems "were out of their realm" when they asked her to "PLEASE DO ANYTHING YOU CAN WITH THIS STUDENT!"

Sharon began to reframe Mike's behaviors for these teachers as she shared the results of her assessments with them. When she explained that although Mike was

11 years old his visual-motor skills were more like those of a kindergartner, the teachers said, "Oh! No wonder he can't write!" Based on this information, they then were able to modify their expectations for him and reduce the amount of his written work. Over time, and with Sharon's help, the teachers made other classroom modifications that enabled Mike to meet the demands of the classroom more efficiently and comfortably.

Laurie, another expert occupational therapist, told a story about Justin, a severely handicapped preschooler, who Laurie first observed as "laying on the floor, self-stimming between two fluorescent lights." Laurie simply sat Justin up and showed the team how, with more upright and functional positioning, structure, and more appropriate expectations for his behavior and functional performance, Justin could participate much more effectively in school and his family life. In a very short period of time, with relatively simple therapeutic modifications, this severely handicapped preschooler learned to feed himself, to scribble with a crayon, and to participate in other preschool activities.

Laurie's intervention resulted in a reframing of Justin's behavior for team members. By demonstrating Justin's potential to team members, through positioning him and trying new activities with him, Laurie served as a catalyst for new interventions by other team members. She enabled them to see more potential in Justin and to raise their expectations for his functional performance in school and at home. As a result of occupational therapy intervention, this student was able to fit into his learning situation more easily and to benefit more from his special education program.

Dawn, a third therapist, served as an advocate for a young student who had been mislabeled as having cerebral palsy. The team, including Jeremy's parents, felt that Jeremy just wasn't trying hard enough to walk. Dawn noticed, as she was treating him, that Jeremy's functional performance was deteriorating in many areas; she recognized that this should not be happening if, in fact, Jeremy had cerebral palsy. Dawn encouraged Jeremy's parents to pursue further medical testing and, when these tests confirmed a diagnosis of a degenerative neuromuscular disease, she interpreted the meaning of this diagnosis for the team, including Jeremy's parents. Dawn's medical background enabled her to intervene with Jeremy by advocating for him and guiding and supporting his parents and the other members of his team as they developed an understanding for the impact that this new diagnosis would have on Jeremy's abilities and needs. This reframing resulted in Jeremy's parents and teachers developing more appropriate expectations for his performance. In short, they did not accuse him of not trying hard enough and began to adapt the demands on him in such a way that he could meet their expectations. They did not give up on him, they merely viewed his performance through new lenses. Through her reframing of Jeremy's problems, Dawn was able to enhance the fit between this student and his learning environment.

Some special education students, like Mike, Justin, and Jeremy, do not fit easily into the educational system. A mismatch between a student and his or her educational environment (Royeen & Marsh, 1988) often is the impetus for team members to seek the services of OTs. The practice stories of these therapists illustrated ways in which they were able to help team members make sense of students' performance discrepancies and to assist teachers or other team members to adjust their expectations to improve the student-environment fit.

Throughout the stories of these expert school system OTs, there is a sense that an explanatory model of practice is emerging (Good & Good, 1981; Kleinman, 1988). Therapists sought to understand, and to help others to understand, the nature of students' performance discrepancies. Therapists' stories illustrated the power and diversity of the process of reframing. Simply naming students' problems differently, and reframing them for others within particular educational environments, often made substantial differences for the students.

Sometimes reframing seemed to occur almost accidentally as a result of simple therapeutic interventions. Sometimes reframing occurred in preparation for such consultative services as suggesting environmental adaptations, alternative teaching strategies, or adaptive equipment. Often dramatic changes occurred as therapists reframed students' behavior for team members by serving as student advocates.

These stories, told by expert therapists, demonstrated that reframing students' behavior and improving the fit between students and their educational environments is neither easy nor straightforward. It requires considerable energy and expertise. When it can be accomplished, it has a powerful effect on the life of a student and, seemingly, on the lives of the many people surrounding him or her.

SITUATEDNESS AND UNTOLD STORIES

Therapists contrasted their successes against a background of "other times." Therapists' "untold" stories revealed dark threads of regret, of feeling both personally and professionally *unknown,* and of being perceived as a disruption to, rather than a facilitator of, the educational process. Therapists noted times when routine strategies had not worked well, when it had not been possible to develop collaborative relationships with other team members, and times when they felt "stuck."

Perhaps, because they had been asked to relate a success story, therapists alluded only briefly to these times in practice when things went wrong. However, by providing these comments about difficult or unsuccessful situations within their practices, therapists creatively wove a background that provided a sharp contrast for these stories of success. These untold stories seemed to reflect some of the stresses and feelings surrounding therapists' attempts to develop situatedness (Benner & Wrubel, 1989) in schools and offered glimpses into the practice worlds these therapists have shaped. In each story, one could see both a "snapshot" of the stress involved with practicing within school settings, and practical ways that these expert therapists coped with, and overcame, some of the stress.

Nancy spoke about how, unlike other times in practice, her success story was "a time when the teaming worked well and ... [there] was a good working relationship with the consultative type of program going on between therapist and teacher." Nancy contrasted this time with the thread of an untold story, an earlier time when she had *not* been able to intervene with a student because she had not had a good working relationship with the team. She said, "It was sad, because you, I felt, I really felt that had [this student] had the services the year before, [when an OT evaluation] was originally initiated, he really maybe could have even gone without the DFG [developmental first grade] placement."

Nancy felt this student might have avoided being placed in a special education program if teachers or team members had known more about the services an OT could have provided for the student. Nancy spoke only cursorily of being sad about this situation and the fact that this student had not received occupational therapy services earlier, before he needed to be placed in a special education program. That was the untold story.

On the other hand, Nancy felt that this time when she had intervened with this same student at a later date, she *had* been successful. She had been able to not only collaborate with the teacher to effect changes in the student, but also to share information with this teacher about the nature of occupational therapy services available in public schools.

These untold stories seemed to serve some very important role for the therapists. Possibly, by working through the situation referred to in the untold story, and by reflecting on her own actions, Nancy was able to intervene more effectively the second time. Perhaps as a result of her first experience, she was able to come up with other, more effective intervention strategies for the next time in practice. Or, perhaps intuitively, rather than consciously, she just handled the situation differently and, on reflection, noticed how her interventions had been different when she felt she had been successful. Perhaps the situations truly *were* different. That is, perhaps the individuals involved were more open to participating in the intervention process with this therapist. In any case, something different happened in these two stories and Nancy chose to express this difference by contrasting the success story with the thread of an earlier time when the outcome had been less successful.

Being perceived as a disruption to, rather than a facilitator of, the educational process, was another dark thread that appeared in several therapists' stories. One therapist said that this time in practice (when she felt successful with her interventions) the situation had been different from times when she felt she had been perceived as disruptive to a teacher's classroom routine. Laurie said, "It wasn't like, 'Oh, there's that lady again, please don't work in my classroom, you're disruptive.' It's like we're doing something!"

Gail, another expert therapist, also included this thread of disruption in her story. She said, "You tippy-toed in, you grabbed your kid, and you tippy-toed out. You did not disrupt [the teacher's] routine."

Both Laurie and Gail must have reflected on this feeling of being perceived as disruptive because they shared strategies that they had developed to deal with this difficulty. Laurie's strategy had to do with doing something a little extra to *demonstrate* to a teacher, for example, that if you darken ditto sheets, visually impaired students can perform fine motor tasks better because they can see the tasks better.

Laurie said sometimes the therapist has to be the one to darken the dittos; she called this "garbage work," done to "get your foot in the door" with a teacher, to get a teacher to listen to the suggestions an occupational therapist can make to enhance a student's ability to learn in school.

Gail, on the other hand, dealt with the sense of being perceived as disruptive, first, by waiting until a new teacher came into the classroom (rather than by disrupting the current teacher's routine) and, then, by gradually "edging into the classroom, seeing what the kids looked like when they were working in the room, ...and then doing more and more consultation." Within therapists' untold stories it was possible to see how these OTs had devised strategies to work through barriers to their attempts to become situated (Benner & Wrubel, 1989) in this practice setting. Given the dark threads of untold stories, the remarkable stories of success each expert OT recounted became all the more brilliant in contrast. These therapists seemed to weave together both the dark threads of difficulty and the brilliant threads of success in ways that enabled them to view their practice of occupational therapy from new, and perhaps, more insightful perspectives.

AMBIVALENCE AND PARADOX

As these five OTs shared their stories of success, they also shared considerable ambivalence concerning a perceived mismatch between occupational therapy services provided within a medical context and occupational therapy services provided within an educational context. It seemed that the interventions the therapists' observed as successful in school settings did not always match their implicit understanding of what constitutes real therapy. That is, although their stories demonstrated how they have begun to adapt their professional beliefs and practices to better match the needs of the educational setting in which they work, they had difficulty labeling some of their interventions with students as being real therapy. This ambivalence may stem, in part, from a discrepancy between what therapists have learned in their professional preparation and previous professional experience constitutes occupational therapy, and what they have experienced as being meaningful intervention for students who require their assistance to be successful in school.

In response to the demands of the educational setting, this indeterminant zone of practice (Schon, 1987), these therapists seemed to ask themselves, "What can I do to help *this* student in *this* situation?" (Fisher, 1989). They responded to this question by applying their knowledge and skills to exploring and interpreting the meaning of students' "disabilities" in light of the demands of their educational settings and then by intervening. Throughout the stories the therapists related, it appeared that the most meaningful and effective interventions they provided for students resulted in changes to the students' educational environments. That is, the major part of the success stories of these therapists related to their reframing of students' behaviors, employing consultative strategies, and developing collaborative efforts between team members (Bundy, in press) rather than direct, hands-on treatment with students designed to remediate physical or learning deficits.

One therapist said that the most important result of her intervention was that it "got people off [the student's] back!" Another therapist said that her intervention had resulted in a student's being able to return from a self-contained program for the deaf to a regular classroom with minimal resource assistance. A third therapist said that her intervention had "made a very picturesque difference" in a student; he had changed from a child who would avoid playground equipment at all cost to a student who could self-challenge on the playground and be so confident in his skills that he could ask to play soccer with peers.

When asked directly, however, all of these therapists either attributed their successes with students to direct, hands-on therapy or they questioned the effects of their interventions; they said they didn't really know whether their therapy made the difference, whether it was something else like "just" building up the student's confidence, whether it was "just" that the teachers were able to look at a student differently, or whether these changes would have occurred anyway, "just" developmentally.

These stories strongly suggest that expert OTs feel real ambivalence about the value of the services they provide to students in public schools. Entering an indeterminant zone of practice—the public schools—has forced these therapists to examine their practice and change their world view of occupational therapy, to enlarge it beyond the scope of the medical model. Although expert OTs have done this successfully, they have not become fully situated in this arena, that is, they continue to question whether or not their interventions, successful as they have been, can be considered to be within the boundaries of real therapy.

One important question that must be raised is, what will encourage OTs to embrace all of the types of interventions they provide to enhance student performance in school as real therapy? More specifically, what can be done to demonstrate to therapists that providing other team members with access to the knowledge contained in practice theories of occupational therapy, thus enabling those team members to understand students differently and develop new and more effective strategies for teaching these students, is a bona fide and important role for therapists practicing in schools?

Conclusions

The discrepancy between what therapists seem to believe they *should* be doing and what they *actually* do is reminiscent of the problem experienced by the students with whom those therapists intervene in schools. Like the occupational therapists, these students experience a discrepancy between what the educational team thinks they should be able to do and what they actually are accomplishing at school. Perhaps the parallel that we have drawn here can be extended further to offer a means for eliminating the discrepancy facing OTs practicing in schools.

In the stories these expert practitioners related they were able to eliminate or minimize the discrepancies the students faced. Most often they did this by providing a new frame through which parents, teachers, and the students themselves were able to view the students' performance. This frame showed the student in a new light and served as a catalyst for the parents and teachers to change their expectations so that they were more in line with the capabilities of the student. Sometimes these therapists intervened directly with a student to enable that student to develop new skills so that he or she was able to meet the expectations that had been set by the educational team. In all the stories they recounted, the therapists assumed the role of the wise person (Goffman, 1963), helping to reduce the stigma of being different and enabling the student to reach his potential in school.

If this parallel can in fact be drawn, therapists practicing in public schools need wise people who can help them to see their roles differently and who can teach them new skills that will enable them to be increasingly effective in these new roles. Given that many OTs practice essentially alone in schools, without access to mentoring from experienced supervisors, who are these wise people to be? That question is beyond the scope of this investigation, but we offer it as a challenge to the profession of occupational therapy. Toward that end, we also offer the stories that have been shared by these expert therapists as a frame through which therapists might begin to see themselves—differently.

Implications for Practice and Further Study

This exploratory study has raised several issues of significance for OTs practicing in public schools and for the profession as a whole. There are implications for the nature of training for therapists who currently practice, or plan to practice, in school settings. Therapists need to develop explicit strategies for becoming situated to enhance our effectiveness in settings outside of the medically oriented hospital or clinic. Second, it is important for us to match our roles to the settings in which we practice; we must carefully and systematically establish and examine the expected outcomes of our various models of service delivery. Third, although this was a small, exploratory study it demonstrated the rich, descriptive data that can be elicited through narrative interviewing. The results of this study offer a glimpse of the potential value of qualitative research methods in generating and developing greater understanding for the nature of occupational therapy practice.

References

American Occupational Therapy Association. (1985). *Occupational therapy manpower: A plan for progress.* Rockville, MD: Author.

American Occupational Therapy Association. (1989). *Guidelines for occupational therapy services in school systems* (2nd ed.). Rockville, MD: Author.

Benner, P. (1984). *From novice to expert: Excellence and power in clinical nursing practice.* Menlo Park, CA: Addison-Wesley Publishing.

Benner, P., & Wrubel, J. (1989). *The primacy of caring: Stress and coping in health and illness.* Menlo Park, CA: Addison-Wesley Publishing.

Bogdan, R., & Taylor, S. (1984). *Introduction to qualitative research methods.* New York: John Wiley.

Bundy, A., Lawlor, M., Kielhofner, G., & Knecht, H. (1989, April). *Educational and therapeutic perceptions of school system practice.* Paper presented at the American Occupational Therapy Association annual conference, Baltimore.

Bundy, A. C. (in press). Consultation and sensory integration theory. In A. G. Fisher, E. A. Murray, & A. C. Bundy (Eds.), *Sensory integration: Theory and practice.* Philadelphia: F. A. Davis.

Coles, R. (1989). *The call of stories.* Boston: Houghton Mifflin.

Education for All Handicapped Children Act of 1975. (Public Law 94–142), 20 U.S.C. 1401.

Fisher, A. (1989, March). *Framing function from the perspective of the professional discipline.* Paper presented at the Maternal and Child Health conference, University of Illinois at Chicago, Chicago.

Gartner, A., & Lipsky, D. K. (1987). Beyond special education: Toward a quality system for all students. *Harvard Educational Review, 57,* 367–395.

Gilfoyle, E., & Hays, C. (1979). Occupational therapy roles and functions in the education of the school-based handicapped student. *American Journal of Occupational Therapy, 13,* 565–576.

Glaser, B., & Strauss, A. (1967). *The discovery of grounded theory.* New York: Aldine Publishing.

Goffman, E. (1963). *Stigma: Notes on the management of spoiled identity.* New York: Simon & Schuster.

Good, B., & Good, M. (1981). The measuring of symptoms: A cultural hermeneutic model for clinical practice. In L. Eisenberg & A. Kleinman (Eds.), *The relevance of social science for medicine* (pp. 165–196). Boston: D. Reidel Publishing.

Guba, E. G. (1981). Criteria for assessing the trustworthiness of naturalistic inquiries. *Educational Resources Information Center Annual Review Paper, 29,* 75–91.

Hopkins, H. (1988). An historical perspective on occupational therapy. In H. Hopkins & H. Smith (Eds.), *Willard & Spackman's occupational therapy,* (7th ed.), (pp. 16–37). Philadelphia: J. B. Lippincott.

Kielhofner, G. (1982). Qualitative research: Part one. Paradigmatic grounds and issues of reliability and validity. *Occupational Therapy Journal of Research, 2,* 67–79.

Kielhofner, G., & Miyake, S. (1983). Rose-colored lenses for clinical practice: From a deficit to a competency model in assessment and intervention. In G. Kielhofner (Ed.), *Health through occupation* (pp. 257–266). Philadelphia: F. A. Davis.

Kleinman, A. (1988). *The illness narratives: Suffering, health and the human condition.* New York: Basic Books.

Knafl, K., & Breitmayer, B. J. (1989). Triangulation in qualitative research: Issues of conceptual clarity and purpose. In J. Morse (Ed.), *Qualitative nursing research: A contemporary dialogue* (pp. 193–203). Rockville, MD: Aspen.

Krefting, L. (in press). Rigor in qualitative research: The assessment of trustworthiness. *American Journal of Occupational Therapy.*

Lincoln, Y. S., & Guba, E. A. (1985). *Naturalistic inquiry.* Beverly Hills, CA: Sage.

Mattingly, C. F. (1989). Thinking with stories: Story and experience in a clinical practice. Unpublished doctoral dissertation, Massachusetts Institute of Technology, Boston.

Mattingly, C. F. (in press). Narrative reflections on practical actions. In D. Schon (Ed.), *The reflective turn: Case studies of reflection and on practice.* New York: Teacher's College Press.

Miles, M. B., & Huberman, A. M. (1984). *Qualitative data analysis: A sourcebook of new methods.* Beverly Hills, CA: Sage.

Ottenbacher, K. (1982). Occupational therapy and special education: Some issues and concerns related to Public Law 94–142. *American Journal of Occupational Therapy, 36,* 81–84.

Patton, M. Q. (1990). *Qualitative evaluation and research methods.* Newbury Park, CA: Sage.

Rowles, G. D. (1988). Themes and challenges. In S. Reinharz & G. Rowles (Eds.), *Qualitative gerontology* (pp. 3-33). New York: Springer.

Royeen, C. (1986). Nationally speaking—Evaluation of school-based occupational therapy programs: Need, strategy, and dissemination. *American Journal of Occupational Therapy, 40,* 811–813.

Royeen, C., & Marsh, D. (1988). Promoting occupational therapy in the schools. *American Journal of Occupational Therapy, 42,* 713–717.

Ruby, D. (1980). Exposing yourself: Reflexivity, anthropology and film. *Semiotica, 30,* 153–179.

Schatzman, L., & Strauss, A. (1973). *Field research.* Englewood Cliffs, NJ: Prentice-Hall.

Schon, D. (1979). Generative metaphor: A perspective on problem-setting in social policy. In A. Ortany, (Ed.), *Metaphor and thought* (pp. 254-283). New York: Cambridge University Press.

Schon, D. (1987). *Educating the reflective practitioner.* San Francisco: Jossey-Bass.

Illustrative Example 11–1: Questions

1. What is the purpose of the research?
2. Does the literature review provide you an understanding of how and why this investigation is important?
3. Do you think the investigation is important? Why or why not?
4. What is the theoretical or conceptual basis of the investigation?
5. How was the research conducted?
6. What type or kind of research is it and why?
7. What were the research questions or hypotheses?
8. What were the variables or phenomena under study?
9. Who were the subjects or units of study? How many were there?
10. How were the subjects or units of study obtained?
11. What information or data were collected?
12. If specific evaluation tools were used, what were they? Was information on the reliability and validity of the evaluation tools provided?
13. How was the information or data collected?
14. Will data collected be able to answer or address the research question or problem under study?
15. How was the information or data analyzed?
16. What were the criteria for interpreting the data?
17. What were the findings?
18. What were the limitations of the study? Was there a critical flaw?
19. Are the conclusions of the study warranted?
20. How can these research findings be used in occupational and physical therapy?

Illustrative Example 11–2: Answers

1. *What is the purpose of the research?*

To study school-based occupational therapy practice.

2. *Does the literature review provide you an understanding of how and why this investigation is important?*

Yes. The need and importance of such a study is carefully presented in a very readable format.

3. *Do you think the investigation is important? Why or why not?*

Clearly this is a bias of my own. I firmly believe we really need to address school-based practice.

4. *What is the theoretical or conceptual basis of the investigation?*

This is more or less a study to find out more about what is. Because only two major studies have been done in this area, there is a critical need to explore it more. Also, the investigators have based the study on work done by expert school-based practitioners.

5. *How was the research conducted?*

The in-depth interview method was used and, notably, the authors identify methods on which the process was based (see the Procedures section). Interviews took about 1–2 hours, and five therapists were interviewed. Specific instructions were given to the therapists to anchor them in a situational format.

6. *What type or kind of research is it and why?*

This is the in-depth interview technique of qualitative research.

7. *What were the research questions or hypotheses?*

There were not set up a priori, which is consistent with qualitative research.

8. *What were the variables or phenomena under study?*

The variables being studied were the phenomena of how school-based therapists viewed their roles as service providers, and the practice knowledge expert therapists have developed.

9. *Who were the subjects or units of study? How many were there?*

Five therapists served as subjects. All subjects had practiced at least 5 years in the schools. The designation of expert was made from identification by two or more peers.[2] Subjects were volunteers.

10. *How were the subjects or units of study obtained?*

This is not exactly clear from the Subjects section.

11. *What information or data were collected?*

Thorough in-depth interviews of the subjects.

12. *If specific evaluation tools were used, what were they? Was information on the reliability and validity of the evaluation tools provided?*

None provided as none was needed. It may be helpful, however, in replication studies to provide a rationale and validation of verbal instructions provided to the subjects.

13. *How was the information or data collected?*

Through audiotape and subsequent transcription.

14. *Will data collected be able to answer or address the research question or problem under study?*

Certainly it will.

2. Just what does expert mean? The criteria of expert could be better developed and defined in subsequent studies.

15. *How was the information or data analyzed?*

The researchers used many of the methods identified earlier in this chapter. A summary of their analysis is

1. use of expert occupational therapists to develop themes
2. use of constant comparative method
3. generation of theoretical perspectives.

See "Data Analysis and Interpretation in Qualitative Research."

16. *What were the criteria for interpreting the data?*

The researchers pulled in concepts from a variety of theoretical perspectives to provide a framework for data interpretation.

17. *What were the findings?*

The following theme emerged: (a) a collaborative intervention process, (b) therapists integrating themselves within the special education setting, and (c) therapist conflict over what constitutes therapy in this setting.

18. *What were the limitations of the study? Was there a critical flaw?*

The selection of criteria of expert witness is not fully developed. The same applied for the therapists used as experts in data analysis.

19. *Are the conclusions of the study warranted?*

Yes.

20. *How can these research findings be used in occupational and physical therapy?*

They can be a foundation for training and further research into school-based practice.

Overview of Qualitative Research

Because of its elegance and simplicity, an overview of qualitative research previously published in the occupational therapy literature is provided as a summary for this chapter.

Reprinted from *American Journal of Occupational Therapy,* Vol. 35, Number 2, February, 1981, pp. 105–106. Used with permission.

ILLUSTRATIVE EXAMPLE 11–2

Qualitative Research and Occupational Therapy

Harriet Schmid

Among health professionals there has been a growing interest in a research paradigm that is responsive to questions of a holistic nature, questions that generate complete knowledge about how an individual, for example a client, perceives himself and the environment in which he selects his mode of life and adapts to it. Such a paradigm exists within the research tradition of the social sciences, namely, anthropology, sociology, and to some extent, social psychology, where emphasis is placed on understanding the meaning of human behavior in social and cultural settings. This research tradition has been variously referred to as qualitative, ethnographic, or phenomenological. Because qualitative research differs from natural science or quantitative research, it is important to understand that research assumptions, strategies, and processes associated with this tradition.

Research Assumptions

A qualitative research approach involves the study of the empirical world from the perspectives of the subjects under investigation. As such, it is based on two assumptions. The first assumption is that human behavior is influenced by the physical and psychological context or environment in which it occurs. Consequently, to understand this contextual influence, the researcher must observe the subjects in their natural context (e.g., home, neighborhood, school, hospital, place of employment). Second, a qualitative approach is based on the assumption that human behavior goes beyond that which can be observed; it lies in the perspectives and meanings held by the individuals in a context. This assumption is amplified in the distinction between "inner" and "outer" perspectives influencing research. The "inner" perspective assumes that understanding is dependent upon active participation in the life of the observed while gaining insight through introspection. The "outer" perspective assumes that knowledge about social life is obtained through the study of Man's behavior. Knowledge of Man is achieved through both "outer" and "inner" perspectives, that is, an understanding arises both from observation of Man's behaviors and information about his perspective of the world. The "inner" perspective, which is emphasized in qualitative research, is known as *verstehen* or subjective understanding (1).

Research Strategies

Qualitative research includes a variety of strategies; for example, participant observation, in-depth interviews, enumerations, and sampling. The foremost of these is participant observation. In sharing the world of the observed for the purpose of gaining understanding, the researcher as observer can assume a variety of social roles. Gold describes four roles on a continuum from complete participant to complete observer (2). Much has been written concerning the advantages and disadvantages of each role (2, 3, 4). The role of the observer requires both detachment and personal involvement. The observer's interests are independent of the cultural life of the observed (3). The role assumed will be one that is deemed plausible within the context of the observed. It will further be determined by the research design and the framework of the culture of the observed. Critical to the participant observer role is recognition that the researcher himself or herself is the key instrument in observing a setting and collecting and analyzing the data.

For several reasons, the researcher, in addition to direct observation, must rely on indirect observation. First, the phenomenon being observed usually occurs in several places, which prevents the researcher from observing more than one setting at a time. Second, the researcher usually studies a phenomenon that has had a previous history, one with which the researcher would be unfamiliar and that would not be available through direct observation. Finally, many perceptions are not adequately inferable by direct observation. Consequently, the researcher adds to his or her information indirect observation from informants and respondents. Informant information takes the form of documents or records and reports of persons present in the setting. Both serve the purpose of providing information to the observer about settings in which he or she could not be present. Respondent information results frequently from interviewing members of the setting concerning their motives, intents, and interpretations of events. In the former, the person or document substitutes for the observer's presence, whereas in the latter, the person acts for and as himself. The use of multiple methods to collect information is known as triangulation and is an attempt by the researcher to rule out rival interpretations and to overcome the intrinsic bias that may occur as a result of single approaches used to gain understanding.

The Research Process

The researcher enters the field, the environment of the observed, with general ideas of assumptions concerning the nature of the setting to be observed; however, no a priori hypotheses guide the research. The researcher is knowledgeable and has a theoretical frame of reference, which is "bracketed" in order to gain an inner perspective. In other words, a theoretical framework may guide the research but it does not govern it. Further, the design is said to be "temporally developing," that is, the researcher does not enter the field with a highly structured design; rather, there is a certain fluidity in decision making by the researcher. Several dimensions or stages of the research process have been identified.

Strauss described three phases, essentially (5). During the initial phase, the specific problems or foci have not been identified and emphasis is placed on observation. Temporary hypotheses begin to emerge from the data as the researcher begins to make sense of the accumulating information. These hypotheses, which may even be conjectures, are tested for relevance as continuing observations are made. Classes of information are developed and the researcher returns to observation and data to look for disconfirmation, qualification, or confirmation. The process is reiterated until hypotheses are confirmed. Characteristic of the research process is the relationship between observation, description, and the reiterative cycle involved in inductive generation of hypotheses. Strauss considers this process necessary for the discovery of grounded theory, theory generated from data (5).

Analytical descriptions generated from qualitative research studies in which the goals of research may be to gain an understanding of the meaning of human behavior in social and cultural settings, may contribute to a body of knowledge in several ways. Existing conceptual frameworks may be expanded, and models that may lead to theory construction can be developed.

Implications for Occupational Therapy

There has been an increasing focus, in occupational therapy, on developing a theoretical body of knowledge to support its practice. Occupational therapy has long been concerned with adaptation of persons to their environment. The development of a theoretical basis for a practice that facilitates adaptation will rely on answers to holistic research questions that seek an explanation for Man's ability to adapt to the world in which he lives. Researchers seeking an answer to such a question will need to expand their research paradigm to include qualitative research methodologies in which understanding arises both from observation of a person's behavior and from information about that person's perspective of the world.

Qualitative research methodologies are not compatible with all research questions, but the fact that this research approach is available enables the researcher to ask questions concerning the complexity of human phenomena. However, before engaging in such a course, the researcher will need to gain the sophisticated knowledge and skill necessary to conduct qualitative research. In summary, as occupational therapy researchers move toward the generation of a theoretical base for occupational therapy practice, they should consider modifying their research paradigms to include qualitative research methodology.

References

1. Weber M: A subjective interpretation in the social sciences. In *Verstehen: Subjective Understanding in the Social Sciences.* Reading, MA: Addison-Wesley Publishing Company, 1974 pp 18–37

2. Gold RL: Roles in sociological field observations. In *Sociological Methods: A source book.* NK Denzin, Editor. Chicago: Aldine Publishing Company, 1970, pp 370–380

3. Bruyn S: *The Human Perspective.* Englewood Cliffs, NJ: Prentice-Hall, Inc., 1966

4. McCall GT, Simmons JL: *Issues in Participant Observation.* Reading, MA: Addison-Wesley Publishing Company, 1969

5. Strauss A: The process of field work. In *Issues in Participant Observation,* GT McCall, JL Simmons, Editors. Reading, MA: Addison-Wesley Publishing Company, 1969, pp 24–27

References

Burns, N., & Grove, S. K. (1987). *The practice of nursing research: Conduct, critique and utilization.* Philadelphia: W. B. Saunders.

Campbell, D. T., & Stanley, J. C. (1979). *Experimental and quasiexperimental designs for research.* Chicago: Rand McNally.

Carlson, M. E., & Clark, F. (1991). *American Journal of Occupational Therapy, 45,* 235–241.

Goetz, J. P., & LeCompte, M. D. (1985). *Ethnography and qualitative design in education research.* Orlando, FL: Academic Press.

Hasselkus, B. R. (1991). Ethical dilemmas in family caregiving for the elderly: Implications for occupational therapy. *American Journal of Occupational Therapy, 45,* 206–212.

Kielhofner, G. (1982a). Qualitative research: Part one. Paradigmatic grounds and issues of reliability and validity. *Occupational Therapy Journal of Research, 2(2),* 80–88.

Kielhofner, G. (1982b). Qualitative research: Part two. Methodological approaches and relevance to occupational therapy. *Occupational Therapy Journal of Research, 2(3),* 150–164.

Kreftig, L. (1991). Rigor in qualitative research: The assessment of trustworthiness. *American Journal of Occupational Therapy, 45,* 214–222.

Krueger, R. A. (1988). Focus groups: A practical guide for applied research. Beverly Hills, CA: Sage.

Mathison, S. (1988). Why triangulate? *Educational Researcher, 17,* 13–17.

McCuaig, M., & Frank, G. (1991). The able self: Adaptive patterns and choices in independent living for a person with cerebral palsy. *American Journal of Occupational Therapy, 45,* 224–332.

Miles, M. B., & Huberman, A. M. (1984). *Qualitative data analysis: A sourcebook of new methods.* Beverly Hills, CA: Sage.

Niehues, A. N., Bundy, A. C., Mattingly, C. F., & Lawlor, M. C. (1991). Making a difference: Occupational therapy in the public schools. *Occupational Therapy Journal of Research, 11,* 195–212.

PSI International. (1989). Evolving methodology in disability research. *Rehab Brief, 12.*

Schmid, H. (1981). Qualitative research and occupational therapy. *American Journal of Occupational Therapy, 35,* 105–106.

Short-Debroff, M. (1994). Critical assessment of qualitative research (editorial). *Occupational Therapy Journal of Research, 14,* 75–77.

Smith, J. K. (1988). Quantitative versus qualitative research: An attempt to clarify the issue. *Educational Research, 3,* 6–13.

Stiley, J. (1988). Physics for the rest of us. *Educational Research, 17,* 7–10.

Yerxa, E. J. (1991). Seeking a relevant, ethical, and realistic way of knowing for occupational therapy. *American Journal of Occupational Therapy, 45,* 199–204.

Recommended Readings

Crabtree, E. F., & Miller, W. L. (Eds.). (1992). *Doing qualitative research.* Beverly Hills, CA: Sage.

Glaser, B., & Strause, A. L. (1967). *The discovery of grounded theory.* New York: Aldine.

Hammick, M. (1995). Qualitative and quantitative research: Adjuvants and alternatives. *British Journal of Therapy and Rehabilitation, 2,* 341–342.

Marshall, C., & Rossman, G. B. (1989). *Designing qualitative research.* Beverly Hills, CA: Sage.

Miles, M., & Huberman, A. M. (1984). *Qualitative data analysis: A sourcebook of new methods.* Beverly Hills, CA: Sage.

Morese, J. M. (Ed.). (1991). *Qualitative nursing research: A contemporary dialogue.* Beverly Hills, CA: Sage.

Straus, A., & Corgin, J. (1990). *Basics of qualitative research.* Beverly Hills, CA: Sage.

Yerxa, E. J. (1991). Special issue on qualitative research. *American Journal of Occupational Therapy, 45,* 199–281.

Learning Activities

1. Imagine that you are planning a research investigation. Consider the pros and cons of a qualitative versus a quantitative investigation.
2. Define and give examples of all key words from this chapter.
3. What are the fundamental differences between qualitative and quantitative research?

CHAPTER 12

The Research Proposal

KEY WORDS

Constant comparative method

Data verification

Dissemination

Evaluation plan

Formative evaluation

Iterative interpretation

Management plan

Project impact

Project outcomes

Research proposal

Stakeholders

Summative evaluation

Conducting a research investigation requires careful planning and management. For many researchers it requires obtaining funding from an agency or committee. Whether you are applying to an agency for potential funding or trying to put together an organized investigation, you need to go through the process of writing a **research proposal**. This process, which starts with a prospectus and can end with a polished comprehensive plan detailing how your research will be carried out, is crucial in both focusing and organizing your investigation and in obtaining funding. Also, it may help your understanding as a research consumer if you are aware of what goes into launching a research investigation.

This chapter describes and presents examples of the components of a research proposal.

The Research Prospectus

A research prospectus is not an official part of a proposal that would be submitted to an agency or committee. It is, however, an excellent first step to take in preparing to write a fully developed proposal. You create a research prospectus when you have an idea, but not a fully developed plan, for a research investigation. A prospectus is an effective way of getting feedback as you develop the concepts that will be the basis of your research. It allows you to share preliminary ideas with a large number of people to get general feedback.

Often, investigators will write a one- to three-page prospectus to share with potential funding agencies to determine if the agency considers the scope of the research to be within their funding guidelines. Example 1 (Royeen & Berkowitz, 1990) is a research prospectus developed during the initial phase of generating a research proposal for a federally funded research competition.

You can see that the researchers presented an overview of the research idea. Details of the investigation, however, are lacking. The purpose of the research prospectus is to give readers a general idea of the proposed investigation, enough so they can react to the proposed project. This particular prospectus was actually used in meeting with government representatives in the National Institute of Disability Research and Rehabilitation (NIDRR), part of the U. S. Department of Education. The use of such a prospectus is significant. It allows potential grant applicants to share preliminary ideas to revise and refine them for a fully developed research proposal. Example 2 shows another research prospectus (Royeen, 1992).

Again, as you can see, the purpose of the prospectus is to gather preliminary reactions, interest, and information about the proposed project. It is a way of "testing the waters" and obtaining necessary feedback. Note again that substantial detail is lacking.

EXAMPLE 1

Research Prospectus.

Implementing the IFSP: Investigating the Partnership between Parents and Professionals

Submitting Agency: The Reginald Laurie Center for Infants and Young Children (formerly the Regional Center for Infants and Young Children), Rockville, Maryland

Targeted Competition: Field Initiated Research, National Institute of Disability Research and Rehabilitation (CFDA No. 84.133G) 34 CFR Parts 350 and 357

Importance of the Proposed Study: Congress has recently legislated (P.L. 99-457, Part H) that parents or guardians of infants who are handicapped participate in developing, implementing and monitoring plans and programs for their children's development. In brief, parents are now to be full and equal partners in the development of the Individualized Family Service Plan (IFSP), which will delineate what and how services will be provided to the infant and family.

Yet, little empirical data exists addressing key issues about implementing this mandate from Congress. Most importantly, there is very little research about how to incorporate parents as full and equal partners in this process. Such research is especially important since few professionals received any preparation in their training or on-the-job experience for working with parents in this new and innovative way. It is critical, therefore, to explore aspects of implementing the IFSP with both parents and professionals so that empirical data can further guide the process. This research, therefore, addresses a problem which is significant to infants with disabilities, their families, and those who treat them. Additionally, this research will generate new and useful knowledge about the problems confronting implementation of the legislated IFSP process as well as about perceived solutions to those problems.

Anticipated outcomes from the research are (1) knowledge about perceived problems in implementing the IFSP across three distinct yet interacting levels (parents, professionals and state and local administrators); (2) knowledge about perceived difficulties in fostering the partnership between parents and professionals during the IFSP process; (3) knowledge about field-based solutions to perceived problems in fostering the partnership between parents and professionals; and (4) instrumentation and protocols for use by others for exploration of the partnership between parents and professionals in other sites and settings.

Conceptual Model: The conceptual model underlying the research investigation is one of action research. In using this model, one assumes that organizational change (facilitation of effective partnerships between parents and professionals) can be best brought about when vested parties (administrators, professionals and parents) are used to explore their interpretation and analysis of the situation, as compared to imposing existing theory references or preconceived judgments about the process. Thus, use of an action model allows for generation of objective (bias free, judgment free) data about the nature of the partnership between parents and professionals.

Design of the Project: Three years of programmatic research are proposed for the project. The key tasks of the three years are presented below.

Year One. Development, Refinement and Pilot Testing of Data Collection Methodology. This study will have many components to assure validity and reliability of data collection procedures. The majority of the work in year one can be done on site at The Reginald Laurie Center for Infants and Young Children in Rockville, Maryland.

- Study One. Use of Delphi Groups (one of state administrators, one of regional administrators, one of professionals, one of parents) to finalize basic questions and categories of issues, concerns, and questions these various stakeholder groups have regarding interpretation of the law, concerns about implementation of the law, attitudes of the various stakeholder groups about one another, perceived problems which could negatively affect the IFSP process, and perceived solutions to foster effective partnerships between key stakeholder groups. Use of these Delphi groups assures the validity of the questions to be addressed in the project.
- Study Two. Development of three categories of structured, open-ended interviews for use with each of the three key stakeholder groups (administrators, professionals and parents).
- Study Three. Development of training procedures for interviewers.
- Study Four. Development of attitude scales for use with each of the three key stakeholder groups. These will be used in years two and three to measure attitude changes before and after involvement with the IFSP process.

Data analysis will be conducted using traditional measures and standards for development of survey and scaling methodology.

Year Two. Field-Based Research in Three Sites. Year Two will consist of three separate investigations in three sites using instrumentation and data collection procedures developed from Year One. Potential sites are as follows:

- Study One. Field-based data collection from Anne Arundel County, Maryland.
- Study Two. Field-based data collection from the District of Columbia.
- Study Three. Field-based data collection from Montgomery County, Maryland.

Collectively, these three studies will address research questions refined from Study One in Year One. Anticipated research questions, however, may center upon understanding of the law, perceived problems and solutions in implementing the IFSP process, how to increase effective partnerships between parents and professionals, and attitude changes before and after IFSP involvement.

Data analysis will be conducted according to guidelines for qualitative data analysis put forth by Miles and Huberman (1984), and by using descriptive statistics.

Year Three. Replication Across Sites and Conditions. Year Three will be used to replicate studies from Year Two in various cross-cultural sites. In this way, the robustness of the findings across conditions can be ascertained, and variations of the partnership between parents and professionals across conditions can be explored. Potential sites are as follow:

- Study One. Replication with Native Americans (Choctaw Tribe, Mississippi: Hopi Tribe, Arizona).
- Study Two. Replication with Hispanic Americans (Miami, Florida).
- Study Three: Replication with Indo-Chinese Americans (Arlington, Virginia).
- Dissemination. (1) Write-up of instrumentation and protocols for possible commercial publication. (2) Articles submitted to journals based upon findings in journals for each respective stakeholder group. For example, parent's publication in *Exceptional Parent.*

EXAMPLE 2

Prospectus for Educational Research Proposal

BACKGROUND

Shenandoah University, a Methodist-affiliated liberal arts institution of 1700 students in Winchester, Virginia, is beginning a master's level program in occupational therapy.[1] Shenandoah University's developing program offers a unique opportunity to research, develop, implement and evaluate an innovative program in occupational therapy based upon answering, "What is excellence in occupational therapy education?"

Inquiry into this arena is critically important considering that the status quo of education in occupational therapy specifically, and the U.S. generally, has been undergoing rapid change due to

1. the prevalence of new programs of occupational therapy being implemented in small, private institutions;[1]
2. the demise or significant reorganization of existing programs of occupational therapy housed in medical schools;
3. overall manpower shortages in occupational therapy in Virginia and the entire U.S.;[2]
4. the transformation of American society from a white majority to pluralistic minorities by the year 2000;

1. A master's level program in physical therapy was started in 1990.

5. the dwindling pool of college-level students due to demographic trends;[3]
6. the need for scholars, critical thinkers, faculty and "movers and shakers" in the discipline of occupational therapy; and
7. the transformation of practice from a medical-model, hospital-driven intervention with the disabled to varied community and systems-driven interventions with the disabled and the normal populations.

STATEMENT OF THE PROBLEM

The future occupational therapist must not only know how to assess and intervene with individuals, but also how to assess and intervene at levels well beyond a single individual. The occupational therapist of the future must apply principles, theories and approaches to new and ever-changing functional problems encountered by those who are disabled and those who are experiencing "deviancy" that is within normal range. And, the occupational therapist of the future must work within the context of a society undergoing rapid changes in values, technology and organizational systems.

PROJECT OVERVIEW

The proposed project will consist of three phases. Phase One includes exploration of what constitutes excellence in occupational therapy education and, based upon the results, articulation of a conceptual and practical model for implementation. Phase Two consists of evaluation of the model for worth and value. Phase Three will be replication of the model or components thereof across sites to provide for a test of the robustness of the model across settings and conditions.

The objectives of the project are presented in Figure 12–1.

FIGURE 12–1
OBJECTIVES OF THE PROJECT

Phase	Year	Objective
One	1	to answer the question, "What is excellence in occupational therapy education?"
One	1	to develop a conceptual and practical model for occupational therapy education based upon the findings
Two	2–5	to implement the model
Two	2–5	to evaluate the worth, value and effectiveness of the model
Three	4–5	to test the robustness of the model or components thereof across settings

This project will be built upon the methodologies of

- historical research,[4]
- qualitative research,[5]
- program development and implementation,[6] as well as
- evaluation research.[7]

Project outcomes will consist of

- a theoretically and empirically tested model program for occupational therapy education;
- an articulated description of the program model for use by others;
- a beginning data base of educational research in occupational therapy, and
- educational policy papers for use by governmental and institutional agencies as well as associations.

Due to the long-term, programmatic nature of what is proposed, only Phase One (Objectives One and Two) are addressed in the following Methods sections.

METHODS

PHASE ONE, OBJECTIVE ONE, PART ONE
MONTHS 1–6

This series of studies is designed to answer the question, "What is excellence in occupational therapy education?"

Study One. Definition of Terms

This study will address the difficult task of revising terminology and constructs used in the project. Terms to be defined are listed in Appendix A. Steps in the process follow.

1. Identify the terms.
2. Define the terms.
3. Submit definition to review panel.
4. Revise and redefine.
5. Resubmit to review panel and submit to new reviewers.
6. Revise.

Study Two. Identification of Assumptions

This study will address identification of what assumptions underlie the conceptualization and implementation of the project. Preliminary assumptions are listed in Appendix B. Steps in the process follow.

1. Identify the assumptions.
2. Define the assumptions.
3. Submit definitions to review panel.
4. Revise and redefine.
5. Resubmit to review panel and submit to new reviewers.
6. Revise.

Study Three. Literature Synthesis

The literature of occupational therapy, education, business and related fields will be reviewed for identification of what constitutes excellence in education.[8] Steps in the process follow.

1. Identify disciplinary literature for review (education, business, occupational therapy).
2. Work with Mary Binderman, AOTF librarian for key terms.
3. Conduct computerized literature search.
4. Obtain literature and read.
5. Identify key citations in literature, obtain them and read.
6. Conduct synthesis.[9]

Study Four. Document Review

1. Confirmation of necessary documents for review. These may be, but are not limited to, AOTA files on curriculum, AOTA essentials, essentials for related organizations (APTA, ASHA).
2. Develop and refine document review form. Submit to Advisory Board for comment. Revise.
3. Review of documents.

Study Five. Focus Groups With Stakeholders

1. Identify stakeholder groups (university administration, occupational therapists, consumers, government agencies, third-party payers, etc.). Plan for homogeneous discussion groups up to five.[10]
2. Transcribe tapes.
3. Analyze tapes.
4. Conduct analysis.
5. Draft preliminary interview for in-depth exploration of issues identified in groups.

Study Six. Interview

1. Pilot-test interview with representative of stakeholder group.
2. Conduct five interviews per stakeholder group.
3. Transcribe.
4. Analyze.

PHASE ONE, OBJECTIVE ONE, PART TWO
MONTHS 3–6

Data Interpretation and Analysis

Study Seven. Ongoing, Iterative interpretation

Using a qualitative approach, patterns, issues and themes will be identified using logical interpretative and subjective judgment during each of the previously identified studies. This will be kept track of over time as each study progresses.[11] An outline of the data analysis, interpretation and verification plan is

a. data reduction using summary forms
b. identification of patterns and themes

c. matrix rating of importance
d. matrix of clustering by group
e. inductive reasoning
f. reflective remarks
g. developing propositions
h. matrix of explanatory effects
i. estimate representativeness
j. triangulation
k. check meaning of outliers
l. replication
m. getting feedback from stakeholders
n. validity check

Study Eight. Triangulation of the Data[12]

Results will be compared across studies, allowing for comparison by sources (literature, stakeholders, experts, and documents). Similarities across sources will be identified. Differences will be identified and explored. Preliminary explanations and interpretations will be rendered and submitted to Advisory Board. Explanations and interpretations will be revised.

Study Nine. Constant Comparative Method

Using another qualitative interpretation strategy, explore the emergence of patterns of themes across studies using a matrix format and logical interpretation.[13]

PHASE TWO, OBJECTIVE TWO
MONTHS 6–10

Study Ten. Develop Conceptual Model

This study is designed to develop a conceptual and practical model for occupational therapy education based upon the results of Study One, Two and Three in Phase One.

1. Initial conceptualization of the model will be based upon the preliminary model presented in Figure 12–2. Figure 12–2 will be revised based upon the outcomes of studies 1–6.
2. The preliminary model will be submitted to the Advisory Board for review and comment.
3. The model will then be revised based upon feedback. The revised model will then be submitted to all stakeholder group members for review and comment.
4. Based upon their feedback, the model will again be revised.
5. The final model will be drafted. Implementation plans will be developed along with a plan for formative evaluation.

FIGURE 12–2

PRELIMINARY CONCEPTUAL MODEL OF EXCELLENCE IN OCCUPATIONAL THERAPY EDUCATION

Variables	Process	Product
Culture	Mentorship	Critical thinker
Regional		
Occupational therapy		
Scholarly		
Clinical		
Curriculum	Learn by doing	Clinical reasoner
Theory		
Environment	Student responsibility	Research consumer
Physical		
SES		
Rural/Urban		
Service	Faculty responsibility	Practitioner
Community		
Expectations		
Research	County agent model	Advocate
Practice		
Leadership	Tutorial	Policy analyst
Policy	Cultural immersion	Lobbyist
Supports		
Study Body		
AOTA essentials		
History		
Class size		

REFERENCES

1. Personal communication with Truby LaGarde, Education Department, American Occupational Therapy Association, Rockville MD (July 13, 1992).
2. Personal communication with Truby LaGarde, Education Department, American Occupational Therapy Association, Rockville, MD (July 13, 1992).
3. Personal communication with Truby LaGarde, Education Department, American Occupational Therapy Association, Rockville, MD (July 13, 1992).
4. Best, J. W., and Kahn, J. V. (1989). Chapter 3, "Historical Research," (pp.57–75) in *Research in Education.* Englewood Cliffs, Prentice Hall.
5. Goetz, J. P., and LeCompte, M. D. (1986). *Ethnographic methods in educational research.* Florida: Orlando Press.
6. Royeen, C. B (1986). Evaluation of school based occupational therapy programs: Need, strategy and dissemination. *American Journal of Occupational Therapy, 40(12),* 811–813.
7. Henry, G. T., Dickey, K. C., and Areson, J. C. (1991). Stakeholder participation in educational performance monitoring systems. *Educational Evaluation and Policy Analysis, 13(2),* 177–188.
8. Cooper, H. M. (1982). Scientific guidelines for conducting integrative research review. *Review of Educational Research, 52(2),* 291–302.
9. ibid.
10. Kreuger, R. A. (1988). *Focus groups: A practical guide for application.* Beverly Hills: Sage Publishing Co.
11 Miles, M. B., and Huberman, M. (1984). *Qualitative data analysis: A synthesis of new methods.* Beverly Hills: Sage.
12. Mathison, S. (1988). Why triangulate? *Educational Research, 17(21),* 13–17.
13. Miles and Huberman, op. cit.

A Research Proposal: Components

Once you have gathered enough feedback to develop a hypothesis to test, you are ready to write a research proposal. The research proposal is a comprehensive document that contains both a research and a management plan. One is a step-by-step delineation of how the research will be conducted, and the other is a description, containing both prose and pictorial material, of how the investigation will be administrated. The typical research proposal will run anywhere from 100 to 200 pages, including all appendices and accompanying information material.

Each agency (or dissertation committee) has its own preferred format for preparing a proposal for submission. And your proposal needs to be specifically developed for their unique format, whatever it may be. Your first step, then, is finding out the specifications and format requirements of the agency to which you are submitting it.

Next, you need to create your research plan. Both quantitative and qualitative research is based on a research plan. The plan for either should let the reader know who will do what, and when and how it will be done. When writing the research plan, keep in mind that the plan is subject to revision based on findings as the research progresses. The research plan, like a treatment plan, can be revised as needed throughout the investigation.

THE QUANTITATIVE RESEARCH PLAN

The quantitative research plan should include, but not be limited to

- purpose and need for the study
- theoretical and conceptual basis underlying the investigation
- directional hypotheses where knowledge or experience permits
- description of the research design, including a sampling plan that specifies the units of analysis and sample definition and selection
- specification of the independent and dependent variables
- plans for data analysis and conceptual rules for interpreting data consistent with research issues and questions being addressed
- measurement tools including psychometric qualities thereof
- timeline of the study
- task analysis of who will be doing what
- feasibility analysis of the investigation that provides supporting evidence from the literature as to design, measurement tools, and so on, and, as required, a plan for pilot studies to establish feasibility of the investigation.

Addressing these issues provides any reader of the research plan with the foundation to understand the nature and scope of the investigation.

THE QUALITATIVE RESEARCH PLAN

It is more difficult to provide a schematic overview of exactly what is covered in the qualitative research plan, as the strategies used can be so varied, and so many different types of research designs fall under the rubric of qualitative research. One still, however, must give some idea of who is going to do what and when. The qualitative research plan should include the following:

- the variables; that is, identify what is to be explored, investigated, or described
- research strategy; that is, delineate how the phenomenon, event, or group will be studied
- selection criteria, or a description of how selection criteria were developed and how they will be applied

- data analysis and interpretation, or the type of data to be collected, and how it will be analyzed and interpreted
- validity check; that is, delineate how validity checks will be made
- a timeline or a projected timetable.

The following example is of a research proposal submitted to the NIDRR (DeGangi & Royeen, 1990).

Note the inclusion of a timeline at the end of the proposal specifying tasks by month. This gives the reader a clear idea of what project tasks will be done at what point in the project.

EXAMPLE 3

B. Research Proposal: Overview

A one-year research fellowship for exploring aspects of the Americans With Disabilities Act (ADA) is proposed. The year-long research fellowship will (1) identify and explore problems perceived by the key stakeholder groups in implementing the ADA, (2) identify actual problems encountered by key stakeholder groups during initial implementation of ADA, and (3) generate field-based methods and solutions for implementing the ADA. Additionally, the year-long research fellowship would allow me the luxury of in-depth study and further learning in qualitative research methodologies, the foundation of the research strategy for the fellowship year.

The dissemination component of this project will consist of three strategies: (1) outreach to NIDRR and Justice Department-funded projects on ADA, (2) dissemination to involved stakeholders, and (3) dissemination to the academic community.

B.1 Research Proposal: Importance

The ADA affects five main areas, i.e., employment, transportation, public accommodations, state and local government, and telecommunications. Due to the wide scope of the law, the current fellowship research will be limited to primarily address the area of employment as discussed in ADA. The employment section of ADA, Title I, prohibits certain employment practices which discriminate against individuals with disabilities. The ADA takes effect July 26, 1992, for employers with 25 or more employees and July 26, 1994, for employers with 15 or more employees. Title I provides that

- Employers may not discriminate against a person with a disability in hiring or promotion if that person is otherwise qualified for the job.
- Employers can ask about an applicant's ability to perform a job, but cannot inquire if that person has a disability or subject applicants to tests that tend to screen out people with disabilities.
- Employers will need to provide "reasonable accommodation" to persons with a disability. This includes steps such as job restructuring and equipment modification.
- Employers do not need to provide accommodations that would impose an "undue hardship" on business operations (p. 2, Jurk, 1991).

There is much in ADA which is unclear, such as "reasonable accommodation" and "undue hardship" (P. L. 101–336). It is assumed, therefore, that ADA could potentially result in considerable litigation between business and industry and those who are disabled as well as advocacy groups representing them. It is further assumed that by (1) identifying the expectations, views, and visions of the different stakeholder groups about ADA, and (2) promoting understanding of the different views on ADA as well as providing guides on implementation of ADA, conflict and resulting litigation could, potentially, be reduced or minimized, thereby saving American businesses, individual taxpayers and those who are disabled time, money and frustration.

DEFINITIONS

For purposes of the proposed fellowship research, the following stakeholder groups are defined.

1. *Individuals who are disabled:* These are individuals who have one or more mental or physical impairments which significantly interfere with life activities.
2. *Associations representing providers:* These are groups such as the American Physical Therapy Association, American Psychological Association, American Speech–Language and Hearing Association, etc.
3. *Associations representing individuals who are disabled:* These are groups such as United Cerebral Palsy, Epilepsy Foundation, Paralyzed Veterans Association, etc.
4. *National business associations:* These are associations which represent businesses, such as better business bureaus, chambers of commerce, etc.
5. *National associations of industry:* These are associations which represent industries such as the hotel and motel industry or food worker industry.
6. *Small businesses:* These are defined as those businesses employing 25 or fewer employees.

A listing of anticipated outcomes from the project are presented in Figure 12–3.

The products to be developed during the course of the project are listed in Figure 12–4.

In summary, the research fellowship being proposed will allow for exploration of a new and important legislative initiative, the ADA, which will have significant influence over American life over the coming decade. And, it will allow me as the research fellow to further immerse myself in the process of qualitative research.

B.2 Research Proposal: Research Objectives, Methods and Design

DESIGN OF THE PROJECT: CONCEPTUAL MODEL OF THE RESEARCH

This project will employ an approach to theory building based upon grounded theory (Glaser and Strauss, 1966; Glaser and Strauss, 1967; Simms, 1981) which allows theory to evolve out of the data collected. Grounded theory is especially useful in situations where little is known about a phenomenon (Hutchinson, 1985). Substantive theories, based upon the data collected, can then be formulated which address a specified, limited area of investigation such as proposed for this research fellowship (Hutchinson, 1985). Thus, the conceptual model underpinning this research is identified in Figure 12–5.

RATIONALE FOR THE RESEARCH METHODOLOGY

Use of focus groups, a qualitative research methodology appropriate for evaluation of new programs, has been selected (Hare, 1984; Higgonbotham and Cox, 1979). This "...phenomenological approach is concerned with everyday knowledge from the shared perceptions of particular respondent subgroups" (p. 418, Basch, 1987). Thus, this research methodology is consistent with the long-range strategy of NIDRR to promote participatory action research.

FIGURE 12–3
LIST OF ANTICIPATED OUTCOMES

No.	Outcome
1.	Knowledge about perceived problems in implementing ADA across stakeholder groups.
2.	Knowledge about actual problems in implementing ADA across stakeholder groups.
3.	Knowledge about solutions to perceived problems in implementing ADA.
4.	Knowledge about solutions to actual problems in implementing ADA.
5.	Guidance for providers and business people on implementation of employment-related aspects of ADA.

FIGURE 12–4
PRODUCTS TO BE DEVELOPED

Product	Description and Dissemination Target
Monograph "Self Study Guide to ADA"	A "user friendly", i.e., practical and readable, 75–100 page monograph portraying theviews of different stakeholder groups on ADA, developed from the research data. The "Self Study Guide" would also be application oriented, including specific comments about implications for each stakeholder group. Potential publisher: American Occupational Therapy Association. This product is targeted toward the involved stakeholder groups.
Journal publication	A scholarly article on the research and results from the focus groups would be submitted to *Archives of Physical Medicine and Rehabilitation.* This product is targeted toward the academic community.
Summary Sheets	These summary sheets will summarize the main points or findings of the research. It will be disseminated to the Justice Department and NIDRR-funded ADA projects, listed in Appendix B.

FIGURE 12–5
CONCEPTUAL MODEL OF THE INVESTIGATION

Data Collection	Data Interpretation	Generation of Hypotheses on Implementation of ADA	Theory Building on Implementation of ADA

Basch further states:

> Another example of how focus groups could be used...would be for studying implementation of innovative programs, which is of great importance and has been neglected. If effective, focus group interviews with various stakeholders could reveal important concerns and barriers to implementation that must be addressed if the program under study is to have an impact. Increasing...understanding of those who are responsible for policy, those responsible for implementation, and those who are the target populations...Group interviews could help to clarify the perspective of the various vested interest groups regarding many relevant issues: Reasons why change efforts are successful and unsuccessful, perceived barriers to change and ways to overcome barriers, and key concerns felt by various stakeholders at different stages of the change process that must be reconciled if progress is to continue (p. 438, Basch, 1987).

Furthermore, the precedent of using focus groups to study stakeholder views related to legislative mandate has already been set by Summers, Dell-Oliver, Turnball, Benson, Santelli, Campbell and Siegel-Causey (1990). They employed focus groups to study aspects of P. L. 94–457, specifically the Individualized Family Service Plan process. Additionally, research funded by the National Institute of Disability Research and Rehabilitation to further study the collaborative process between parents and professionals mandated by P. L. 94–457 using focus groups is currently under way in my project, codirected with Dr. Georgia DeGangi.

The focus group methodology was similarly used to identify feelings and perceptions of parents of medically fragile children (Diehl, Moffett, and Wade, 1991). This methodology, therefore, appears innovative yet reliable in revealing critically important information about participant groups' viewpoints affecting implementation of legislative mandate.

Thus, the current research will build upon these precedents by using focus groups to study stakeholder views regarding aspects of the ADA.

RESEARCH PLAN

Focus groups will be used to explore attitudes, experiences and anticipated problems regarding implementation of ADA. An advisory board of national experts has been gathered to guide the investigator during the year of fellowship study. The experts are listed with their respective area of expertise. Most communication with these experts will be by telephone, FAX and mail to keep costs low. As needed, however, meetings will be held with the two local advisors.

ADVISORY BOARD

John Baber, OTR, Employer Development Representative for Michigan Rehabilitation Services, 501 Municipal Office Center, 100 McMorran Blvd., Port Huron, MN 48060

Susan Pewitt, JD, OTR, Attorney in private practice and occupational therapy consultant to business and industry. Miami, FL

Wiley Borg, PhD, OTR, Specialist in Qualitative Research Methodology, Director of Education and Research, Occupational Therapy Section, Walter Reed Army Medical Center, Washington, DC 20307–5000

Jack Smith, M.Aud., CCC-A, Project Director, Communication Disabilities and the ADA: The A, B, C's. American Speech-Language-Hearing Association, Rockville, MD

STUDY ONE. PILOT STUDY

Summary. The purpose of Study One is to pilot the focus groups' material prior to actually conducting the focus groups with subjects. Additionally, a pretest of data collection methodology and provisional interpretation criteria will be accomplished during the pilot study. A questionnaire for obtaining information about participants' level of knowledge and experience with ADA will be pretested. A draft version of this questionnaire is included in Appendix C.

Research Questions: The research questions addressed in the focus groups will also be pretested and revised based upon feedback. The provisional questions for use in Study One were developed after personal communication with Judith Jurk and Barbara Kornblau, and are consistent with length and content recommendations for focus group methodology (Krueger, 1988), and are presented in Figure 12–6.

FIGURE 12–6
PROVISIONAL QUESTIONS FOR USE IN STUDY ONE

1. What is your vision of the employment section of the ADA?
2. What are anticipated beneficial effects of implementing the ADA?
3. What are perceived and actual problems with implementing the employment provision of ADA?
4. How can an employer determine essential job functions?
5. How can an employer appropriately ask about the ability of an applicant, who happens to be disabled, to do the job?
6. What is your interpretation of "reasonable accommodation"?
7. What is an example of "reasonable accommodation" an employer must provide someone who is handicapped?
8. What is your interpretation of "undue hardship"?
9. What is an example of "undue hardship" an employer could experience due to accommodating an individual who is handicapped?
10. What is the single biggest problem you see with ADA?
11. What three things can best facilitate implementation of ADA?
12. Is there anything else about ADA you wish to share?

Subjects: Personnel from the American Occupational Therapy Association will be used for the pilot study:[1]

- Jane Smith, Technology Program Manager
- Joe Brown, Pediatric Program Manager
- Linda Green, Director of Division of Continuing Education
- Sue Jones, Geriatric Program Manager
- Anne Kline, President-Elect, AOTA

1. It is acknowledged that a hallmark of focus group methodology, use of strangers as group participants, will be violated by using personnel from one agency for the pilot study (Krueger, 1988). Since this meeting is a pilot study to evaluate procedures and questions, however, this violation of assumptions is deemed acceptable.

- Molly White, Director of Professional Practice
- Larry Katz, Program Manager of Legislative Affairs

Procedures. The pilot focus group will meet during the third month of the project at the American Occupational Therapy Association. The focus group will be scheduled for three hours and be run by the principal investigator. The first part of the focus group will consist of a presentation on the nature and plan of the project. The second part of the focus group will consist of asking the participants to react to the proposed research questions and issues and to generate additional research questions and issues deemed appropriate. A sample script and Participant Field Note Form is included in Appendix D.

Data Collection Methods: The entire meeting will be taped and transcribed. Additionally, participants will be asked to write out any recommendations they have about the focus group's at the end of the pilot study. Dr. Matin Royeen, a specialist in group dynamics and cross-cultural counseling, will serve as cofacilitator during this and all subsequent focus groups.

Data Analysis and Criteria for Interpretation: Recommendations of the focus groups members will be analyzed using criteria of (1) consistency with intent of the research, (2) consistency with procedures of focus groups, and (3) practicality. If these criteria are met, then the recommendations will be incorporated.

Revision. The script, including the questions, for the focus group will be revised. Data collection sheets will also be revised. Revised materials will be sent to the Advisory Board for review and confirmation.

STUDIES TWO, THREE, FOUR AND FIVE. FOCUS GROUPS WITH VESTED STAKEHOLDERS

Summary. The purpose of Studies Two, Three and Four is to collect data from vested stakeholders, i.e., business and industry representatives, individuals who are disabled, providers of services to the disabled, on their respective views and visions of the ADA.

Research Questions: The research questions addressed by this study are "What are the differing views and expectations of those affected by the ADA?" The revised research questions developed in the pilot study will be used in the focus groups. Additionally, at the end of each focus group participants will be asked to rank the three most important issues or ideas from each question. This is an innovation in focus group methodology which has been successfully developed during my current NIDRR-funded project and which guides interpretation of the importance of the issues.

Subjects: Three main subject groups will be used. They are listed below:

I. Representatives from national associations that provide services to the disabled

- American Occupational Therapy Association
- American Physical Therapy Association
- American Speech-Language-Hearing Association
- American Association of Rehabilitation Specialists
- American Psychological Association
- American Association of Psychiatrists
- RESNA

II. Representatives from national consumer associations, i.e., associations that represent groups of individuals who are disabled:

- United Cerebral Palsy
- Epilepsy Foundation
- Paralyzed Veterans Association

III. Consumers directly affected by ADA, i.e., individuals who are disabled. These individuals will be solicited with the cooperation of

- American Retarded Citizens Association
- United Cerebral Palsy
- American Occupational Therapy Association
- American Physical Therapy Association
- National Rehabilitation Hospital

IV. Representatives from Business and Industry.

- International Association of Machinists
- National Restaurant Association
- American Hotel and Motel Association

Demographic data will be collected on each participant, including their knowledge of and experience with ADA, through the pretest questionnaire. The demographic and experience data will assist in grounding interpretation of the data to the unique experience of the subjects.

Procedures: Each focus group will consist of 6 to 10 subjects (Krueger, 1988), from one of the four main stakeholder groups. As recommended by focus group methodology, the groups will be homogeneous and individuals from differing stakeholder groups will not be mixed. This facilitates disclosure among participants. Focus groups will be scheduled during the sixth to tenth months of the project. The focus group will be scheduled for three hours and be run by the principal investigator. A detailed script of how to run the focus groups, as developed from the pilot study, will structure them. Generally, though, the first part of the focus group will consist of a presentation on the nature and plan of the project. The second part of the focus group will consist of asking the participants to respond to the questions posed. Focus groups will be held at the American Occupational Therapy Association or at a centrally located region in downtown Washington, D.C.

Data Collection Methods: The entire meeting will be audiotaped for transcription. Additionally, participants will be asked to complete a Participant Field Note Form (See Appendix D).

Data Analysis and Criteria for Interpretation: A summary view of the data analysis plan is presented here. More detail can be found in Appendix E. Comments from each focus group member will be analyzed accordingly to standard methodology (Krueger, 1988; Miles and Huberman, 1984) in the following manner:

1. Data verification and clean-up of transcribed tapes.
2. Analysis of demographic data of subjects using descriptive statistics and prose summaries.
3. Content analysis of recurring themes, patterns and issues using logical interpretation of the data.

4. Frequency analysis of themes and issues.
5. Importance of themes and issues analyzed by logical interpretation.
6. Descriptive statistics on ranking of issues by participants.
7. Data interpretation summary and hypotheses generation.
8. Validity and reliability check of the data. Data interpretation will be submitted to group participants for review and comment. This step helps to assure the validity and reliability of the data.

   In order to obtain information regarding the robustness of these findings related to other stakeholder groups, as well as its trustworthiness overall (Guba, 1981; Kreftig, 1991), the findings will also be submitted to the following groups for review and comment:

   1. Job Accommodation Network of America, Inc. 800-526-7234
   2. Project Officer, NIDRR
   3. President's Committee on Employment of People with Disabilities, 1111 20th Street, NW, Ste 636, Washington, DC 20036–3470. (202) 635-5044

9. Incorporation of participants' comments and data interpretation revision.
10. Data interpretation summary.
11. Data interpretation format for use in subsequent focus groups. This is a form of constant/comparative data analysis which allows for increased validity of the research.
12. Comparison and contrast of findings across all four focus groups.

DISSEMINATION

Please refer to Figure 12–4 for specification of the products to be developed, including development of a "Self Study Guide to Implementing ADA"

The finished manuscript will be complete with "mini-assessments" which assist the reader in directly linking the material to his or her situation.

Formative Evaluation: Included in the first 500 copies of the "Self Study Guide to Implementing ADA" will be an evaluation and a stamped, preprinted envelope to return the evaluation to the publisher. The formative evaluation data will be analyzed and any necessary changes made in the "Self Study Guide to Implementing ADA." Revisions will be made and a second version of the "Self Study Guide to Implementing ADA" printed. The formative evaluation would be negotiated with the publisher as an author contract condition.

DEVELOPMENT OF THE SUMMARY SHEETS

Summary sheets, similar to a "user-friendly" executive summary, will be developed. It is anticipated that there will be four summary sheets (one per stakeholder group) and an overall summary sheet, making a complete set of five. These will be mailed to the project directors listed in Appendix B.

DEVELOPMENT OF THE JOURNAL ARTICLE

The Editor of *Archives of Physical Medicine and Rehabilitation* will be contacted to discuss possible article submission and to solicit any editorial recommendations. An article will be drafted and submitted.

CONFERENCE PRESENTATION

A paper will be submitted on the fellowship research for presentation at the Research Forum of the American Occupational Therapy Association Annual Conference for 1993 in Seattle, Washington. A schematic of the timeline is presented in Figure 12–7.

FIGURE 12–7
PROPOSED TIMELINE

Mo	Action
1	Submit research plan to advisory board for review and comment.
2	Finalize research plan based upon feedback.
2	Contact target organizations to recruit subjects for Studies Two, Three and Four.
3	Conduct pilot study.
3/4	Conduct data analysis of pilot study and revise materials as needed.
4	Conduct Study Two.
4	Conduct preliminary data analysis/interpretation of Study Two.
5	Conduct Study Three.
6	Conduct preliminary data analysis/interpretation of Study Three.
6	Conduct Study Four.
6	Conduct preliminary data analysis/interpretation of Study Four.
7	Conduct data analysis/interpretation across all studies.
7	Submit preliminary analysis/interpretation to advisory board and external reviewers.
8	Revise based upon feedback.
9	Finalize data analysis and interpretation.
10/11	Prepare conference presentation.
10/11	Prepare Self Study Guide to ADA. Review and comment by advisory board. Render final draft.
10/11	Prepare journal article. Review and comment by advisory board. Render final draft.
10/11	Prepare summary sheets. Review and comment by advisory board. Render final draft.
12	Prepare final report.

REFERENCES

Americans With Disabilities Act of 1990 (P. L. 101–336), 42 U.S.C., 12101.

Basch, C. E. (1987). Focus group interview: An under-utilized research technique for improving theory and practice in health education. *Health Education Quarterly,* Vol. 14, No. 4, 411–448.

Diehl, S. F., Moffett, K. A., & Wade, S. M. (1991). Focus group interviews with parents of children with medically complex needs. *Children's Health Care,* Vol. 20, No. 3, 170–178.

Glaser, B. G., & Strauss, A. L. (1966). The purpose and credibility of qualitative research. *Nursing Research,* Vol. 15, No. 1, 56–61.

Glaser, B. G., & Strauss, A. L. (1967). *The discovery of grounded theory: Strategies for qualitative research.* New York: Aldine Publishing Company.

Guba, E. G. (1981). Criteria for assessing the trustworthiness of naturalistic inquiries. *Educational Communication and Technology Journal,* Vol. 29, No. 2, 75–91.

Hare, R. D. (1984). The focused group interview: An examination of the use of a research method. University of Michigan International Dissertation Services, Ann Arbor, MI.

Higgonbotham, J. P., & Cox, K. K. (1979). *Focus group interviews: A reader.* Chicago: American Marketing Association.

Hutchinson, S. (1985). Chapter 6, "Grounded Theory: The Method." In *Qualitative approaches in nursing research.* New York: Grune and Stratton.

Jurk, J. K. (1991). The Americans With Disabilities Act: An opportunity to link occupational therapy with business and industry. *Physical Disabilities Special Interest Section Newsletter,* Vol. 14, No. 3, 1–2.

Kreftig, L. (1991). Rigor in qualitative research: The assessment of trustworthiness. *American Journal of Occupational Therapy,* Vol. 45, No. 3, 214–222.

Krueger, R. A. (1988). *Focus groups: A practical guide for applied research.* Newbury Park, CA: Sage Publishing Co.

Miles, M. B., & Huberman, A. M. (1984). *Qualitative data analysis: A summary of new methods.* Beverly Hills, CA: Sage Publishing Co.

Simms, L. M. (1981). The grounded theory approach in nursing research. *Nursing Research,* Vol. 30, No. 6, 356–359.

Summers, J. A., Dell-Oliver, C., Turnball, A. P., Benson, H. A., Santelli, E., Campbell, M., & Siegel-Causey, E. (1990). Examining the Individualized Family Service Plan process: What are family and practitioner preferences? *Topics in Early Childhood Education,* Vol. 10, No. 1, 79–100.

THE MANAGEMENT PLAN

Once you have specified how you will conduct your research, you need to describe, through prose, charts and graphs, how you will manage or administrate the investigation. The **management plan** should address how the overall project will be supervised; it should clearly show who will do what and when. One common method of identifying who will do what when is through a chart presenting key project personnel and their job responsibilities. Figure 12–8 contains such a chart (DeGangi & Royeen, 1990), which shows the percentage of time key project personnel will devote to the project. It also gives a brief description of their qualifications and job responsibilities.

FIGURE 12–8

Key Project Personnel

	Qualifications, Time and Job Requirements		
Position	**FTE**	**Qualifications**	**Job Responsibilities**
Coprincipal Investigator, Georgia DeGangi, Ph.D.	15%	Registered Occupational Therapist Doctor of Philosophy Research Psychologist Expertise in clinical assessment Expertise in research, psychometrics and teaching	Design and implementation of research Supervision of project staff Data Analysis and evaluation of project
Co principal Investigator, Charlotte Royeen, Ph.D.	15%	Registered Occupational Therapist Doctor of Philosophy Administrator Research Analyst Computer Specialist	Development and implementation of data collection Design of research Data Analysis and evaluation Dissemination of results
Project Coordinator, Albert Berkowitz, Ed.D.	60%	Doctor of Education Educational Psychologist Expertise in administrative functions Trainer and editor	Supervision of project staff Coordination of project activities Administration of subject selection, materials development and project evaluation
Assessment Specialist, Shirley Wietlisbach	50%	Registered Occupational Therapist Expertise with learning-disabled youngsters Master of Science	Assessment of study subjects, including selection/development of measures coordination of assessments, intervention recommendations, and data collection

Figure 12–9 (DeGangi & Royeen, 1991) presents what is called a person loading chart (PLC). The PLC here shows the number of days each person will devote to the proposed project tasks in a calendar year. A PLC is often required by funding agencies in proposals.

The research management plan should also give the conceptual basis for project administration, usually in prose format. Most funding agencies require you to present a plan that addresses how the overall project will be evaluated. Example 4 shows an evaluation plan submitted in a recent research grant application.

FIGURE 12–9

Person Loading Chart

(Days of Effort for Year One)

Personnel	Subject Select/ Assessment	Devel of Material	Data Collect	Data Analysis	Dissemination	Project Evaluation	Total Year
Georgia DeGangi, Ph.D., Co-Principal Investigator				15	9	15	39
Charlotte Royeen, Ph.D., Co-Principal Investigator	9	8		13		10	39
Albert Berkowitz, Ed.D., Project Coordinator	10	10	30	15	40	40	156
Shirley Wietlisbach, M.S., Assessment Specialist	19	60	40	20			130

EXAMPLE 4

Evaluation Plan

The Evaluation Plan consists of three mechanisms: (1) review and feedback from experts and OSEP project officer, (2) formative evaluation, and (3) summative evaluation. These mechanisms of evaluation are explained below and detailed in Figure 12–10.

Review and Feedback

Expert review and feedback will be derived from meetings with the National Advisory Board, Local Advisory Board and the OSEP project officer as described in detail in the Management Plan section of this proposal.

Formative Evaluation

Formative evaluation will be achieved using criterion- or objective-based evaluation. The mechanisms for criterion evaluation of the programmatic research are (1) administrative review on the part of the co-principal investigators regarding adherence to timelines, (2) determination of accomplishment of project goals and objectives, and (3) semiannual self-study sessions. Evaluation procedures to assist informative evaluation are presented in Figure 12–10.

Administrative review based upon timeline management will allow for identification completion or slippage of project tasks. The project secretary will monitor this process under supervision of the co-principal investigators.

Determination of accomplishment of project goals and objectives will be achieved using monthly reports. Each participating staff member will submit monthly summaries of progress to date regarding their work related to project goals and objectives. Additionally, staff will be requested to identify anticipated future problems which may hinder accomplishment of their project tasks in the future one to two months. In this way, the co-principal investigators may be able to identify and solve project problems before they actually occur.

In the semiannual self-study sessions, the co-principal investigators will meet for one full day to review and discuss progress and accomplishments to date of the programmatic research, as well as monitor and check implementation of the dissemination plan detailed earlier in the management plan. The co-principal investigators will use evaluation questions delineated by Royeen (1989) and

FIGURE 12–10
EVALUATION PLAN

Evaluation Area	Evaluation Questions	Evaluation Scores
Project Management and Administration	How successfully does the project adhere to the timeline?	Review of management plan on a monthly basis to document achievement of activities and to establish plan for achieving upcoming activities.
	How successfully does the project complete its objectives?	Documentation of the number of completed activities and the date on which they were completed. Documentation of the number of activities adjusted or added objectives. Documentation of the dates on which the adjusted activities were accomplished.
Project Impact	What was the overall impact of the project on researchers and practitioners?	Documentation of the numbers of individuals and organizations who have requested information and/or who have attended presentations and sessions. Records of people requesting information. Questionnaires distributed to all individuals/organizations to whom training manuals were distributed.

apply them to each separate study of the programmatic research as the foundation for each self-study analysis.

SUMMATIVE EVALUATION

Summative project evaluation will be accomplished using outcome evaluation applied to each specified study of the plan of research. Outcome evaluation will be the primary responsibility of one co-principal investigator (Dr. Royeen) and will be based upon the empirically derived qualitative and quantitative data the different research studies will yield.

In this chapter I described the process of putting together a research proposal and gave descriptions and examples of the components of a research proposal. This chapter was not meant to take you through the process of actually writing such a proposal, but should give you an idea of the information you would need to gather and the steps you would have to take to write a proposal. Knowing what is involved in the process should help you if you decide to conduct an investigation; and knowing the process should also enhance your understanding as a research consumer.

References

DeGangi, G. A., & Royeen, C. B. (1990). *Investigating the Individual Family Service Plan.* Submitted in the Field Initiated Research Competition. National Institute of Disability Research and Rehabilitation.

DeGangi, G. A., & Royeen, C. B. (1991). Submitted to the U.S. Department of Education.

Miles, M. B., & Huberman, A. M. (1994). (2nd Ed.). *An expanded sourcebook: Qualitative data analysis.* CA: Sage.

Royeen, C. B. (1992). *Prospectus for educational research in occupational therapy.* Unpublished manuscript.

Royeen, C. B., & Berkowitz, E. (1990). *Prospectus for a study on parent–professional collaboration.* Unpublished manuscript.

Recommended Readings

Stein, F. (1989). *Anatomy of clinical research* (Appendix A.7). Thorofare, NJ: Slack.

Burns, N., & Grove, S. K. (1987). *The practice of nursing: Conduct, critique and utilization* (pp. 363–382). Philadelphia: W. B. Saunders.

CHAPTER 13 Where Do You Go From Here?

KEY WORDS

Concurrent validity
Domain specification
Effectiveness
Efficacy
Efficiency
Journal club
Peer review
Replication
Research profile

You have now completed 12 chapters of this book; and you should have the foundation skills to be a research consumer—an increasingly important focus for therapists (Domholdt & Malone, 1985). Having learned the basics of reading and understanding research literature, you are now ready to proceed to the next step. So, where do you go from here?

How do you continue as you finish this book? And how do you grow beyond the level of a research consumer? How do you become a participant in the exciting process of research? These questions will be addressed in chapter 13 of this research primer. Ideas for sustaining your interest and participating as a research consumer after completing this book will be put forth in the form of action plans. Approximately half of the action plans focus on things that research consumers can do. The second half of the action plans present feasible research ideas for the beginning research practitioner.

For even though it was stated in chapter 1 that this book will only train you as a research consumer, this is the perfect opportunity for me to identify for you things you could realistically do to contribute to the practice of research. Now, look at the action plans, consider what interests you, and decide which of them you wish to pursue. Pick and choose the action plan(s) that best

FIGURE 13–1. REVIEWING RESEARCH ARTICLES (ABBREVIATED VERSION)

Author(s): ______________________________

____

Publication: ______________________________

Date: ______________________________

Volume, pages: ______________________________

____

Problem addressed:

____

____

____

Theoretical/Conceptual basis:

____

____

____

Research plan or design:

____

____

____

Sample:

____

____

____

Variables:

____

____

____

Findings:

____

____

____

Limitations:

____

____

Applications:

____

____

____

____

Note. This format was developed and used for the article, "Use of Neurodevelopmental Treatment as an Intervention: Annotated Listing of Studies 1980-1990" (Royeen & DeGangi, 1992). Used with permission.

fits your time, money, and interests. But do select at least one of them to continue your participation as a therapist committed to research.

Action Plans for the Research Consumer

ACTION PLAN 1: DEVELOP A RESEARCH PROFILE

What is your special area of interest? Is there something in your clinical practice that especially intrigues you? Are you certified in sensory integration testing and diagnosis or neurodevelopmental treatment? Are you apt in technology? Think a moment and select an area that interests you. This can serve as the foundation of a **research profile** you develop. Now that you have selected the topic area, carefully monitor your professional literature for articles related to that topic. Each time a research article is published, read it and carefully interpret it using the interpretation questions used throughout this book. Or if you are beginning to feel more of an expert in using that questionnaire, you may prefer to use the abbreviated version provided in Figure 13–1.

Following are reviews of neurodevelopmental treatment intervention studies by me and Georgia DeGangi that appeared in *Perceptual and Motor Skills.* Review the following examples and complete the abbreviated questionnaire.

Reprinted from *Perceptual and Motor Skills,* *75,* pp. 175–194. Used with permission.

ILLUSTRATIVE EXAMPLE 13–1

Use of Neurodevelopmental Treatment as an Intervention: Annotated Listing of Studies 1980–1990[1]

Charlotte Brasic Royeen and Georgia A. DeGangi
Reginald S. Lourie Center for Infants and Young Children, Rockville, MD

Neurodevelopmental treatment (NDT) is a technique originally developed by the Bobaths (Bobath, 1967, 1980; Valvano & Long, 1991) specifically to enhance large motor skills, balance, quality of movement, hand use, eye-hand coordination, self-care skills, and perceptual skills of those with movement disorders. Such therapy typically consists of direct physical handling techniques, parental education, home or classroom programming, and a positioning program for daily care and functional activities. Physical handling is directed towards developing the components of movement that underlie functional motor performance (i.e., neuromotor maturation, balance, postural alignment and stability, mobility skills, weight bearing, and weight shifting). This approach is widely used by physical and occupational therapists, speech and language therapists, and educators in the habilitation and rehabilitation of infants, toddlers, and children having cerebral palsy (d'Avignon, 1981; Gorga, 1989; Kluzik, Fetters, & Coryell, 1990; Laskas, Mullen, Nelson, &

1. Address correspondence to Georgia DeGangi, Reginald S. Lourie Center for Infants and Young Children, 11710 Hunters Lane, Rockville, MD 20852.

Willson-Broyles, 1985), Down syndrome (Harris, 1981a, 1981b), developmental delay, or a high-risk profile (Goodman, Rothberg, Houston-McMillan, Cooper, Cartwright, & Van Der Velde, 1985; Piper, Kunos, Willis, Mazer, Ramsay, & Silver, 1986; Piper, Mazer, Silver, & Ramsay, 1988).

In spite of the widespread use of NDT treatment in pediatric and adult rehabilitation and educational settings, evidence of its effectiveness is inconclusive (Ottenbacher, Biocca, DeCremer, Gevelinger, Jedlovec, & Johnson, 1986; Palisano, 1991; Parette & Hourcade, 1984; Parette, Hendricks, & Rock, 1991; Stern & Gorga, 1988). To understand better the scope of the related literature, a research synthesis was commissioned by the NeuroDevelopmental Treatment Association, Inc., and conducted on NDT literature published in peer-reviewed journals for the period 1980-1990. Literature was identified through a comprehensive literature search which included a computerized Medline search. A panel of 16 physical and occupational therapists serving on the NDTA Research committee reviewed the listing of literature for its comprehensiveness, adding articles that had been omitted. Detailed information on the research synthesis can be found elsewhere (Royeen & DeGangi, 1992). Review of all published literature during this time period (41 articles) yielded some interesting phenomena.

First, only one quantitatively based literature review existed. Ottenbacher, et. al. (1986) conducted a quantitative literature review (meta-analysis) on the use of NDT procedures with a pediatric population. Statistical analysis showed that the effect size for NDT intervention is small because samples are small, changes in quality of movement and posture are difficult to measure, and research designs lack rigorous control. Their findings suggest that those pediatric clients receiving NDT-based treatment or some combination of NDT and other related therapy performed better than about 62.2% of the subjects who did not receive such services.

Second, qualitative literature reviews on NDT-based treatment were many (Harris, 1988; Hourcade & Parette, 1984; Keshner, 1981; Olney, 1990). In fact, almost one-quarter of all NDT-related literature published in peer-reviewed journals during 1980–1990 were qualitative literature reviews on effectiveness of NDT procedures. Such a high percentage of qualitative literature reviews suggests great interest in and controversy over this treatment.

Third, there appeared to be pervasive flaws in research design and implementation throughout the experimentally based literature. And, the prevalence of such flaws could account, in our opinion, for the inconsistent nature of the findings on effectiveness.

The call for more rigor in research on effectiveness (Harris, 1988; Olney, 1990) requires an understanding of the strengths and limitations of existing literature on the topic. An annotated listing of NDT-related research on effectiveness, therefore, is critically important for research investigators and program developers.

The annotated listing presented in this article represents 19 of the 41 studies from the medical, therapy, and special education literature using experimental designs. Only those articles presenting experimentally based research were included. They fell in the three categories of experimental research, single-subject experiments, and quasi-experimental research.

Illustrative Example 13–1. Annotation

I. EXPERIMENTAL RESEARCH

Basmajian, J. V., Gowland, C. A. Finlayson, A. J., Hall, A. L., Swanson, L. R., Stratford, M. S., Trotter, J. E., & Brandstater, M. E. (1987). Stroke treatment: Comparison of integrated behavioral-physical therapy vs traditional physical therapy programs. *Archives of Physical Medicine and Rehabilitation, 68,* 267–272.

Problem: What are the relative effects of an NDT-based physical therapy intervention program compared to a program of behavioral and cognitive training in the rehabilitation of stroke victims?

Theoretical/Conceptual Basis: This study sought to examine the effectiveness of therapeutic exercise with the hemiplegic upper limb.

Plan/Design: A pretest-posttest randomized clinical trial was used. Treatment was over a 5-week period, 3 times weekly for 45 minutes per session. Treatment A was cognitively based including biofeedback and cognitive training. Treatment B was NDT-based physical therapy. Measures consisted of the Upper Extremity Function Tests, the Finger Oscillation Tests, the Health Belief Survey, the Beck Depression Inventory.

Sample: 29 subjects, 19 men and 10 women, ranging in age from 30 to 79 years. Severity of stroke was controlled. Subjects were well defined.

Variables: The independent variable was type of intervention. The dependent variables were upper extremity function and emotional/social status.

Findings: Repeated-measures analysis of variance indicated significant effects from therapies but no difference between therapies. Both interventions were effective, but one was not more effective than the other.

Limitations: Numerous statistical tests were conducted when the total sample size was only 29. Also, multivariate techniques assume characteristics of data which were not confirmed.

Applications: This paper suggests the effectiveness of NDT-based therapy as well as of a cognitively based therapy for assisting in the rehabilitation of stroke victims. The authors include a description of how they monitored therapy to assure the validity of the two different interventions which is often lacking in most research articles. Although no measures of reliability and validity of assessment of therapist's compliance with each therapeutic approach were reported, the fact that compliance was attempted is important.

D'Avignon, M. (1981). Early physiotherapy *ad modum* Vojta or Bobath in infants with suspected neuromotor disturbance. *Neuropediatrics, 12,* 232–241.

Problem: What are the relative effects of Vojta and Bobath based treatments in early intervention?

Theoretical/Conceptual Basis: The authors stated that there are relatively few data on the relative effects of different types of physical therapy for infants suspected of having cerebral palsy.

Plan/Design: This study's design is loosely based upon a pretest, posttest, control group design.

Sample: Subjects from the participating physicians' clinics were selected using Vojta principles (age less than six months, primitive reflexes, and six pathological postural reflexes). These criteria diagnostic standards were double checked using blind evaluators. Subjects were randomly assigned to Vojta or Bobath treatment groups. A third group of subjects for control were obtained from another clinic.

Variables: The independent variables were treatment condition (Vojta, Bobath, or none). The dependent variables were motor performance as assessed by physicians.

Findings: Simple frequency counts were used in analysis. No statistically significant difference between the treatment groups was reported. The control group was judged by the author to give an invalid comparison.

Limitations: It is difficult to evaluate the study since the reader does not know how children were evaluated for outcome measures.

Applications: The authors identify the need to consider the implications of early intervention on the family.

Harris, S. R. (1981). Effects of neurodevelopmental therapy on motor performance of infants with Down's syndrome. *Developmental Medicine and Child Neurology, 23,* 477–483.

Hypothesis: Infants with Down syndrome will show significantly greater motor gains than infants not receiving NDT.

Theoretical/Conceptual Basis: This investigation studied the effects of NDT on motor and mental processes in a sample of infants having Down syndrome.

Plan/Design: This was a pretest, posttest, two-group design. Infants were pretested with the Bayley Scales of Infant Development (standardized forms of mental and motor) and the Peabody Developmental Motor Scales (nonstandardized). Also, four individualized therapy goals were written for each infant and were NDT-oriented. Subjects were randomly assigned to groups. Therapy lasted for nine weeks. Blind evaluators rated whether subjects met objectives. All treatment was delivered at home except for one subject receiving therapy at the school. Therapy sessions were approximately 40 minutes, three times weekly for nine weeks. The control group received their usual, weekly infant learning program. Description of the therapy delivered in NDT terms is provided.

Sample: Twenty infants, aged 2.7 to 21.5 months, with Down syndrome participated. Of these, 18 subjects were from an educational center associated with the University of Washington. Two additional subjects were from a similar program. This was essentially a sample of convenience. Subjects were randomly assigned to groups. Statistical analyses of groups prior to intervention gave no significant differences.

Variables: Intervention (treatment group and no treatment group) was the independent variable and posttest measures from the Peabody and Bayley were the dependent measures.

Findings: Interrater reliability was 100% for evaluation of subjects' objectives or individualized therapy goals. There was no statistically significant difference between groups on the Bayley or the Peabody. The NDT treatment group attained more objectives than the control group at a statistically significant rate.

Limitations: Generalizability is limited due to restricted, nonrandom sampling. Replication can provide insight into generalizability. Use of multiple t tests increased likelihood of a Type I error.

Applications: Individualized objectives might more likely show effectiveness of NDT intervention than the Bayley and Peabody standardized scores.

Harris, S. R. (1981). Physical therapy and infants with Down's syndrome: The effects of early intervention. *Rehabilitation Literature, 42,* 339–343.

Problem: The author explored the effectiveness of NDT with infants and toddlers having Down syndrome.

Theoretical/Conceptual Basis: The first part of this article provided a justification and rationale for using NDT with children having Down syndrome. The second part of the article was a brief report on a research investigation into NDT with infants having Down syndrome.

Plan/Design: A pretest, posttest, two-group design was used (experimental and control). Subjects were blocked on the variables of age, sex, and pretest scores and were then randomly assigned to groups. Groups were then randomly assigned to treatment conditions. For nine weeks the treatment group received home-based, individualized NDT programs three times per week for 40 minutes from a registered physical therapist. The control group received no special intervention. Both groups continued in a weekly infant program at the center. At the onset of the study, infants were pretested. After pretesting, four individualized and behavioral measurable objectives were generated for each subject.

Sample: Twenty infants from a center at the author's university participated in the study. Infants ranged in age from 2.7 mo. to 21.5 mo. Eleven were female and nine were male.

Variables: Infants were pretested on the Bayley Scales of Infant Development and the Peabody Developmental Motor Scales. The dependent measures were attainment of the individualized objectives, and the standardized test scores on the posttest.

Findings: Percentages of individualized goals achieved by group are reported (experimental reached 80% of objectives whereas control group reached 57.5% of objectives). The author reported a significant difference between groups ($p<.05$), but none on pre- and posttest standardized scores.

Interpretation of Findings: The author states that the findings "... lend support to the hypothesis that neurodevelopmental therapy will improve motor performance in infants with Down's syndrome" (p. 342). The author further suggests that the lack of between-group differences on standardized testing may result from (1) small sample, (2) short intervention period, and (3) inability of these tests to measure motor changes with this population.

Limitations: The design would improve if the control group received some sort of intervention rather than contrasting therapy with no therapy. There was no control for the effect of home-based intervention, that is, this study may support inclusion of home setting as much as support of NDT. A sample of convenience, in spite of random assignment to groups, limits generalizability. Inadequate specification of procedures in analysis limits analysis of observations.

Applications: The study does provide preliminary evidence that a home-based program of NDT for infants with Down syndrome will help in attainment of individualized objectives.

Jenkins, J. R., Sells, C. J., Brady, D., Down, J., Moore, B., Carman, P., & Holm, R. (1982). Effects of developmental therapy on motor impaired children. *Physical and Occupational Therapy in Pediatrics, 2,* 19–28.

Problem: The problem addressed is the lack of data on effectiveness of therapy services.

Theoretical/Conceptual Basis: There is a lack of empirical data from well-controlled studies regarding effectiveness of physical and occupational therapy services for children having motor delays.

Play/Design: A pretest, posttest, three-group, experimental design was used. Subjects were assessed prior to intervention and after 15 weeks of intervention. Examiners were blind to the severity of subjects' delay as well as to the treatment condition assigned. The following measurements were used: Pediatric Screening Tool (PS) for evaluation of the need for services in the public schools, the Peabody Developmental Motor Scales, and an instrument designed specifically for this study to assess quality of movement of basic motor activities. Subjects were randomly assigned to one of three groups: (1) therapy one day per week, (2) therapy three days per week, and (3) no therapy. Fifteen subjects were assigned to each group, controlling for severity of need for therapy. Each therapy session lasted 40 minutes and was individually provided. Therapy consisted of a "combination of procedures drawn from sensory integrative therapy and from neurodevelopmental therapy…" (p. 14). Two occupational therapists and one physical therapist provided the interventions.

Sample: No information about the total possible sample provided (subjects used were a sample of convenience from an educational program associated with the University of Washington). A total of 112 children were screened using the Pediatric Screening Tool for possible inclusion in the study. The 45 subjects in this study had to score about 40 on the Pediatric Screening Tool and be judged by a pediatrician and a therapist to be motor delayed. Subjects with known disorders such as muscular dystrophy and cerebral palsy were excluded.

Subjects ranged in age from 3 to 15 years. IQs ranged from 35 to 116; 19 were mentally retarded, 6 were also diagnosed as autistic, and 20 had severe communication problems.

Variables: Independent variables were frequency of therapy and presence or absence of therapy. Dependent variables were subjects' performance on posttest measures of motor performance.

Findings: On the Peabody Developmental Motor Scales, treatment groups performed significantly better than control on gross motor functions but not on fine motor. All groups made significant improvement in quality of postural responses posttest, but no differences between groups noted. Frequency of therapy did not affect outcome. Therapy one time per week appeared to be as effective as therapy offered three times per week.

Limitations: The investigators assumed that physical therapy and occupational therapy are the same intervention, "developmental therapy" (p. 24). The investigator assumed that NDT and sensory integration are provided in the same manner by physical and occupational therapists. The actual interventions are inadequately described. Since the control group received no intervention, the design could have been significantly strengthened by offering them some sort of intervention like a regular gym class. The generalizability of findings is questionable due to lack of random sampling.

Applications: This study documented significant improvement in gross motor skills for both treatment groups. The basic design appears solid and could serve as a foundation for replication studies.

Mulder, T., Hulstijn, W., & Van Der Meer, J. (1986). EMG feedback and the restoration of motor control. *American Journal of Physical Medicine, 65,* 173–188.

Problem: The relative effectiveness of EMG vs NDT techniques for improving dorsiflexion of the foot of hemiparetic subjects was investigated.

Theoretical/Conceptual Basis: None was specified.

Plan/Design: Training lasted five weeks, three times per week. Subjects were randomly assigned to one of the two treatment conditions (EMG vs NDT). Measures of range of motion, EMG activity, and gait velocity pre- and posttest were made.

Sample: Twelve subjects aged 34 to 68 years participated. All subjects had previously received unsuccessful rehabilitation for foot dorsiflexion.

Variables: The independent variable was treatment condition. The dependent variable was dorsiflexion of the foot as measured by gait, EMG, and range of motion.

Findings: Only on the measurement of EMG did the NDT subjects perform better than the EMG feedback group. The authors concluded that there was no significant difference between the two methods.

Limitations: The NDT treatment was not described.

Applications: The authors identified the fact that the long time span needed for recovery influences research using a short-term model.

Palmer, F. B., Shapiro, B. K., Wachtel, R. C., Allen, M. C., Hiller, J. E., Harryman, S. E., Mosher, B. S., Meinert, C. L., & Capute, A. J. (1988). The effects of physical therapy on cerebral palsy. *Physical Therapy and Cerebral Palsy, 318,* 803–808.

Problem: This study investigated NDT-based physical therapy as compared to a program of infant stimulation for infants having cerebral palsy.

Theoretical/Conceptual Basis: There is little research using clinical trials to investigate the effectiveness of NDT-based physical therapy with children who have cerebral palsy.

Plan/Design: Infants (n = 48) were assigned to a random order of Group A (NDT-based physical therapy) and to Group B (infant stimulation). Therapy was done for six months, and infants were followed up after one year. Infants were assessed pre- and posttest on a variety of measures. The NDT group had lower mean motor and mental scores on standardized tests.

Sample: Infants aged 12 to 19 months coming to the Kennedy Institute for Handicapped Children served as subjects. Enrollment criteria were delineated; all subjects were diagnosed spastic diplegia.

Variables: The independent variable was type of treatment. Dependent variables were motor and mental skills.

Findings: Infants receiving stimulation performed significantly better than those receiving NDT-based therapy. Evidence for effectiveness of NDT-based physical therapy was not found.

Limitations: The therapy provided was not described adequately. Reliabilities of the nonstandardized measures were not provided, so measurement of status and change were thereby compromised. Equivalency of groups at onset may have been compromised, with the NDT group being more neurologically involved.

Applications: Use of nonparametric statistics was exemplary.

Piper, M. C., Kunos, I., Willis, D. M., Mazer, B. L., Ramsay, D. P., & Silver, K. M. (1986). Early physical therapy effects on the high-risk infant: a randomized control trial. *Pediatrics, 78,* 216–224.

Problem: The primary research question addressed differences, if any, appearing at age one year between a group of high-risk infants who received NDT-based physical therapy intervention compared to a group of infants who did not receive such intervention.

Theoretical/Conceptual Basis: The lack of research documenting the effectiveness of physical therapy, and NDT-based therapy specifically, prompted conduct of this study. The authors maintain that early NDT-oriented physical therapy is almost routinely offered to high-risk infants without a data base to support the action.

Plan/Design: A two-group, pretest, posttest, quasi-experimental design was used. Infants were assessed prior to intervention to stratify their random assignment to groups. Groups were compared on 25 independent variables to assure comparability of groups. Intervention consisted of weekly NDT-oriented physical therapy for the first three months and biweekly for the subsequent nine months. For the first 30 minutes of each session, treatment of the infant involved direct contact; in the last 30 minutes demonstration and instruction to parents were given. It appears that the same physical therapist delivered all treatment but this is not clear. Measures employed for evaluation at 12 months (corrected for prematurity) were Wolanski Gross Motor Evaluation, Wilson Developmental Reflex Profile, Milani-Comparetti

Motor Development Screening Test, Griffiths Mental Development Scale, and Neurological Examination of the Collaborative Perinatal Project. Measures of weight, height, and other attribute variables were made. Outcome measures were made by independent evaluators blind to group assignment.

Sample: 134 (115 completed the protocol) infants participated. Detail is provided regarding subjects available for the study, who participated as well as who dropped out and why. Subjects were from neonatal intensive care units of two Montreal hospitals.

Variables: The main independent variable was group assignment (treatment or no treatment). Numerous other independent variables were considered in evaluating subjects. Dependent variables were scores from the administered tests plus status of attribute variables measured.

Findings: Overall, the investigators found no significant differences between the experimental and the control groups. Efficacy of NDT-oriented physical therapy for high-risk infants in the first year of life was not demonstrated.

Limitations: No psychometric data on any test used in the investigation are provided. The actual NDT-oriented intervention is not described sufficiently for replication. Self-report was used to assess home programming, yet no validity checks were employed. No outcome measures of functional activities of the infants or measures of parental/family status or satisfaction were employed. No check of assumptions underlying use of statistical analysis procedures were rendered, so statistical results cannot be adequately evaluated. Some subjects in the control group did receive therapy, possibly compromising the internal validity of the study.

Applications: Aspects of the quasi-experimental design are very strong and, consequently, this study could be used as a foundation for designing subsequent replication studies with improved measurement of independent and dependent variables. Weight of less than 750 grams at birth emerged as the only variable clearly related to performance at 12 months.

Sommerfeld, C., Fraser, B., Hensinger, R. N., & Beresford, C. V. (1981). Evaluation of physical therapy service for severely mentally impaired students with cerebral palsy. *Physical Therapy, 61,* 338–344.

Problem: What is the effect of physical therapy services in the public schools with severely impaired subjects having cerebral palsy?

Theoretical/Conceptual Basis: The authors addressed their concern about how to provide the "most beneficial" (p. 338) form of therapeutic services to the target group of subjects in the schools. The research is considered to be NDT related since the therapists administering the intervention had post graduate training in NDT techniques, among other things; however, this study addressed physical therapy as an intervention and not NDT per se.

Plan/Design: Pretest, posttest, quasi-experimental design. Of the subjects 19 were paired and randomly assigned to either the treatment group or the group receiving an alternative therapy of supervised management. Ten subjects were in a control group receiving no physical therapy. Groups were pretested for equivalence. Students in treatment received two 30-min. sessions a week in the classroom for five months. Students in supervised management had a program developed by the physical therapist carried out by the teacher and classroom aide, with the therapist checking the program one week after onset, and follow-up instruction every six weeks.

Test reliability was estimated by retesting a random sample of 15 subjects from the two intervention groups two weeks after pretest.

Sample: There were 29 students aged 3 to 22 years who were matched in groups of age, severity and type of cerebral palsy. Fifteen were male and 14 were female. Criteria for selecting subjects were classification, diagnosis, age, history of school attendance, and little or no physical therapy outside of school.

Variables: The independent variable was intervention (physical therapy, supervised management, or no treatment). The dependent variables were developmental reflexes, gross motor skills, and joint range of motion measured by the Wilson Developmental Reflex Test, a gross motor evaluation and range of motion test.

Findings: No significant differences between groups pretest or posttest. The authors suggest that supervised management may be as effective as direct treatment.

Limitations: No major limitations noted.

Applications: The attempt to ensure test reliability by retesting two weeks after the pretest is relatively novel and could easily be replicated in other studies to ensure some aspect of psychometric soundness.

II. SINGLE SUBJECT RESEARCH

Campbell, P. H., & Stewart, B. (1986). Measuring changes in movement skills with infants and young children with handicaps. *Journal for the Association for Persons with Severe Handicaps, 11,* 153-161.

Problem: The article addresses how to measure movement, both quantitatively and qualitatively, in this target group.

Theoretical/Conceptual Basis: The article had two purposes: (1) to define and illustrate a process for measuring change in movement skills of infants and young children linked to functional outcomes, and (2) to illustrate use of the measurement process with an actual group of subjects using an NDT-based intervention.

Plan/Design: A modification of single-subject research design was used to illustrate procedures of measurement. The authors first reported the process of setting intervention targets for each subject based upon functional areas and clinical observations. Then, baseline assessments were obtained for each subject. Intervention consisted of either NDT or NDT combined with behavioral analysis methods. Subjects received two 45-min. treatment sessions per week. Parents and other professionals were trained for follow-through. Treatment sessions consisted of individually designed treatment coupled with measurement of functional outcome.

Sample: The article does not provide specific information on how many subjects were treated and their responses analyzed using these procedures.

Variables: The quantitative (functional outcome) and qualitative (how movement was accomplished) aspects of movement were investigated.

Findings: The authors purport to illustrate a system of measurement for evaluating treatment and changes in movement. Limited reliabilities are available for this approach.

Limitations: This article is only illustrative of use of a particular measurement approach and, as such, cannot be readily applied to other settings and situations without careful analysis, which includes pretesting.

Applications: The message here is to use appropriate measurement systems when attempting to evaluate the effects and interactions of treatment, posture, and movement.

DeGangi, G. A., Hurley, L., & Linscheid, T. R. (1983). Toward a methodology of the short-term effects of neurodevelopmental treatment. *American Journal of Occupational Therapy, 37,* 479–484.

Problem: The authors stated that methodological problems have limited research into the effectiveness of NDT intervention. The authors' purpose was to develop a methodology for measurement of short-term effects of NDT. The authors hypothesized that NDT would be more effective than nonspecific play for qualitative motor performance of children having cerebral palsy.

Theoretical/Conceptual Basis: The authors stated that NDT is used extensively in occupational and physical therapy. Although the theoretical foundation of NDT appears valid, evidence of effectiveness is needed. Research to date is compromised by methodological problems, so a solid data base supporting NDT intervention is lacking. The authors state that one methodological problem centers upon the lack of a reliable and valid way to measure qualitative changes in movement, postural tone, and automatic responses.

Plan/Design: A single-subject design was replicated with four subjects. Each subject was seen eight times for two treatment conditions (25 min. of NDT therapy and 25 min. of nonspecific play) over a five-week period. Three repeated measures of subjects' performance were videotaped and evaluated by the scorers blind to treatment conditions. Repeated measures were focused upon two or three goals within the areas of postural tone, weight shift and bearing, transitional movements, and functional gains, and were individually developed for each subject.

Sample: Four females diagnosed as having cerebral palsy and aged 10 to 22 months were tested. Purposive sampling was employed.

Variables: The independent variable was treatment condition (NDT or nonspecific play). The dependent variable was the quality of movement specified as a subject's individualized goal.

Findings: Interobserver agreement was .86. The sign test indicated to significant differences between treatment conditions. In the short term, neurodevelopmental treatment was not more effective than nonspecific play. The authors suggest that duration of therapy (5 weeks) may have been too short for qualitative motor changes to occur and that the measures of change may not have been sensitive enough.

Limitations: Replications were across subjects but not sites.

Applications: The high reliability suggests that qualitative motor performance can be reliably measured for research in this area.

Laskas, C. A., Mullen, S. L., Nelson, D. L., & Willson-Broyles, M. (1985). Enhancement of two motor functions of the lower extremity in a child with spastic quadriplegia. *Physical Therapy, 65,* 11–16.

Problem: The hypothesis was that administration of four NDT treatment activities would increase dorsiflexor muscle activities during posterior equilibrium reaction and increase the frequency of heel contact during movement to a standing position.

Theoretical/Conceptual Basis: The authors stated that clear and extensive documentation of NDT effectiveness is sparse. This research is a replication of Mullen's work.

Plan/Design: This is an A-B-A, single-subject design. Muscle activity was measured using a Cyborg J53 EMG biofeedback instrument. Behavioral measurement consisted of frequency counts of the number of times a subject's heel touched the floor during movement to a standing position. Baseline measures were taken for the first seven days at the subject's home in the morning (A). Treatment occurred for the next nine days in the morning (B). The final seven sessions were Baseline 2 (A).

Sample: One subject was selected based upon age, diagnosis, and level of motor function, an example of purposive sampling.

Variables: The dependent variables were muscle activity in the dorsiflexor muscles and frequency of the heel touching the ground. The independent variables were treatment (A) (four NDT activities) and no treatment (B) conditions.

Findings: Significant differences between baseline and treatment were found. The authors stated that analysis demonstrated immediate changes in dorsiflexor muscle activity during a posterior equilibrium reaction after administration of four NDT activities.

Limitations: Routine physical therapy was provided the subject during all phases of the study. Effects of this are unknown. Investigator bias could have influenced the outcome since the researcher administered treatment as well as measured change.

Applications: The method of EMG recordings coupled with behavioral observation effectively documented neurodevelopmental treatment over the short term.

Lilly, L. A., & Powell, N. J. (1990). Measuring the effects of neurodevelopmental treatment on the daily living skills of 2 children with cerebral palsy. *American Journal of Occupational Therapy, 44,* 139–145.

Problem: The authors explored effects of NDT procedures on two subjects.

Theoretical/Conceptual Basis: The authors remarked that control-group designs have not shown a strong effect of neurodevelopmental treatment, so they explored single-subject research as an alternative research strategy.

Plan/Design: Two single-subject research protocols were run with girls ages 27 and 32 months and diagnosed as having spastic diplegia. Subject 1 received NDT once per week for 12 weeks. Subject 2 received neurodevelopmental treatment twice per week for 12 weeks. For six sessions, subjects received a combined NDT/play intervention and pre- and posttesting. For the other six sessions, subjects received a full 45 min. of NDT therapy.

Sample: Not applicable.

Variables: Pre- and posttest measures before and after therapy were given each session. Tests were administered by the therapist in the study. Measurement criteria for dressing skills for each subject were stated.

Findings: No significant differences between pre- and posttesting times were found. NDT and nonstructured play had similar effects on functional activity of these subjects.

Limitations: Potential examiner bias exists since the test administrator was involved in treatment. Authors suggest limitations of measurement influenced results.

Applications: A series of recommendations for research are presented. Some of these are to (1) refine testing procedures related to NDT, (2) establish high interrater reliability, (3) increase the number of data points, and (4) provide longer NDT sessions.

III. QUASIEXPERIMENTAL RESEARCH

Dickstein, R., Hocherman, S., Pillar, T., & Shaham, R. (1986). Stroke rehabilitation: Three exercise therapy approaches. *Physical Therapy, 66,* 1233–1238.

Problem: The authors addressed the question, "What are the relative effects of NDT vs exercise with functional activities vs proprioceptive neuromuscular facilitation for stroke victims?"

Theoretical/Conceptual Basis: Various forms of therapeutic exercise are used in rehabilitation but little empirical information supports "a specific therapeutic benefit" (p. 1233).

Plan/Design: A three-group, pretest, posttest design was used. Subjects were assigned to treatment condition on a sequential basis over a period of 18 months. Treatment lasted for 6 weeks.

Sample: Of a possible 169 subjects, 131 completed the study. This was a sample of convenience—all subjects were from the same hospital.

Variables: The independent variable was treatment condition (NDT, neuromuscular facilitation, functional orientation). The dependent variables were activities of daily living, motor control and gait measured, all measured by different assessments.

Findings: No significant differences obtained between the three groups. The findings were consistent with previous studies.

Limitations: Loss of subjects may have affected the outcome: Who were the subjects who dropped out of the study? Most important, however, is the fact that each therapist provided all three interventions with inadequate measurements of the fidelity of treatment. In fact, the reader does not know how different the therapies were in actual delivery. This may have confounded the treatment condition and compromised the validity of the study.

Applications: This study employed pilot exploration which is a model of "pretesting" that could be beneficial for NDT-oriented investigations.

Goodman, M., Rothberg, A. D., Houston-McMillan, J. E., Cooper, P. A., Cartwright, J. D., & Van Der Velde, M. A. (1985). Effect of early neurodevelopmental therapy in normal and at-risk survivors of neonatal intensive care. *Lancet, 2,* 1327–1330.

Problem: The authors investigated whether NDT procedures significantly affect performance of low birthweight, high-risk infants as indicated by the neurodevelopmental score.

Theoretical/Conceptual Basis: The authors stated that there is confusion about what constitutes appropriate intervention for low birthweight, high-risk infants. The study investigated whether NDT procedures affect development of a group of low birthweight, high-risk infants.

Plans/Design: A repeated-measures, four-group design was applied. Low birthweight, high-risk infants were first divided into a normal and an at-risk group based upon their scores on neurodevelopmental assessment. These two groups were further subdivided into treated and nontreated groups. Thus, the four groups were Group 1: normal infants without treatment; Group 2: normal infants with treatment; Group 3: those at risk without treatment; and Group 4: those at risk with treatment. Subjects were first assessed at 3 months (corrected age) and retested at 6, 9, and 12 months.

Sample: A sample of convenience (N = 80) with 20 subjects assigned to each group were tested. Subjects were alternately assigned to treated or nontreated groups.

Variables: The independent variables were intervention (treatment and no treatment) and subjects' characteristics (high-risk and normal). The dependent variable was motor performance as indexed by the neurodevelopmental score.

Findings: No significant differences between groups were indicated by two-tailed t test or Kruskal-Wallis analysis of variance. No actual values of statistics or p were provided, however.

Limitations: The psychometric quality of the instrument used to measure change was not specified so one cannot evaluate what the authors measured (change in subjects or fluctuations in instrumentation). Lack of random selection of subjects limited generalizability. The same instrument was used to diagnose and measure change, compromising internal validity. No rationale was provided for why treatments were scheduled monthly (how often must treatment be provided in order to have an effect?).

Applications: The number and severity of the limitations compromised the validity of the study and possible applications.

Kluzik, J., Fetters, L., & Coryell, J. (1990). Quantification of control: A preliminary study of effects of neurodevelopmental treatment on reaching in children with spastic cerebral palsy. *Physical Therapy, 70,* 65–76.

Problem: Will reaching movements of children diagnosed with spastic cerebral palsy change after one neurodevelopmental treatment session?

Theoretical/Conceptual Basis: Research on intervention in individuals with cerebral palsy has concentrated on functional or gross motor skills with limited success in measuring change. The current study focused on objective measurement of factors more associated with the quality of movement.

Plan/Design: A one-group pretest, posttest design was used.

Sample: Five subjects, aged 7 to 12 years and diagnosed with spastic cerebral palsy, participated. Information on age, sex, hand preference, and muscle tone was presented for the 12 subjects. Criteria for inclusion of subjects were understanding verbal directions, ability to localize an object visually, adequate passive range of motion to reach the target, and informed consent. Subjects were selected from a school in Massachusetts.

Subjects first performed a reaching task. A 35-min. NDT-oriented therapy session was provided by an NDT-certified therapist. The reaching task was then repeated. Reaching tasks were videotaped.

Variables: The independent variable was the NDT intervention. The dependent measures were quality of reaching movements measured by the Waterloo Spatial Motion Analysis and Recording Techniques (WATSMART ©) and videotape.

Findings: Movement time for the reaching tasks decreased significantly. Length of path and associated reactions did not significantly differ.

Limitations: How subjects were selected was not identified.

Applications: The authors set $p = .10$ as the level of significance since samples were small and they wanted to reduce the likelihood of Type II error, i.e., they wanted to increase chances of finding a significant difference if one existed. This level may be more appropriate for NDT research than $p = .05$, especially when small samples are used. Emphasis on aspects of reaching behavior for measuring change was innovative and effective.

Logigian, M. K., Samuels, M. A., Falconer, J., & Zager, R. (1983). Clinical exercise trial for stroke patients. *Archives of Physical Medicine and Rehabilitation, 64,* 364–367.

Problem: This study addressed whether there are differing effects between the Bobath and Rood facilitation approach compared to a traditional approach for therapeutic exercise with stroke patients.

Theoretical/Conceptual Basis: "The conflict in the evaluation of neuromuscular facilitation techniques results from insufficient evidence to justify intensive and protracted treatment" (p. 364). The authors proposed to explore this issue by conducting an intervention study.

Plan/Design: Pretest and posttest were given in a two-group design.

Sample: Adults with an average age of 61.6 yr. (24 men and 18 women) participated.

Variables: The independent variable was condition of therapeutic exercise. The dependent variables were functional performance and muscle strength as measured by the Barthel Index and manual muscle testing.

Findings: Both traditional and facilitation types of therapeutic exercise improved functional and motor performance as measured by the Barthel Index and the manual muscle testing. The authors reported that the results were consistent with previous studies.

Limitations: No psychometric data on measures were provided. Description of the interventions was incomplete. No attempt was made to measure fidelity of treatment.

Applications: The authors explored why no differences were found, identifying three possible factors: (1) heterogeneity of the stroke population, (2) small sample, and (3) the particular measurement tools employed. This is one of the few articles to address assumptions underlying use of parametric statistics. Such consideration might also be included in other NDT research.

Piper, M. C., Mazer, B., Silver, K. M., & Ramsay, M. (1988). Resolution of neurological symptoms in high-risk infants during the first two years of life. *Developmental Medicine and Child Neurology, 30,* 26–35.

Problem: This study presented the developmental history of high-risk infants over the first 24 months of life to document the neurological symptoms and to examine the role of physical therapy in affecting outcomes.

Theoretical/Conceptual Basis: None were presented.

Plan/Design: The subjects were followed from birth to 24 months. Infants had neurological assessments at 12 and 24 months and developmental assessments at 6 and 12 months. The design is somewhat confusing since these subjects were also part of another study the first author was conducting. It appears that 56 of the subjects were in a treated group (receiving physical therapy) and 59 in the control group. Treatment consisted of teaching parents to use NDT principles. For the first three months the infants received weekly, hour-long physical therapy sessions. For the next nine months, the treated group of infants were seen every two weeks.

Sample: 115 high-risk infants were the subjects and had been identified from participation in another study. Only 96 infants were available for the 24-month follow-up.

Variables: Diagnostic categories, age, and presence or absence of therapy were the independent variables. Dependent variables were outcome performance areas.

Findings: About 25% of the infants were at-risk at 12 months, and of those a little more than 50% were "normal" at 24 months. Children who were diagnosed normal or abnormal at 24 months were diagnosed similarly at 112 months. There was an inverse relationship between birthweight and neurological outcomes. Physical therapy did not affect outcomes.

Limitations: No psychometric data on the neurological examination were provided and none on the examination of mental status used to assess subjects. Treatment was inadequately described for replication to be undertaken.

Applications: None were presented.

Watt, J., Sims, D., Harckham, F., Schmidt, L., McMillan, A., & Hamilton, J. (1986). A prospective study of inhibitive casting as an adjunct to physiotherapy for cerebral-palsied children. *Developmental Medicine and Child Neurology, 28,* 480–488.

Problem: "The hypothesis tested was that a three-week course of inhibitive casting in conjunction with neurodevelopmental therapy (NDT) would improve the static tonus, developmental skills, passive range of motion of the ankles, and the gait pattern" (p. 493).

Theoretical/Conceptual Basis: Inhibitive casting consistent with Bobath principles can be an effective adjunct to more traditional neurodevelopmental therapy.

Plan/Design: Pretest and posttest in a one-group design were planned. The single group of subjects were provided three weeks of inhibitive casting and neurodevelopmental therapy. Subjects were tested for muscle tone, developmental skills, the passive range of ankle dorsiflexion, and gait pattern before therapy, two weeks after treatment, and five months after treatment.

Sample: Purposive sampling was employed. The size of the population was not identified, but 32 children were selected to participate by applying five qualifying criteria. Participants were 17 boys and 11 girls, ages 18 months to five years. Four subjects were unable to complete the study.

Variables: The independent variable was the intervention, i.e., NDT therapy plus inhibitive casting.

Findings: No significant improvement was observed in developmental skills. Improved passive ankle dorsiflexion in these spastic children was the most significant improvement and followed by foot-floor contact during walking at the testing two weeks posttreatment. After five months the improvements were not evident. Lack of significant improvement in motor skills might reflect the inadequacy of the assessment scale and the short duration of treatment. The authors concluded that three weeks of treatment was not adequate to change motor milestones since the effects of therapy and casting were not long lasting.

Limitations: The size of the population from which the sample was purposively selected was not identified.

Applications: The authors identified use of nonparametric statistics for data not appropriate for parametric analyses. This type of careful application of statistical analysis, i.e., matching the type of analysis to the level at which the data are measured, would be useful in further NDT research. Also, this is essentially a clinical population which was followed and written up for research purposes. There was no comparison or control group. This article may serve as a model for clinically based research operating as part of routine procedures.

Resumé

A major problem confronting therapists and teachers who provide services to children with neuromotor handicaps is identifying the most appropriate therapeutic program to address the child's multiple needs. Is one therapeutic approach more effective than another and with which children? Such documentation is important to justify the need for therapy to referring physicians, administrators, and third-party reimbursement agencies.

In this annotated bibliography, several problems were identified in the NDT literature. These include the following five: (1) Instruments have tended to focus on child-outcome measures (e.g., developmental performance) and are often not sensitive as indicators of change in motor performance (Ottenbacher, et al., 1986; Palisano, 1991; Parette & Hourcade, 1984; Stern & Gorga, 1988). (2) The vast majority of early intervention studies have been based on subjective, clinical observations with only 48% yielding statistical evidence of effectiveness (Palisano, 1991; Simeonsson, Cooper, & Scheiner, 1982). (3) Statistical significance is often low because sample sizes are small. (4) Children often progress in domains not measured by the dependent variables (i.e., management areas rather than gains in developmental milestones). (5) Subjects' characteristics are often not examined or considered in the research design (i.e., environment, parents' and families' traits, severity of child's handicap, and etiology).

What is needed are studies that investigate the *efficacy* of specific sensorimotor interventions, e.g., NDT (Parette et al., 1991). Studies of efficacy would answer the question: are gains or benefits obtained over time when an intervention is provided? Once efficacy of treatment has been established, research should focus on the *effectiveness* of treatments. Such studies answer the question whether one treatment approach is more beneficial than another and for which clinical populations.

The first step in research is to address efficacy using questions adapted from Olney (1990). Such a study would investigate the following features: What is the treatment? When should treatment be initiated? When should treatment be ended? At what frequency and duration should therapy be provided to obtain positive effects? Who should provide the therapy and how? Issues such as discipline of provider (i.e., occupational therapist, physical therapist, speech and language pathologist, teacher), how therapy is delivered (i.e., direct treatment, consultation, parental involvement), and setting (i.e., home, clinic, school setting) need to be assessed. How do different disciplines providing NDT differ in their application (i.e., emphasis on activities of daily living, feeding, play skills, mobility, etc.)?

Through developing a systematic data base on variables related to treatment, it would be possible to answer these questions. The task that lies ahead is certainly a challenging one; however, this research is needed to establish the most effective ways of intervening with individuals with neuromotor handicaps.

References

Bobath, B. (1967) The very early treatment of cerebral palsy. *Developmental Medicine and Child Neurology,* 9, 373–390.

Bobath, K. (1980) *A neurophysiological basis for the treatment of cerebral palsy.* London: Heinemann.

d'Avignon, M. (1981) Early physiotherapy *ad motum* Vojta or Bobath in infants with suspected neuromotor disturbance. *Neuropediatrics, 12,* 232–241.

Goodman, M., Rothberg, A. D., Houston-McMillan, J. E., Cooper, P. A., Cartwright, J. D., & Van Der Velde, M. A. (1985) Effect of early neurodevelopmental therapy in normal and at-risk survivors of neonatal intensive care. *Lancet, 2,* 1327–1330.

Gorga, D. (1989) Occupational therapy treatment practices with infants in early intervention. *American Journal of Occupational Therapy, 43,* 731–735.

Harris, S. R. (1981a) Effects of neurodevelopmental therapy on motor performance of infants with Down's syndrome. *Developmental Medicine and Child Neurology, 23,* 477–483.

Harris, S. R. (1981b) Physical therapy and infants with Down's syndrome: The effects of early intervention. *Rehabilitation Literature, 42,* 339–343.

Harris, S. R. (1988) Early intervention: does developmental therapy make a difference? *Topics in Early Childhood Special Education, 7,* 20–32.

Hourcade, J. J., & Parette, H. P. (1984) Motoric change subsequent to therapeutic intervention in infants and young children who have cerebral palsy: Annotated listing of group studies. *Perceptual and Motor Skills, 58,* 519–524.

Keshner, E. A. (1981) Reevaluating the theoretical model underlying the neurodevelopmental theory. *Physical Therapy, 61,* 1035–1040.

Kluzik, J., Fetters, L., & Coryell, J. (1990) Quantification of control: A preliminary study of effects of neurodevelopmental treatment on reaching in children with spastic cerebral palsy. *Physical Therapy, 70,* 65–76.

Laskas, C. A., Mullen, S. L., Nelson, D. L., & Willson-Broyles, M. (1985) Enhancement of two motor functions of the lower extremity in a child with spastic quadriplegia. *Physical Therapy, 65,* 11–16.

Olney, S. J. (1990) Efficacy of physical therapy in improving mechanical and metabolic efficiency of movement in cerebral palsy. *Pediatric Physical Therapy, 2,* 145–154.

Ottenbacher, K. J., Biocca, Z., DeCremer, G., Gevelinger, M., Jedlovec, K. B., & Johnson, M. B. (1986) Quantitative analysis of the effectiveness of pediatric therapy. *Physical Therapy, 66,* 1095–1101.

Palisano, R. J. (1991) Research on the effectiveness of neurodevelopmental treatment. *Pediatric Physical Therapy, 3,* 143–148.

Parette, H. P., Hendricks, M. D., & Rock, S. L. (1991) Efficacy of therapeutic intervention intensity with infants and young children with cerebral palsy. *Infants and Young Children, 4(2),* 1–19.

Parette, H. P., & Hourcade, J. J. (1984) A review of therapeutic intervention research on gross and fine motor progress in young children with cerebral palsy. *American Journal of Occupational Therapy, 38,* 462–468.

Piper, M. C., Kunos, I., Willis, D. M., Mazer, B. L., Ramsay, D. P., & Silver, K. M. (1986) Early physical therapy effects on the high-risk infant: A randomized control trial. *Pediatrics, 78,* 216–224.

Piper, M. C., Mazer, B., Silver, K. M., & Ramsay, M. (1988) Resolution of neurological symptoms in high-risk infants during the first two years of life. *Developmental Medicine and Child Neurology, 30,* 26–35.

Royeen, C. B., & DeGangi, G. A. (1992) *Annotated bibliography of NDT peer-reviewed literature 1980–1990, inclusive.* Oak Park, IL: NeuroDevelopmental Treatment Association, Inc.

Simeonsson, R. J., Cooper, D. H., & Scheiner, A. P. (1982) A review and analysis of the effectiveness of early intervention programs. *Pediatrics, 69,* 635–641.

Stern, F. M., & Gorga, D. (1988) Neurodevelopmental treatment (NDT): Therapeutic intervention and its efficacy. *Infants and Young Children, 1,* 22–32.

Valvano, J., & Long, T. (1991) Neurodevelopmental treatment: A review of the writings of the Bobaths. *Pediatric Physical Therapy, 3,* 125–129.

Illustrative Example 13–1: Discussion

Start regularly reading articles using the abbreviated questionnaire, and keep a file of your summaries of articles on a particular area of research; you are functioning as a well-organized research consumer. You may find your reviews helpful in talking about what you do with families and administrators. Reading the articles, writing up your summaries, and maintaining the file will reinforce your understanding of the research in your chosen topical area. This approach to being a research consumer is appropriate for (a) those newly engaged in the process of being a research consumer, and (b) those who choose to work alone in the process of being a research consumer.

ACTION PLAN 2: USE RESEARCH

When I was doing my third internship out of undergraduate school, I had the good fortune to be placed with Virginia Scardina in the Cincinnati Public Schools. What was so exciting about that internship was that the entire experience was predicated on using the research literature in sensory integration, that is, it was founded on using research. Research use is the process of applying research results to the practice setting.

Sounds good, right? But why is it done so little? Be honest with yourself—when was the last time you read your professional journal and tried to use the research results presented there? We all have busy lives and busy professions. It is imperative, however, that we renew our commitment to research as a foundation of our professional demeanor. And that means *reading* and *using* the research literature in your profession.

It is no longer acceptable to shun personal responsibility for using the research findings presented in *Physical Therapy* or the *American Journal of Occupational Therapy.* Rather, we must accept the personal and professional challenge to wade through difficult reading (recall the "Why is Research Boring and Hard to Read?" section in chapter 5) as a part of our professional conduct. I suggest that you set a personal goal to identify, for each issue of your professional journal, at least one research finding that you can apply in your daily practice (Smith, 1975). In fact, why not start a journal of research use as a part of the documentation of your professional development?

In that journal, record the following

1. monthly issue of professional journal
2. research finding identified for use (include specification of the article, author, pages, etc.)
3. identification of how that finding is being used, that is, in your practice (assessment, intervention or administration)
4. differences in practice or administrative outcomes because of using of the research data.

If at all possible, build this process into your professional development plans at work. That way, you can earn or achieve recognition from your supervisor for making use of research. Your journal of research use will be the foundation of your achievement.

In fact, I suspect it would be a fascinating conference presentation (annual, regional, or local) to hear a clinician share his or her research use journal. Wouldn't you like to hear how your colleagues used research results over the past year? Such activity should be required of all therapists who supervise interns. We should require it of ourselves to model exemplary professional practice, and using research is one component of this.

ACTION PLAN 3: PARTICIPATE IN A JOURNAL CLUB

Do you work alone? If so, it may be difficult to share your enthusiasm for research with your colleagues. In this case, it may be best to form a journal club with occupational and physical therapy colleagues outside of your work setting. If you are in a rural setting with no other colleagues in physical proximity, you may need to form an "E-mail Journal Club."

A **journal club** should ideally consist of five to ten members. Each member should agree to read, review, and critique one article for the year. Club members should then sign up for a month in which to present their review. All journal club members should read the article prior to the meeting. After the lead reviewer presents his or her interpretation, all members should participate in the ensuing discussion. The E-mail journal club should do the same, only sending their reviews and comments through the E-mail system. Such a journal club could easily be formed as a component of existing local or regional organizations, such as the local district of your state organization. Reviews could then be written up by each presenter and shared with others at a regional meeting in a poster presentation session or through a mailing with other organizational materials.

ACTION PLAN 4: DO PEER REVIEW

Do journal articles seem too esoteric and not related to your area of practice? If you think this, have you done anything to change it? **Peer review** is the process of reading and critiquing papers or proposals anonymously. One way to get started is to volunteer to review paper proposals for conference presentations. Almost all professional associations (the American Physical Therapy Association, the American Occupational Therapy Association, TASH, ARC) have annual conferences. Usually there is some sort of review of paper proposals by clinicians in practice. You can write to the organization of your choice and volunteer to participate in this process.

If you feel pretty confident of your research knowledge, it may be appropriate to write to a journal you read on a regular basis and nominate yourself as a reviewer for that journal. You are probably thinking, "Oh, I couldn't do that!" Why not? There is nothing like on-the-job training to teach you more about research. Maybe you have some practice-based insight and experience that would be critical to offer: common sense goes a long way as a background tool for evaluation of any manuscript or research project.

The previous action plans all relate to participation in some form of research use. Let's now look at action plans for participating in research development or scholarly activity.

Action Plans for Research Development and Scholarly Activity

You may now want to go further in developing your skills in research beyond that of research consumer. You may wish to develop beginning-level research practitioner skills. Or you may wish to further enhance your skills as a research consumer. The next two action plans will help you do both.

As a prelude to actually conducting research, some of you may prefer instead to participate in what we will call scholarly activity. That is, it may not be what some would call true research per se (based on quasiexperimental or experimental design), but it is a form of descriptive research.

ACTION PLAN 5: READ RESEARCH LITERATURE

There are any number of excellent books available for those wishing to further develop their skills as a research consumer or to develop beginning-level skills as a research practitioner. The following resources are recommended for those choosing this action plan.

Bailey, D. M. (1991). *Research for the Health Professional.* St. Louis, MO: F. A. Davis.

This book presents a workbook approach to learning more about actually conducting research.

Burns, N., & Grove, S. K. (1987). *The Practice of Nursing Research: Conduct, Critique and Utilization.* Philadelphia: W. B. Saunders.

This excellent resource provides the research consumer with advanced-level information about how to look at and understand research. For the beginning researcher, it is a valuable overview of just about everything. This is not light reading, and is more of a reference resource than a book one would sit down and read all at once.

Royeen, C. B. (1988). *Research Tradition in Occupational Therapy: Philosophy, Process and Status.* Thorofare, NJ: Slack.

This book is nontechnical, and the first chapter covers much of what is in this text. The other chapters, however, introduce and discuss the concepts of humanism in research, the similarity to research and clinical practice, and an analysis of current and future trends in occupational therapy research.

Fetterman, D. M. (Ed.). (1988). *Qualitative Approaches to Evaluation in Education.* New York: Praeger.

For the therapist learning more about qualitative approaches in research, this is an excellent and highly readable resource.

Stein, F. (1989). *Anatomy of Clinical Research: An Introduction to Scientific Inquiry in Medicine, Rehabilitation and Related Health Professions.* Thorofare, NJ: Slack.

This book provides a solid overview of the fundamentals of quantitative research including research design and introductory concepts of data analysis.

Finally, I strongly encourage you to read the Recommend Readings at the end of each chapter in this primer.

ACTION PLAN 6: TAKE A COURSE

The other option for increasing skills and knowledge is to take a course at a local university. I recommend the following types of courses:

- introduction to research
- educational research and evaluation
- introductory statistics
- qualitative methods
- program and policy evaluation
- research methods.

Different institutions name their courses differently. Obtain a course description of any given course or talk to the instructor before enrolling. Make certain to take courses within education, psychology, nursing, therapy, public health, or comparable departments.[1] Participating in such courses will open up an entirely new world for you.

ACTION PLAN 7: WRITE FOR PUBLICATION

There are two general types of publications: scholarly and popular press. Not only is there a real need for more scholarly publications in occupational and physical therapy, but we also need more information and articles about what we do and how in the popular press. The popular press consists of newspapers, magazines, association newsletters, and so on. A review of a research article written well and for the layperson may be of interest to readers of *Parents, Redbook,* or other types of magazines.

You may ask, What does writing for the popular press have to do with research? Well, when was the last time you looked at a publication like *Redbook* or *Parents*? Often a psychologist or a physician presents a meaningful discussion of recent research findings and states what the findings mean for the readership. We can do the same thing. There are certainly parents and family members interested in information and research findings from occupational and physical therapy.

If you choose this route, there are five rules to follow:

1. Determine what it is you wish to write. What do you have to say of interest to others?
2. Locate the publication to which you wish to submit. It could be the *NDTA Newsletter.* Or it could be *Redbook.* Find out who the editor or manager is and call them with your preliminary idea. Find out page requirements, style suggestions, and so on. Most publications have some sort of information sheet or style guide for contributors that they can send you.
3. Make it professional. Do not submit handwritten documents. They should be typed according to the publication's requirements.
4. Ask a friend, colleague, or mentor to read what you write and comment on it prior to submission. Writing always needs an objective second look before being submitted.
5. Don't give up. Do not let yourself get discouraged. Remember the maxim: Success is 1% inspiration and 99% perspiration!

"Parent/Professional Collaboration in the IFSP" is an example of an article written for public dissemination. It is an excellent example of a research project description that could have been academic and very boring. But Ms. Stein had the knack for making the project description interesting. After seeing it, I suggested she submit it to *OT Week* for publication, and it's in press. Following are just a few examples of the kinds of topics on which therapists could write for the popular press:

- an intervention strategy used with a particular client
- how families and therapists work together
- rewards and frustrations of being a therapist
- increased sensory needs in normal aging
- joint protection techniques for kitchen activities
- a review of current research with subjects in a particular disability group.

My personal goal is to someday publish in *Reader's Digest.* There is a lack of understanding of occupational and physical therapy in the United States. We can change that by writing for popular publications.

1. I do not recommend that you take courses out of departments of mathematics or statistics.

ILLUSTRATIVE EXAMPLE 13–2

Parent/Professional Collaboration in the IFSP

Elizabeth Stein

The Reginald S. Lourie Center for Infants and Young Children, located in Rockville, Maryland, has completed a three-year grant funded by the National Institute on Disability and Rehabilitation Research (NIDRR). The focus of this research was the parent–professional collaboration during the IFSP process. The ultimate outcome of the grant was a self-assessment guide for centers using the IFSP. This guide will help centers evaluate how the IFSP process is working, as perceived by all those involved—parents, professionals and administrators.

Research efforts included focus groups as well as individual interviews with parents, professionals and administrators involved in the IFSP process to find out how they view the process, especially the collaborative relationship between parent and professional. We asked participants in the IFSP to describe any perceived problems or barriers to the IFSP process, as well as any solutions that they may have to offer. The information collected has been interesting because, while many of the parents and professionals agree on what the problems were, they offered very different solutions!

On the whole, the IFSP has been a wonderfully successful collaboration model for parents. Most of the parents I interviewed seemed very pleased with the way the entire IFSP process worked. Many parents described their case managers as "members of the family."

However, as a parent working on this study, I observed some factors that, I believe, affected the early part of the collaborative effort. The issues of bereavement and of parenting experience can profoundly affect the way in which professionals and parents share information.

As soon as a child is identified as needing the services of an IFSP program, a very intensive parent–professional effort begins. In less than three months, the child should be fully involved in an early intervention program designed by professionals and parents together. And yet, these are very difficult times for both the families and the professionals involved.

The early weeks of any parent–professional collaboration are crucial to the development of trust and communication. However, it is a time when hope and possibility clash with the limitations inherent in the system.

The underlying concept of the parent–professional collaboration in the IFSP process is an assumed equality of involvement. However, parents and professionals may bring to this relationship very different perceptions and experiences. Equal participation assumes that both parties involved have arrived at this collaboration with the same knowledge, understanding of their roles in the IFSP experience, similar values and goals, as well as a willingness to be involved. In practice, this is not always the case.

The importance of the IFSP collaborative experience must not be underestimated. This is the first experience a parent of a child with disabilities may have in working with professionals. It is also formative in developing most of the skills he or she will need for life—in becoming the advocate the child so desperately needs.

And yet, the parents' bereavement and differences in parenting experiences may affect what information is shared by families as well as how they perceive their responsibilities toward the child. In one focus group both of these issues came up very clearly.

One parent felt very guilty about her child's cerebral palsy because she had received hormone treatments during her pregnancy and was so sure that the CP was her fault that she never questioned anything the professionals said to her, even when she did not understand what they were saying, because she felt so consumed by guilt. Another parent was afraid to mention parenting concerns because she was afraid that the professionals would be angry with her for not setting more limits around certain behaviors.

Another parent described her problem this way:

> Sometimes I find it is hard to believe that he does have a disability. I wonder what's wrong with him?... I don't know. I guess I'm not around children that much to know what they should be doing at a certain age.

This parent said that she was too intimidated by the professional's knowledge to even ask about normal development so that she could understand how her child was delayed.

Some parents expressed their feeling that professionals assume that they have already accepted their child's disabilities, when in fact, they still have a lot of grieving and acceptance to go through.

Another parent summarized many parents' experiences when she said:

> A lot of children here are premature. When you come out of the intensive care unit, you are just so grateful that your child is alive. They can say that your child's going to be mentally retarded, severely. You don't want to hear it. You *don't* hear it. You don't hear it because you are just so thankful that he is alive and breathing on his own. I'm sure they told me a million things and I just said, "Fine."

But how do you help parents who are vulnerable because of their grief—as their life is suddenly thrown into a state of chaos? How do you reach parents who don't—or can't—articulate their needs because of their exhaustion, because of their guilt, because of their inexperience as parents? How do you help parents—in only 45 days—become the aggressive, articulate, knowledgeable collaborators that professionals so often depend on?

One solution would be to leave room in the collaborative process to discuss the frustrations and fears shared by both sides of the collaboration. This is an extraordinary experience—this collaboration. Parents are feeling their worst, yet have to do their best. Many professionals have their doubts too. They may distrust parents. They may be discouraged by the enormity of the task they face. The call for early intervention puts pressure on everyone involved.

There is a tendency in all of us to avoid emotionally charged or painful issues. Emotional content is powerful—not only because it can dramatize a message, but also because it can evoke emotion in the listener. It can deflect attention from the issue under consideration and be seen as intrusive or distracting (perhaps even "unprofessional"). But it doesn't have to. With support, with honesty, with sympathy, it can be a crucial part of the healing process that parents must undergo before they can effectively focus their energies on their child's needs.

Parents from different family or cultural backgrounds may choose to hide their emotional experiences or may have an appropriate outlet for their feelings outside the parent–professional collaboration. Some parents may be unable to hold back their feelings and, in fact, may need to vent them in order to move on to rational planning and decision making.

But it is never the wrong time to help parents allay their guilt, their worry and their grief. Developing an openness to these issues and becoming more sensitive to the particular needs of grieving parents and of inexperienced parents may go a long way toward making this or any parent–professional collaboration a better and more productive experience for everyone involved—especially the children.

Action Plan 8: Write a Letter to the Editor, Book Review, or Commentary

The *American Journal of Occupational Therapy* and *Physical Therapy* both publish book review sections. Do you ever preview tests, texts, or videos for use in your clinic? In essence, you are already doing the type of reviews that appear in these publications. To build on what you are already doing, you could participate in the exciting process of evaluating texts, videos, and software by writing up such a review. This is a service to your colleagues and to the profession overall.

Have you ever read a book review and thought, I could write that. You probably can; so, as the NIKE commercial says, "Just Do It." Below are some sample book reviews.

Reprinted from *Physical Therapy,* Vol. 72, Number 2, February, 1992, p. 93. Used with permission.

ILLUSTRATIVE EXAMPLE 13–3

Marketing Techniques for Physical Therapists

Schaefer, K.
Gaithersburg, MD 20878. Aspen Publishers Inc. 1991, hardback. 194 pp. illus.

Books on marketing that are intended for physical therapists are rare. This book is designed as a "cookbook" to solve marketing problems with minimal effort and to achieve maximum results. It is designed for therapists who do not have formal training in marketing techniques and can be used by therapists in all clinical settings. This well-written book is especially useful for therapists with low budgets and for those who wish to utilize the information without hiring outside consultants.

The book is a must for anyone who wishes to understand the dynamics of marketing as it applies to physical therapy. Marketing theory is presented concisely and is geared toward physical therapy practice. The attitudes that good service sells itself and that word of mouth is the best marketing tool may no longer help a practice position effectively in a market that is ever-changing. A market plan must now target consumers, insurance carriers, and industry. Considerations for positioning oneself in the marketplace are explored, and it becomes very clear that the practitioner must be positioned properly.

The chapter on "strategic marketing planning" outlines an excellent approach to getting started. Suggestions for analyzing data and attitudes are presented that include data collection, community resources, self-assessment, focus groups, surveys, and interviews. Understanding the principles in this chapter will ensure that the plan to be developed will be comprehensive and meaningful.

The chapter on "internal marketing" forces the therapist to take a hard look at himself and at the practice. The importance of an image, both personal and professional, is explored in the context of environment, personnel, attitudes, and policy. A self-assessment of a practice can sometimes shock the owner, but this assessment is vital if a true picture of the practice is to be developed.

Issues in public relations, such as logos, brochures, newsletters, public speaking, and interviews, are explored in detail with excellent suggestions provided for developing and assessing these tools. Chapters on selling and advertising help the reader consider what it takes to be the most effective and open-minded in one's approach. The last chapter clearly states what competition means. The benefits of competition, as well as ways to analyze the competitors, will help one develop winning strategies in dealing with increased competition and increased demands on the profession.

This book will help anyone who wishes to consider a marketing approach or who wishes to analyze and improve existing plans. The depth of coverage is excellent, and the information is most appropriate for helping physical therapists face the challenge in today's health care environment.

Charles Kaplan, PT
Edgewater Rehabilitation Associates, Inc.
Chicago, Illinois

Children's Psychological Testing. A Guide For Nonpsychologists, Second Edition

Reprinted from *Physical and Occupational Therapy in Pediatrics,* Vol. 11, Number 2, February, 1991, pp. 83–85. Used with permission.

Woodrich, DL and Kush, SA.
Baltimore, Paul H. Brookes Publishing Co., 1990

The stated purpose of this text is to help nonpsychologists become informed consumers of psychological tests. The authors select and review typical tests in each of several areas.

The introductory chapter provides a summary of major principles of tests and measurements. The overview presented is a useful introduction to concepts of tests and measurements for the "novice" tester. For the therapist wishing greater detail, these topics are more fully covered in *Developing Norm Referenced Standardized Tests* (edited by L. Miller, 1989). In the second chapter, there is a discussion of factors to consider when making a referral for psychological testing. Practical suggestions are included that can be drawn upon by occupational and physical therapists to enable them to make better referrals to other disciplines and/or help other disciplines such as education make better referrals for OT or PT evaluations.

The next section of the book reviews developmental and IQ assessments in infancy, preschool, and school age. In addition to reviews of specific tests, the authors discuss specific issues in testing. In infancy, the issue of temperament is highlighted; in preschool assessment, the authors examine issues related to diagnosis of mental retardation and learning disabilities. The school age chapter discusses interpretation of patterns of ability/disability and utilization of these patterns in remediation.

Following the presentation of age-specific assessments are reviews of tests that cut across the life span including tests of academic achievement and personality tests. The chapter on tests of academic achievement is of particular relevance to therapists working with children in school systems. The authors include a comparison of criterion-referenced and norm-referenced assessment. Measures of personality are categorized and discussed as objective and projective measures. Disturbed behavior is viewed from three theoretical perspectives: psychoanalytic, biobehavioral, and psychoeducational, and the classification system of emotional disturbance under DSM-III-R is compared with the federal law PL 94-142.

Following a review of the different tests is a discussion of contemporary issues in testing including assessment of minority children and the use of neuropsychological assessment. The final chapter includes a discussion of using and interpreting test findings. The authors emphasize the need for interpretive rather than descriptive reports and provide excellent examples of each type.

Overall, I found the content in this text was consistent with the authors' stated purpose. Although only approximately 25% of the tests reviewed in this text are actually given by occupational or physical therapists, therapists do need to be able to utilize results from other disciplines and the book clearly adds to the therapist's knowledge in this area. The book was easy to read and the issues presented made one give more thought to testing practices. The case studies throughout the text were especially helpful in enabling the reader to better understand the uses and misuses of tests.

The reviewer would identify two criticisms of this book. First, there is a heavy reliance on the views of Sattler in critiquing tests. Second, although some of the typical assessments used by therapists are summarized in an Appendix, the reviews do not reflect knowledge of "state of the art" assessment in OT and PT. For example, the SCSIT rather than the SIPT was presented, and, review of the MAP did not incorporate the published validity studies. Although it is felt that *A Therapist's Guide to Pediatric Assessment* (edited by L. King-Thomas and B. Hacker, 1987) provides a more comprehensive review of tests more frequently used by therapists, the present book includes reviews of tests, the results of which are utilized by therapists. This book is highly recommended as a reference for occupational and physical therapists working in pediatrics.

Sharon A. Cermak, EdD, OTR/L, FAOTA
Associate Professor of Occupational Therapy
Director, Neurobehavioral Rehabilitation Research Center
Boston University, Sargent College

The last item in this action plan is to write a commentary. Commentaries are often invited to be written and published with the article itself. Other times, however, an unsolicited commentary will be considered if (a) it raises valid issues to be discussed, and (b) it is well written. As you keep a research journal, you may find there is an article about which you feel passionate enough to write. Following are two sample commentaries with the article on which they focused.

Note that one commentary is written by two authors. It is often advantageous to team up with a colleague to pursue scholarly activity or research-related interests. Such pairing allows expertise from different viewpoints to be combined for a more powerful approach.

ILLUSTRATIVE EXAMPLE 13–4

Reprinted from *Infants and Young Children,* Vol. 4, Number 2, October, 1991, pp. 1–13. Used with permission.

Efficacy of Therapeutic Intervention Intensity with Infants and Young Children with Cerebral Palsy

Howard H. Parette, Jr., EdD, Mary D. Hendricks, PhD, Stephen L. Rock, PhD

Physical therapy and occupational therapy are two of the most frequently employed means for the provision of early therapeutic intervention with children who have cerebral palsy[1-3] and are integral components of federally mandated services via Public Law 94-142, Education of All Handicapped Children Act of 1975, and Public Law 99-457, Education of the Handicapped Act, Amendments 1986. In an era when diminishing fiscal resources seem to be affecting service delivery systems with increasing intensity, school systems and other service providers will, of necessity, begin to examine more closely questions relating to therapeutic intervention effectiveness. Issues such as the efficacy of therapy with specific types of children, the forms of therapy that are most effective, and whether or not the effects of therapy are maintained over time will become critical in decision-making processes.[1,4] In a similar vein, the efficacy of alternative forms of therapeutic intervention service delivery, such as family-focused interventions[5-8] and parent/child groups,[9] will have to be investigated.

The effects of therapeutic intervention strategies have been far from definitive.[2,8,10-12] This has placed considerable pressures on service providers and the scientific community to adhere to rigorous research approaches to determine the efficacy of various intervention approaches with infants and young children who have cerebral palsy. Of particular importance are the contributory effects of specific subject and treatment variables on therapeutic intervention outcomes. Studies have suggested that subject variables such as mental competence,[15-17] age,[18,19] type of cerebral palsy,[20,21] emotional disturbance,[12,22] and degree of involvement[14,23] (also: Parette HP, Hourcade JJ, April 1990. Unpublished data) interact to affect children's responses to the interventions. Similarly, treatment variables such as type of intervention[8,19] have also been reported to have an impact upon children's responses to physical therapy and occupational therapy. One treatment variable that has received relatively little attention in the professional habilitation literature is intensity of treatment.

Intensity and frequency of therapeutic intervention services are terms often used interchangeably in research on outcomes of occupational therapy and physical therapy strategies with children who have cerebral palsy. Earlier reports have typically reflected the prevailing position taken by occupational therapists and physical therapists, that treatment provided to children is highly individualized and depends on the child and his or her individual needs.[24,25] For example, Phelps[26] stated that daily 1-hour treatment sessions for 6 weeks to 3 months should produce results in the child if any are to be obtained. Conversely, Crothers and Paine[27] suggested that rigid, prolonged, and closely supervised therapy is not always necessary but does have its place for some children.

Piper et al[3]. found that high-risk infants receiving physical therapy failed to perform better than a control group of such children. These researchers suggested that their therapeutic intervention (ie, weekly 1-hour sessions) may have been too infrequent to effect positive outcomes. Previous studies conducted with culturally disadvantaged children have also implied that daily intensive intervention is required to derive positive outcomes,[28,29] though comparison groups of children not receiving therapeutic intervention were not included in such studies. Thus, it would seem that intensity of treatment, in a general sense, assumes dual dimensions of frequency and duration, which are inextricably interwoven in ways that are little understood. This lack of understanding is also reflected in the wide variability of how therapists view the manner in which intensity of treatment should be applied to children. Unfortunately, only three articles have addressed the issue of intensity of treatment, two of which failed to include children having cerebral palsy,[30] while the other categorized previous studies by measuring the trustworthiness of therapy efficacy reported.[31]

Lacking both empirical and theoretical structures for establishing treatment levels for children with cerebral palsy, professionals often have little choice but to rely on custom and intuition in making decisions.[1,25] In public school settings, some children may be scheduled to receive therapeutic intervention intermittently, such as once weekly, while others are treated on a daily basis but only for a short duration of time, such as 6 weeks. Public school officials who are charged with the responsibility of making decisions regarding the allocation of scarce resources are becoming concerned about how services such as physical therapy and occupational therapy should be provided under PL 94-142.[32,33] Similarly, PL 99-457 specifies that the public schools are the payers of last resort for early intervention services, such as occupational and physical therapy for children from birth to 2 years,[34] placing even greater importance on justifications for the frequency of therapeutic regimens provided to this population.

Description of the Study

In order to address the need for a better understanding of intensity of treatment, a comprehensive *Index Medicus* and computer search of the therapeutic intervention effectiveness literature published between 1960 and 1989 was conducted. Intensity was defined as occupational therapy or physical therapy that was reported in the context of either frequency or duration of intervention. Duration included both the length of the therapy session and the duration of the intervention study. Included in the review were reports of children with a diagnosis of cerebral palsy, who were 5 years or less in age at the time that therapy was initiated. Reports describing only a single child were not considered, though numerous case studies relating to therapeutic intervention effectiveness have been published. Studies were classified in the following manner:

- ex post facto studies were categorized as no control group or descriptive;
- studies with two or more experimental groups with no control were categorized as contrast; and
- studies that employed control group methodology (both with and without random assignment) were categorized as control group.

Additionally, outcome measures were examined across studies, with an emphasis upon whether therapy intensity was reported to affect children's responses to treatment or whether a relationship was indicated by the data. Finally, studies were examined for suggestions relating to alternative forms of therapy such as therapist-supervised or parent-implemented intervention.

Findings

A review of the literature generated 13 studies that met the categories described previously. A summary of these findings is presented in the Appendix (at end of article following commentaries).

SAMPLE CHARACTERISTICS

As earlier reports have noted,[10,35,36] criteria for inclusion of subjects in studies that examined therapeutic intervention effectiveness have been far from rigid. Samples of infants and young children with various types of cerebral palsy have typically been drawn from only a limited geographic locale or have drawn from children being served at a particular center or facility.

Descriptive studies

Four studies were categorized as descriptive studies. The number of children in the treatment groups evidenced a wide range, with groups as small as three[37] and as large as 114[20] being reported. Those studies that have employed larger groups of children tend to reflect greater heterogeneity of age ranges.[15,20,38]

Contrast studies

Only six studies used a contrast or comparison group research design. Of these studies, sample sizes ranged from 12 children[19] to 48[2] to 194.[39] In all but one of these studies,[40] the types of cerebral palsy under consideration were described.

Control studies

Three studies were control studies. Characteristically, they used smaller groups of children. Parette[41] described the progress of 25 children, and Wright and Nicholson[12] described the progress of more than 40 children. One study investigated results in fewer than 30 children.[17] Of these three studies, only one provided detailed information regarding the types of cerebral palsy represented in the subjects.

THERAPEUTIC INTERVENTION INTENSITY

Descriptive studies

As shown in the appendix, the therapeutic intervention dimension of duration of therapy for groups of children varied from 9 months[37] to 4 years,[15] and the length of therapy sessions was generally unreported in descriptive studies, with the exception of Norton's study,[37] in which 1-hour treatment sessions were provided. The frequency of therapeutic intervention also varied markedly, ranging from once a year[38] to once a week[20] to daily sessions.[37]

Contrast studies

Four of the six contrast studies described specific treatment parameters relating to length and frequency of treatment. These parameters ranged from biweekly 1-hour sessions for 12 months[2] to 6-day-a-week, 1.5-hour sessions for 4 months.[42] Banham[40] specified only the duration of treatment, ranging from 12 to 22 months for respective treatment groups. One study provided only a mean and standard deviation for treatment duration.[39]

Control studies

The three control studies reported shorter periods of treatment. One reported treatment of 12 months[12] but failed to delineate the frequency of therapeutic intervention strategies provided or the length of therapy sessions. One[17] specified both the duration and frequency of intervention services; treatment reported in this study consisted of 30-minute sessions provided twice weekly for 5 months. The third study[41] reported "individualized" treatment sessions being provided to infants over a period of 6 months.

INSTRUMENTATION

Descriptive studies

Typically, these descriptive studies reported the use of nonstandardized assessment instruments, which addressed such aspects of functioning as fine motor skills[38] and general functional skills across several domains.[15,20] Only one study[37] employed a standardized evaluation instrument, though this study was severely limited in sample size.

Contrast studies

Three of the six contrast studies used standardized assessment instruments.[2,19,40] Two studies[8,42] reported the use of clinic-specific assessment instruments for documenting children's responses to therapeutic intervention. One study[39] employed Vojta screening and assessment procedures along with computed tomography scans to examine the severity of brain damage.

Control studies

The three control studies used two or more instruments to document responses to intervention.[12,17,41] One study[12] reported the use of a clinic-specific assessment instrument in combination with norm-referenced tests and clinical appraisals of physical and neurologic functioning. Another study[17] also described the use of a clinic-specific instrument along with a criterion-referenced instrument employing a well-defined system of coding and scoring performance and a noncalibrated set of guidelines developed by a professional organization. A third study[41] used a norm-referenced evaluation instrument in conjunction with a clinic-specific instrument.

RESPONSE TO TREATMENT AND INTENSITY IMPACT

Descriptive studies

In all four descriptive studies reported in the appendix, children receiving therapeutic intervention demonstrated gains in motor functioning. Three studies suggested a relationship between the provision of intense regimens of therapy and positive motor outcomes: greater progress in those children receiving "adequate" treatment[20]; the attainment of higher developmental levels[37]; and a consistent relationship between number of treatments provided and greater motor progress.[38]

Contrast studies

The six studies employing a comparison group research design reported equivocal findings, with two of the studies conducted during the 1970s[40,42] indicating that treatment provided for a longer duration was critical for greater motor gains. A more recent study[2] reported that therapy provided more than twice monthly might not be as efficacious as other types of intervention.

Control studies

The implications of those studies that have used control group methodology are unclear. The authors of the earliest of these studies[12] commented that therapeutic gains subsequent to intense treatment generally are evidenced in nonmotoric areas, though they never addressed the issue of treatment intensity. One study[17] reported that less intense therapy, or other alternatives, may be indicated for this population. Another study[41] suggested that motor milestones measured by standardized assessment instruments might be obscured through the provision of therapeutic intervention strategies, although more subtle changes such as improved quality of motor acts or movement patterns might be observed.

Discussion

A review of the available literature offers some support for the efficacy of therapeutic intervention for infants and young children with cerebral palsy. However, it fails to reveal any consensus relating to the delineation of "intense therapeutic intervention." Further, it reiterates the ongoing need to examine therapeutic efficacy. With increasing attention being placed upon the implementation of PL 99–457 across the country, the effectiveness of related services such as occupational therapy and physical therapy in these and other children will be even more carefully scrutinized. For professionals who will increasingly be called upon to make decisions regarding which children should receive therapeutic intervention, an attempt to clarify the meaning of the variable of intensity/frequency becomes important, because high service levels for some children may mean that other children will receive little or no services.[1]

The review of the existing literature on data collection and analytical tools used in both physical therapy and occupational therapy suggests that inadequate measurement of children's responses to therapeutic intervention is prevalent.[14,43,44] Traditionally, most therapists have relied on semiobjective, anecdotal reports or simple outcome studies for their evaluation of therapeutic programs. Sometimes, a potentially effective treatment strategy may be deemed to be ineffective because of improper behavior selection and definition, poor measurement strategies, or the failure to evaluate environmental factors.[43] Often, children's failure to respond positively to treatment is attributed to their lack of motivation[22] or to the degree of brain damage.[14] Instead of examining variables that relate to the therapist, the child, or the type of therapy provided, therapists many times resort to attributing lack of progress to the child's behavior or organic condition.[14,43]

In addition to case reports and subjective clinical evaluations, a large number of assessment procedures and instruments typically have been employed to study the effects of therapy in young children who have cerebral palsy. Strategies employed that are readily identifiable in the literature include functional inventories and evaluations of activities of daily living,[15,45] skill tests,[46] motor ability tests,[8,47,48] developmental profiles,[49] and pattern analysis charts.[50]

In any given program serving children who have cerebral palsy, it is often unclear as to how decisions are made regarding the intensity of therapy.[51] Of particular concern is the growing impetus toward more creative programming options for the provision of needed related services to infants and young children with cerebral palsy. This has important implications for public school systems from a fiscal ethics perspective (ie, decisions on how resources are to be allocated for related services under PL 94–142 and PL 99–457). Piper[31] suggested that physical therapy must be provided a minimum of twice weekly to be efficacious in promoting motor milestone attainment. Barnett[32] has noted that the resources needed to adequately provide such services to all handicapped children under existing legislation are inadequate, thus suggesting the need for states to develop alternative models of service delivery that might potentially be based on cost, child progress, or other long-term benefits. Greater attention might be focused on alternative approaches to treatment, such as therapist-supervised, parent-implemented therapy, which could be provided at less expense on a more frequent basis to those children in need of services.

As the habilitation professions continue to examine the effectiveness of therapeutic intervention for children with cerebral palsy, alternatives to traditional intervention are likely to emerge. The demand for accountability in all fields of intervention has been perceived as a call for "developmental physical and occupational therapists to provide objective, systematic documentation of the results of our treatment efforts."[52 (p. 30)] Professionals must continue to investigate the process of evaluating treatment effectiveness; defining the parameters of treatment is necessary if firm conclusions are to be made about what works and how much treatment is necessary.[53] The therapeutic intervention literature is replete with calls that greater attention be given to such treatment parameters as intelligence, degree and type of involvement, age at entry into program, emotional disturbance, and type of treatment approach employed. The efficacy of specific treatment methodologies for specific children will remain clouded by uncertainty if occupational therapists and physical therapists do not achieve consensus regarding the variables that guide and direct their research. "Intensity" is a critical variable requiring clarification and careful delineation if the implications of the researcher's treatment effects are to be fully realized.

A newly emerging database is being reflected in the field of early intervention research. Heightened levels of sophistication are consistently demonstrated in reported studies, characterized by the use of experimental designs that minimize threats to internal validity, careful documentation of procedures and outcomes, and approaches that incorporate theories of general child development.[54] Physical and occupational therapy research is similarly affected as calls for accountability become increasingly evident in the professional literature. With such changes transpiring both within these disciplines and in the systems that employ them, changes may be anticipated with regard to how the intensity of therapeutic intervention is viewed and applied.

References

1. Jenkins JR, Sells CJ. Physical and occupational therapy: Effects related to treatment, frequency, and motor delay. *J Learn Disab.* 1984;17:89–95.

2. Palmer FB, Shapiro BK, Wachtel RC, et al. The effects of physical therapy on cerebral palsy. *N Engl J Med.* 1988;318:803–808.

3. Piper MC, Kunos VI, Willis DM, Mazer BL, Ramsay M, Silver KM. Early physical therapy effects on the high-risk infant: A randomized controlled trial. *Pediatrics.* 1986;78:216–224.

4. Goodman M, Rothberg AD, Houston-McMillan JE, Cooper PA, Cartwright JE, Van der Velde MA. Effect of early neurodevelopmental therapy in normal and at-risk survivors of neonatal intensive care. *Lancet.* 1985;2:1327–1331.

5. Ottenbacher K, Petersen P. The efficacy of early intervention programs for children with organic impairment: A quantitative review. *Eval Program Plann.* 1985;8:135–146.

6. Parette HP, Hourcade JJ. Parental participation in early therapeutic intervention programs for young children with cerebral palsy: An unresolved dilemma. *Rehabil Lit.* 1985;46:2–7.

7. Rainforth B, Salisbury CL. Functional home programs: A model for therapists. *Top Early Child Spec Educ.* 1988;7:33–45.

8. Scherzer AL, Mike V, Ilson J. Physical therapy as a determinant of change in the cerebral palsied infant. *Pediatrics.* 1976;58:47–52.

9. Tyler NB, Chandler LS. The developmental therapists: The occupational therapist and physical therapist. In: Allen KE, Holm VA, Schiefelbusch RL, eds. *Early Intervention: A team approach.* Baltimore: University Park Press, 1978.

10. Parette H P, Hourcade JJ. A review of therapeutic intervention research on gross and fine motor progress in young children with cerebral palsy. *Am J Occup Ther.* 1984;38:462–468.

11. Tirosh E, Rabino S. Physiotherapy for children with cerebral palsy. *Am J Dis Child.* 1989;143:552–555.

12. Wright T, Nicholson J. Physiotherapy for the spastic child: An evaluation. *Dev Med Child Neurol.* 1973;15:146–163.

13. Gonella C. Designs for clinical research. *Phys Ther.* 1973;53:1276–1283.

14. Matin JE, Epstein LH. Evaluating treatment effectiveness in cerebral palsy. *Phys Ther.* 1976;56:285–294.

15. Footh WK, Kogan KL. Measuring the effectiveness of physical therapy in the treatment of cerebral palsy. *J Am Phys Ther Assoc.* 1963;43:867–873.

16. Parette HP, Hourcade JJ. How effective are physiotherapeutic programmes with young mentally retarded children who have cerebral palsy? *J Ment Defic Res.* 1984;28:167–175.

17. Sommerfeld D, Fraser BA, Hensinger RN, Beresford CV. Evaluation of physical therapy service for severely mentally impaired students with cerebral palsy. *Phys Ther.* 1981;61:338–344.

18. Brandt S, Lonstrup H, Marner T, Rump KJ, Selman P, Schack LK. Prevention of cerebral palsy in motor-risk infants by treatment ad modum Vojta. *Acta Paediatr Scand.* 1980;69:283–286.

19. Carlsen PN. Comparison of two occupational therapy approaches for treating the young cerebral palsied child. *Am J Occup Ther.* 1975;29:267–272.

20. Karlsson B, Nauman B, Gardestrom L. Results of physical treatment in cerebral palsy. *Cerebral Palsy Bull.* 1960;2:278–285.

21. Zuck FN, Johnson MK. The progress of cerebral-palsy patients under in-patient circumstances. In: American Academy of Orthopaedic Surgeons, eds. *Instructional Course Lectures,* vol 9. Ann Arbor, MI: J. W. Edwards, 1952.

22. Hourcade JJ, Parette HP Jr. Cerebral palsy and emotional disturbance: A review and implications. *J Rehabil.* 1984;50:55–60.

23. D'Avignon MD, Noren L, Arman T. Early physiotherapy ad modum Vojta or Bobath in infants with suspected neuromotor disturbances. *Neuropediatrics.* 1981;12:232–241.

24. Levitt S. *Treatment of Cerebral Palsy and Motor Delay.* Oxford: Blackwell, 1977.

25. Denhoff E, Robinault IP. *Cerebral Palsy and Related Disorders: A Developmental Approach to Dysfunction.* New York: McGraw-Hill, 1960.

26. Phelps W. The cerebral palsy problem. *Postgrad Med.* 1950;7:206–209.

27. Crothers B, Paine RS. *The Natural History of Cerebral Palsy.* Cambridge, MA: Harvard University Press, 1959.

28. Heber R, Garber H. The Milwaukee project: A study of the use of family intervention to parent cultural-familial retardation. In: Friedlander B, Sterritt G, Kirk G, eds. *Exceptional Infant: Assessment and Intervention.* New York: Brunner/Mazel, 1975.

29. Ramey C, Smith BJ. Assessing the intellectual consequences of early intervention with high-risk infants. *Am J Ment Defic.* 1976;81:318–324.

30. Jenkins JR, Sells CJ, Brady D, et al. Effects of occupational and physical therapy in a school program. *Phys Occup Ther Pediatr.* 1982;4:19–29.

31. Piper MC. Efficacy of physical therapy: Rate of motor development in children with cerebral palsy. *Pediatr Phys Ther.* 1990;2:126–130.

32. Barnett WS. The economics of preschool special education under Public Law 99-457. *Top Early Child Spec Educ.* 1988;8:12–23.

33. Smith BJ, Strain PS. Early childhood special education in the next decade: Implementing and expanding P.L. 99–457. *Top Early Child Spec Educ.* 1988;8:37–47.

34. Fox HB, Freedman SA, Klepper BR. Financing programs for young children with handicaps. In: Gallagher JJ, Trohanis PL, Clifford RM, eds. *Policy Implementation & P.L. 99–457: Planning for Young Children with Special Needs.* Baltimore: Paul H. Brookes, 1989.

35. Dunst CJ, Rheingrover RM. An analysis of the efficacy of infant intervention programs with organically handicapped children. *Eval Prog Plann.* 1981;4:287–323.

36. Simeonsson RJ, Cooper DH, Scheiner AP. A review and analysis of the effectiveness of early intervention programs. *Pediatrics.* 1982;69:635–641.

37. Norton Y. Neurodevelopment and sensory integration for the profoundly retarded multiply handicapped child. *Am J Occup Ther.* 1975;29:93–100.

38. Tyler NB, Kogan KL. Measuring effectiveness of occupational therapy. *Am J Occup Ther.* 1965;19:8–13.

39. Kanda T, Yuge M, Yamori Y, Suzuki J, Fukase H. Early physiotherapy in the treatment of spastic diplegia. *Dev Med Child Neurol.* 1984;26:438–444.

40. Banham KM. Progress in motor development of retarded cerebral palsied infants. *Rehabil Lit.* 1976;37:13–14.

41. Parette HP. *The Relationship of Specific Variables to Motoric Gains in Infants Who Have Cerebral Palsy or Motor Delay: A Comparative Treatment Study.* Tuscaloosa, AL: University of Alabama; 1982. Dissertation.

42. Abdel-Salam E, Maraghi S, Tawfik M. Evaluation of physical therapy techniques in the management of cerebral palsy. *J Egypt Med Assoc.* 1978;61:531–541.

43. Carr BS, Williams M. Analysis of therapeutic techniques through use of the standard behavior chart. Implications for physical therapy. *Phys Ther.* 1982;52:177–183.

44. Whitney PL. Measurement for curriculum building for multiply handicapped children. *Phys Ther.* 1978;58:415–420.

45. Ingram AJ, Withers E, Speltz E. Role of intensive physical and occupational therapy in the treatment of cerebral palsy: Testing and results. *Arch Phys Med Rehab.* 1959;40:429–438.

46. Crosland JH. The assessment of results in the conservative treatment of cerebral palsy. *Arch Dis Child.* 1951;26:92–95.

47. Johnson MK, Zuck FN, Wingate K. The motor age test: Measurement of motor handicaps in children with neuromuscular disorders such as cerebral palsy. *J Bone Joint Surg (Am).* 1951;33:698–707.

48. Zausmer E, Tower G. A quotient for the evaluation of motor development. *J Am Phys Ther Assoc.* 1966;46:725–728.

49. Doman GJ, Delacato CH, Doman RJ. *The Doman-Delacato Developmental Mobility Scale.* Philadelphia: The Rehabilitation Center, 1960.

50. Milani-Comparetti A, Gidoni EA. Pattern analysis of motor development and its disorders. *Dev Med Child Neurol.* 1967;9:625–630.

51. Haley SM. Patterns of physical and occupational therapy implementation in early motor intervention. *Top Early Child Spec Educ.* 1988;7:46–63.

52. Harris SR. Early intervention: Does developmental therapy make a difference? *Top Early Child Spec Educ.* 1988;7:20–32.

53. Bailey DB, Simeonsson RJ. Design issues in family impact evaluation. In: Bickman L, Weatherford DL, eds. *Evaluating Early Intervention Programs for Severely Handicapped Children and Their Families.* Austin, TX: Pro-Ed, 1986.

54. Guralnick MJ. Recent developments in early intervention efficacy research: Implications for family involvement in P.L. 99–457. *Top Early Child Spec Educ.* 1989;9:1–17.

Editor's note: The previous article by Parette, Hendricks, and Rock raised several important issues regarding the cost effectiveness of certain interventions. We asked several experts in the fields of occupational therapy and physical therapy to respond. We hope you will find the two contributions provocative.

Commentary

Barbara Hanft, OTR/L, MA, FAOTA, Charlotte Brasic Royeen, OTR, PhD, FAOTA

We welcome the opportunity to comment upon the discussion presented by Parette, Hendricks, and Rock that the intensity (ie, frequency and duration) of therapy is an important issue to study. We believe, however, that the authors' discussion of intensity is too narrow. How much is enough therapy for children with cerebral palsy is a question that can only be considered in the context of each child's profile of abilities and delays, the service setting, and who is providing the care. Before proceeding, however, we wish to discuss three related but distinctly different terms that we have paraphrased from a noteworthy discussion on research by Pless.[1] The terms are **efficacy**, **effectiveness**, and **efficiency**.

- Efficacy refers to documenting that an intervention is more beneficial than it is harmful.
- Effectiveness refers to documenting that an efficacious intervention can be realistically applied to a target population.

- Efficiency refers to documenting the effectiveness of an intervention with the least expenditures of time, personnel, and money.

According to these definitions, we would argue that the body of research related to therapeutic intervention with infants and young children clearly shows it to be efficacious but not efficient (i.e., other interventions may be less expensive and as effective). Parette, Hendricks, and Rock may really be calling for more studies of efficiency rather than efficacy.

Unidimensional vs Multidimensional

Parette et al. asked, "What is the efficacy of therapeutic intervention intensity with infants and young children with cerebral palsy?" This is an important question, but it reflects a unidimensional view that may be too simplistic. Instead, we believe a multidimensional view is required when evaluating the efficiency of services to any population. A multidimensional view of the efficiency of therapeutic intensity with infants and young children with cerebral palsy would have to address (and not just as a limitation) myriad factors in relationship to each other, as follows[2]:

- Entry criteria (who will benefit?).
- What is the intervention?
- What is the frequency of intervention?
- What is the duration of intervention?
- Who provides the intervention (therapist, aide, family member, or combination thereof)?
- Where is the intervention provided?
- What are the expected outcomes of intervention?
- Exit criteria (will continued intervention yield beneficial results?).

Phases of Research

A second issue we wish to address relates to how empirical data on intervention research is developed over time. By discounting all single subject research regarding the efficacy of therapeutic intensity, Parette, Hendricks, and Rock miss an important body of knowledge. We would argue that single case studies provide an opportunity to gather data important to identifying parameters and launching large clinical trials. One of the premier medical journals in the country, the *New England Journal of Medicine,* publishes a case study in each edition.

Gonella described four phases of knowledge development related to clinical trial research, which are instrumental for understanding the importance of single subject research, as well as other nonexperimental research, such as descriptive correlation and intervention studies.[3] The four phases in Table 1 represent the big picture regarding the development of a body of knowledge for a particular intervention.

Table 1 identifies a hierarchical arrangement, with phase 4 research dependent upon information obtained in previous phases. Though single subject research can be executed to address factors related to phases 3 and 4, it is most often employed when developing a database (phases 1 and 2). A rush to execute clinical trials in phase 4, without adequate preparation in the previous phases, assures contradictory and confounded comparative studies.

TABLE 1
FOUR PHASES OF KNOWLEDGE DEVELOPMENT RELATED TO CLINICAL TRIAL RESEARCH

Research phase	Purpose
Phase 1	Identify parameters of interest.
Phase 2	Describe the effectiveness of the intervention with a number of patients.
Phase 3	Estimate the predictability or reliability of the intervention across patients.
Phase 4	Execute comparative clinical trials.

Differences in Clinical Practice

Parette, Hendricks, and Rock treat occupational and physical therapy as though they were interchangeable interventions. While desired outcomes may be similar (ie, that children function at age-appropriate levels) it is a mistake not to acknowledge differences in treatment objectives and modalities of each discipline. The modality, or specific intervention, chosen by each professional will influence the intensity of treatment. Each profession has diverse treatment approaches that cannot be generically grouped together. Moreover, data from "therapy" studies that include both physical and occupational therapy interventions should also not be grouped together without carefully analyzing the specific services provided. Teaching a child to button his or her shirt versus improving postural stability or eye-hand coordination requires differing amounts of therapist involvement. Working through other professionals or parents versus providing "hands-on" therapy to reach the desired outcome is another variable that will influence the intensity of services.

The question of intensity of services, then, is appropriate to raise *only* within a specific treatment context related to the therapist's professional orientation and accepted standards for best practice. Asking how often therapy should be offered without identifying the desired outcomes is similar to asking what the best age or height is—for what purpose? Research regarding the intensity of therapy is multidimensional and must be connected to the purpose for therapy.

Setting and Intensity

We agree with Parette et al. that an important rationale for looking at the intensity of therapy is the interest of school administrators in implementing Public Law 94–142 and Public Law 99–457. However, these laws, their accompanying regulations, and related judicial decisions define how and when therapy can be provided.

Under PL 94–142, physical and occupational therapy can be provided *only as related services* to help a child benefit from special education.[4] In contrast, PL 99–457 identifies physical and occupational therapy as *primary* services (not tied to special education) that can be offered to assist infants and toddlers with disabilities and their family members.[5] Therefore, occupational or physical therapy provided to a preschool child with cerebral palsy in the school system must be educationally relevant. That same child could receive very different services from a physical or occupational therapist in a private clinic or medical setting.

Therefore, any study addressing the intensity of therapy for children must also look at the context or setting in which the therapy is provided. Again, the question of intensity of services is a multidimensional question, that is, how much therapy is needed to reach the desired outcome for a child with a specific condition and ability profile?

Diagnosis and Intensity

By selecting a diagnostic category for studying the intensity of services, Parette et al imposed an arbitrary classification on their analysis. Therapists do not treat cerebral palsy; they treat the limitations in function and mobility accompanying the condition. By reviewing studies whose subjects were children with cerebral palsy, Parette, Hendricks, and Rock imply, incorrectly, that there is a yet-undetermined "correct" number of hours of therapy to provide. Obviously, children with cerebral palsy demonstrate a very wide continuum of abilities and delays.

We agree that grouping children by diagnosis may help differentiate the outcome of therapy for children who have cerebral palsy versus a different condition such as closed head trauma. However, when considering the question of how much therapy to provide, it is equally important to look at the degree of involvement, the profile of the child's functional abilities and limitations, and the desired outcome of intervention.

Recommendations

In reviewing the literature regarding the intensity of therapy for young children with cerebral palsy, Parette, Hendricks, and Rock have raised an important issue for clinicians and researchers to consider. We believe it is vital for future research to address this issue in a multidimensional context, as it relates to the real world in which services are provided for children. Few insights have been provided regarding the functional relationship between methodology and desired outcomes in early intervention programs.[6] It is simply not helpful to ask how often physical or occupational therapy should be provided without framing the questions within a multidimensional framework that address who needs therapy, for what reason, and who will provide it in what setting.

References

1. Pless IB. On doubting and certainty. *Pediatrics.* 1976;58:7–9.
2. Olney SJ. Efficacy of movement in cerebral palsy. *Pediatr Phys Ther.* 1990;—:145–154.
3. Gonella C. Designs for clinical research. *Phys Ther.* 1973;53:1276–1283.
4. Hanft BE. The changing environment for early intervention services: Implications for practice. *Am J Occup Ther.* 1988;42:724–731.
5. Royeen CB, ed. Occupational therapy in the schools. *Am J Occup Ther.* 1988;42:697–750.
6. Dunst C, Snyder S. A critique of the Utah State University early intervention programs with organically handicapped children. *Except Child.* 1986;53:269–276.

Commentary

Susan R. Harris, PT, PhD, FAPT

While I concur with the desire of Parette, Hendricks, and Rock to examine the effects of therapeutic treatment intensity for young children with cerebral palsy, I do not feel that their extensive review of the early intervention efficacy literature adds much to our understanding of the central question: "Is more therapy better than less?" Although the authors are correct in reporting that the issue of treatment intensity has not been addressed in the research literature concerning young children with cerebral palsy, the study conducted by Jenkins and colleagues[1,2] during the early 1980s involving preschoolers with motor delays deserves more than the passing comment that was received in this review. Since the two articles based on this study are the only ones in the therapeutic intervention literature to address the topic of treatment intensity, they warrant further description.

Research on Treatment Intensity

The earlier article by Jenkins and colleagues[1] examined the effects of different intensities of developmental therapy on the gross motor and fine motor performance of 45 preschool and school-aged children with significant motor delays, as indicated by scores on the pediatric screening tool (PST).[3] The children were stratified according to their scores on the PST and then randomly assigned to one of three groups. The developmental therapy intervention was described as a combination of procedures derived from sensory integration and neurodevelopmental treatment (NDT). Children in the first group received treatment three times a week, children in the second group received treatment once a week, and children in the third group served as a no-treatment control. Treatment sessions were 40 minutes in duration and took place over a 15-week period. All of the children were pre- and posttested on the gross motor and fine motor portions of the Peabody Developmental Motor Scales (PDMS)[4] and on a seven-item scale measuring quality and maturity of postural reactions.

Children in the two treatment groups made significantly greater gains on the PDMS gross motor scores than children in the control group. However, there was no significant difference in gains between the group that received treatment three times a week when compared to the once-weekly treatment group. On the fine motor portion of the PDMS, the children in the two treatment groups made greater gains than the children in the control group but the differences were not statistically significant. All three groups showed significant improvements on the postural reactions scale, but there were no between-group differences in gain scores.

In their discussion of these results, the authors made the following comments:

> One of the more remarkable findings in this research relates to frequency and quantity of treatment. On the PDMS gross motor scale there was evidence of a significant therapy effect, but this effect did not vary with the quantity of therapy provided. Children who received therapy one time a week did as well as those who received three times that amount.[1(p27)]

In a follow-up article elaborating on this research, Jenkins and Sells[2] examined the possibility of different effects of the therapy on children at high and low need for therapy based on their scores on the PST and the PDMS pretest. Children who were more delayed initially based on PDMS developmental motor quotients and who received treatment made large and significant gains on the gross motor scale, whereas the less-delayed children made the same amount of gain regardless of whether or not they received therapy. The authors concluded: "Thus, by determining a motor quotient based on PDMS pretest, it was possible to predict which students would benefit from therapy."[2(p92)] There were no differential effects, however, on PDMS fine motor scores. In the final sentence of this important article, published in 1984, the authors made a plea for replication of this study. However, as Parette and colleagues have noted, no such replications have been published in the intervening 7 years.

Consensus Statements on Treatment Intensity

In the proceedings of a recent consensus conference examining the efficacy of physical therapy in the management of cerebral palsy, Piper[5] examined the issue of treatment intensity/frequency by carefully and systematically summarizing results of 14 studies that had evaluated the effects of physical therapy on promoting the rate of motor development for children with cerebral palsy. Based on the three studies that had employed randomized trials and had demonstrated clear-cut results,[6-8] Piper concluded that "Physical therapy, in order to be efficacious in promoting motor milestone attainment, must be offered a minimum of two times a week."[5(p129)] It is important to note, however, that the final consensus statements summarizing the results of this landmark conference decried the use of motor milestone acquisition as the sole or primary outcome measure in most previous efficacy studies, to the exclusion of more important and more relevant treatment outcomes such as prevention of contractures and deformities; improvements in posture, functional independence, family coping and physical management of the child; and cost/benefit analyses.[9]

Directions for Future Research

The issue of *optimal* treatment intensity for infants and young children with cerebral palsy remains to be addressed. Previous studies on children with cerebral palsy[6-8] have suggested that twice-weekly therapy is needed to effect attainment of motor milestones,[5] but none of these studies was specifically directed at examining the effects of different treatment intensities. No studies have been published that have addressed systematically the effects of varying intensities of therapy on outcomes, such as postural control, functional motor skills, and family adaptations for the child with cerebral palsy.

In spite of pleas by Jenkins and colleagues[1,2] for replication of their study examining the effects of treatment intensity on motor milestone attainment and postural responses in young children with motor delays, no replications have been published. In light of their finding that therapy conducted three times a week was no more efficacious than that conducted once a week, it would seem entirely ethical to partially replicate their design using a sample of young children with cerebral palsy. Rather than including a no-treatment control group, the third group could be a contrast group that would receive a developmental stimulation program similar to the Learningames curriculum[10] that was used by Palmer and colleagues.[7]

While the authors of *this* review article are to be commended for raising the important issue of the relationship of treatment intensity to therapeutic outcome, their article falls short in describing and elucidating the existing research on this topic. It is hoped that this commentary will provide additional food for thought on this important topic and will prompt readers to consider the need for replications of previous studies examining the issue of treatment intensity.

Addendum: Subsequent to the submission of this commentary, an article[11] was published that examined the issue of treatment intensity for young children with cerebral palsy. Although the independent and dependent variables were somewhat different than those examined by Jenkins and colleagues,[1,2] the results were surprisingly similar in that the group that received three times as much NDT did not do significantly better than the group that received less intensive treatment. Readers are advised to review this important study and evaluate its implications concerning treatment intensity.

References

1. Jenkins JR, Sells CJ, Brady D, Down J, Moore B, Carman P, et al. Effects of developmental therapy on motor impaired children. *Phys Occup Ther Pediatr.* 1982;2(4):19–28.
2. Jenkins JR, Sells CJ. Physical and occupational therapy: Effects related to treatment, frequency, and motor delay. *J Learn Disabil.* 1984;17:89–95.
3. Taylor D, Christopher M, Freshman S. *Pediatric Screening: A Tool for Occupational and Physical Therapists.* Seattle: University of Washington Health Sciences Learning Resources Center, 1978.
4. Folio R, DuBose RF. *Peabody Developmental Motor Scales.* Revised experimental edition. IMRID Behav Res Mon No. 25. Nashville, Tenn: George Peabody College for Teachers, 1974.
5. Piper MC. Efficacy of physical therapy: Rate of motor development in children with cerebral palsy. *Pediatr Phys Ther.* 1990;2:126–130.
6. Carlsen PN. Comparison of two occupational therapy approaches for treating the young cerebral-palsied child. *Am J Occup Ther.* 1975;29:267–272.
7. Palmer FB, Shapiro BK, Wachtel RC, Allen MC, Hiller JE, Harryman SE, et al. The effects of physical therapy on cerebral palsy: A controlled trial in infants with spastic diplegia. *N Engl J Med.* 1988;318:803–808.
8. Scherzer AL, Mike V, Ilson J. Physical therapy as a determinant of change in the cerebral palsied infant. *Pediatrics.* 1976;58:47–52.
9. Campbell SK. Consensus statements. In: Campbell SK, ed. Proceedings of the Consensus Conference on the Efficacy of Physical Therapy in the Management of Cerebral Palsy. *Pediatr Phys Ther.* 1990;2:175–176.
10. Sparling J, Lewis I. *Learningames for the First Three Years.* New York: Walker, 1979.
11. Law M, Cadman D, Rosenbaum P, Walter S, Russell D, DeMateo C. Neurodevelopmental therapy and upper-extremity inhibitive casting for children with cerebral palsy. *Dev Med Child Neurol.* 1991;33:379–387.

ACTION PLAN 9: CONDUCT A CLINICAL CASE STUDY

A case description is a wonderful way to begin to identify how clients improve as a result of our intervention. Select a client that you are about to treat or have been treating. A profile guide for writing up the case is provided in Figure 13–2.

FIGURE 13–2*

Individual Completing Profile

Your Name: ______________________________

Discipline: ______________________________

(Include degrees and credentials as you would like them to appear in credits)

Place of Employment: ______________________________

Mailing address: ______________________________

City/State/Zip Code: ______________________________

Description of the Client:

1. Age of client when participating in therapy program:

[ ] Infant/toddler (0–2)	[ ] Adolescent (13–19)
[ ] Preschooler (3–5)	[ ] Adult (20–64)
[ ] School age (6–12)	[ ] Elderly (65+)

2. Disability of client:

[ ] Cerebral palsy (give type:)

[ ] Neuromuscular dysfunction

[ ] Mild-to-moderate motor handicap

[ ] Severe motor handicap

[ ] Multiply handicapped

[ ] Orthopedic handicap

[ ] Learning disabled with motor involvement

[ ] Cardiovascular accident (CVA)

[ ] Aphasic

[ ] Other:

* We wish to acknowledge Georgia DeGangi's contributions to the development of the research on which this figure is based.

3. Cognitive level:
   - [ ] Normal I.Q.
   - [ ] Mild retardation
   - [ ] Moderate-to-severe retardation
4. Associated handicaps:
   - [ ] Sensorimotor dysfunction (i.e., sensitivities to touch or movement)
   - [ ] Hearing loss
   - [ ] Visual impairment
   - [ ] Perceptual problem
   - [ ] Speech and language impairment
   - [ ] Feeding and oral-motor problems
   - [ ] Emotional/behavioral problems
   - [ ] Orthopedic handicap
   - [ ] Medically fragile
   - [ ] Other:
5. When were clients' problems first identified and the referral made for treatment?

   ____

6. Sociocultural background of client
   a. Economic:
      - [ ] Poverty or working poor
      - [ ] Middle class
   b. Environment:
      - [ ] Rural
      - [ ] Urban
      - [ ] Suburban
   c. Education level of parents (or client if adult):
      - [ ] Grade school
      - [ ] High school or equivalent
      - [ ] College education or above
   d. Occupation of parents (or client if adult):
      - [ ] Unskilled labor
      - [ ] Skilled labor
      - [ ] Professional

7. Ethnic background

   a. Race:

      [ ] Caucasian

      [ ] Hispanic

      [ ] Black

      [ ] Native American

      [ ] Middle Eastern

      [ ] Asian

      [ ] Other:

   b. Cultural origin:

      [ ] Parents (or adult client) born in United States

      [ ] Parents (or adult client) born in foreign country

   c. Primary language:

      [ ] English, first language

      [ ] English, second language—fluent

      [ ] Other first language:

      [ ] Language used by therapist:

8. Family structure

   a. Family composition:

      [ ] Single parent

      [ ] Mother and father present at home

      [ ] Extended family in home

      [ ] 1–2 children

      [ ] 3–4 children

      [ ] 5 or more children

   b. Child client:

      [ ] Adopted

      [ ] Foster child

      [ ] Biological

Description of the Therapy Program:

9. Setting(s) where therapy was provided:

   [ ] Outpatient clinic   [ ] Home

   [ ] Hospital setting   [ ] School

10. Environment(s) where therapy was provided:

[ ] Individual therapy room

[ ] Shared with other therapists and clients

[ ] Classroom

[ ] Home

[ ] Other

11. Disciplines providing services to client:

[ ] Physical therapy

[ ] Speech and language therapy

[ ] Occupational therapy

[ ] Special education

[ ] Psychology

[ ] Social work

[ ] Psychiatry

[ ] Nursing

[ ] Nutrition

[ ] Other

Of the disciplines listed above, star or check those involved in the NDT management program (e.g., the "NDT team").

12. How long did the client receive NDT?

[ ] Under 6 months

[ ] 7–12 months

[ ] 1–2 years

[ ] 2 years +

13. Give the client's age at the beginning and end of the treatment program that you will be describing.

[ ] Age at start:

[ ] Age at finish:

14. How often did the client receive NDT (this may include all members of team)?

[ ] 2×/mo.

[ ] 1×/wk.

[ ] 2×/wk.

[ ] 3×/wk.

[ ] Daily

[ ] Other:

15. How long were the typical treatment sessions?

[ ] 15 min. [ ] 1 hr.

[ ] 30 min. [ ] > 1 hr.

[ ] 45 min.

16. Which areas were considered an emphasis of the treatment program of the NDT team?

[ ] Quality of movement

[ ] Sensory

[ ] Activities of daily living

[ ] Upper extremity

[ ] Lower extremity

[ ] Feeding/oral-motor

[ ] Vocational/play

[ ] Reflexes, posture

[ ] Tone

[ ] Communication

[ ] Functional performance

[ ] Behavior, motivation

[ ] Other:

17. What were your specific goals for the client?

a. ______________________________

b. ______________________________

c. ______________________________

d. ______________________________

e. ______________________________

f. ______________________________

18. Did other members of the NDT team have different goals?

Yes [ ] No [ ]

If yes, were these discipline specific?

Yes [ ] No [ ]

19. Did the client and/or family have different goals?

Yes [ ] No [ ]

If yes, please explain.

20. In addition to NDT what other treatment techniques did the client receive during the program you are describing?

[ ] Myofascial release

[ ] Cranio-sacral

[ ] Mobilization

[ ] Sensory integration

[ ] Biofeedback

[ ] Resistive exercises

[ ] Developmental

[ ] Technology

[ ] Muscle energy

[ ] Proprioceptive neuromuscular facilitation

21. What equipment and materials did you use in your NDT treatment session?

[ ] Mobile surfaces

[ ] Benches

[ ] Suspended equipment

[ ] Manual vibrators

[ ] Theraband

[ ] Weights

[ ] Vocational training

[ ] ADL training

[ ] Orthotics

[ ] Pictures, books, visual stimuli

[ ] Other:

22. Which therapeutic handling techniques did you use?

[ ] Sustained deep pressure

[ ] Intermittent handling

[ ] Traction

[ ] Weight bearing/shifts

[ ] Vibration

[ ] Mobilization

[ ] Pressure tapping

[ ] Sweep tapping

[ ] Stretching (passive range of motion)

[ ] Active range of motion

[ ] Graded deep pressure with movement

[ ] Other:

Please star those handling techniques that seemed to work best.

23. Which key points did you use in handling?

[ ] Trunk [ ] Lower extremities

[ ] Pelvis [ ] Hands

[ ] Shoulders [ ] Feet

[ ] Upper extremities [ ] Neck

24. Which of the following did you include in the client's NDT program?

[ ] Preparation (e.g., alignment, activating tone, inhibitors, etc.)

[ ] Work on movement patterns (e.g., transitions, components of movement, weight-bearing patterns, etc.)

[ ] Functional skills (e.g., ADL, dexterity, stair climbing, feeding, etc.)

[ ] Positioning program

[ ] Home program

[ ] Other:

25. If a home program was included, what did it involve?

[ ] Positioning

[ ] Stretching

[ ] Practice of movement patterns

[ ] Specific exercises

[ ] Functional skills (i.e., self-care, daily care routines)

[ ] Work/play activities

26. How involved was the client/family in carrying out the home program?

[ ] Very involved [ ] Somewhat involved [ ] Minimally involved

27. How motivated was the client to improve in areas addressed by the NDT program?

[ ] High [ ] Moderate [ ] Low

28. Which elements did your therapy sessions include?

[ ] Physical handling

[ ] Verbal monitoring of client's movements

[ ] Positioning

[ ] Stimulating movement through positioning of materials or selection of activities

[ ] Consultation to family or client

[ ] Consultation to other professional(s)

29. Please describe any other aspects of the treatment program that you feel were important in contributing to the changes that you observed.

____

____

____

30. Outcomes

Using the chart below, please indicate with a "B" where the client's responses fell *before* you began treatment and with an "A" where they fell at the end of your program (or when you made observations of progress).

Areas observed	**Functionally independent or age appropriate**	**Partially dependent; mild lag or dysfunction (i.e., up to 6 mos.)**	**Functionally dependent; moderate to severe dysfunction or lag (over 1 year lag)**
1. Gross motor			
2. Fine motor			
3. Communication/language			
4. Cognition			
5. Perceptual			
6. Work/play			
7. Self-care			
8. Feeding			
9. Social emotional			
10. Other			

31. Please indicate in the appropriate column

a) if a problem was observed in a particular area at the onset of the therapy program;

b) if the problem was still present with little to no progress;

c) if progress was apparent but the problem remains;

d) if the problem has resolved; and

e) when the changes occurred (e.g., two months after therapy program began).

Area Observed	Original Problem	Little to no progress	Gains observed; still problem	Problem resolved	When change observed after beginning of treatment
A. Reflex Maturation: 1. Presence of primitive reflexes 2. Righting and equilibrium reactions					
B. Postural Tone/Control: 1. Postural alignment 2. Postural tone 3. Weight-bearing patterns 4. Postural adjustments 5. Anti-gravity movement					
C. Functional Motor Skills: 1. Fine motor 2. Gross motor 3. Quality of movement 4. Movement patterns					
D. Functional Performance: 1. Self-care (e.g. dressing bathing) 2. Feeding/eating 3. Work/play					
E. Sensory Processing: 1. Somatosensory 2. Vestibular functions 3. Motor planning 4. Bilateral integration					
F. Learning/Communication: 1. Attention/arousal 2. Perception 3. Speech 4. Language/communication 5. Information processing					

Area Observed	Original Problem	Little to no progress	Gains observed; still problem	Problem resolved	When change observed after beginning of treatment
G. Socialization/Emotion: 1. Motivation 2. Social interactions 3. Emotion regulation/behavior					
H. Other Areas:					

32. Please describe the ways in which your client improved in those areas indicated in no. 30.

Area: ______________________________

How Improved: ______________________________

Area: ______________________________

How Improved: ______________________________

Area: ______________________________

How Improved: ______________________________

Area: ______________________________

How Improved: ______________________________

Area: ______________________________

How Improved: ______________________________

Area: ______________________________

How Improved: ______________________________

Area: ______________________________

How Improved: ______________________________

Area: ______________________________

How Improved: ______________________________

33. Please elaborate on any other things that are pertinent to the case that have not been described in this profile.

____

Even simply describing a model program may be a type of case. Such a description is provided in the following example.

"Autistic Adolescents" reveals that sometimes even just a description of an innovative program is worth sharing.

ILLUSTRATIVE EXAMPLE 13–4

Reprinted from *Occupational Therapy in Health Care,* Vol. 2, Number 3, Fall, 1985, pp. 59–68. Used with permission.

Autistic Adolescents: Developmental Milestones and a Model Treatment Program

Charlotte Brasic Royeen, MS, OTR, Linda F. Little, MS, PhD

For most individuals adolescence is a time of major developmental changes.[1] Adolescence starts with the onset of puberty and continues until the ill-defined stage of adulthood. Adolescence is often conceptualized in terms of stages and tasks. The early adolescent is just beginning to assert independence from parents, to think abstractly and ideologically, and to experience sexual arousal.[2] By midadolescence, the young person has moved from interacting with same-sexed crowds, through the stage of opposite-sexed groups, to coupling of opposite-sexed partners who isolate themselves from others and experiment with intimate relationships.[3] It is during midadolescence when thoughts turn to who and what one can become, to exploring one's potential and testing limits for who one might be. Late adolescence is typically the stage of most ambivalence for adolescents and their parents. It has been labeled by Schenk and Schenk as the NQA stage, that is, the not-quite-adult, not-quite-adolescent stage when parent and adolescent fluctuate greatly between perceiving the adolescent as a grown-up peer and an immature child.[4] It is during late adolescence when parents are also faced with developmental tasks of their own: their offspring, who consumed much of their attention and energy since birth, have with the progression of adolescence diminished demands for the parenting role. Parents' thoughts turn to issues surrounding their identity without parenting as a primary role.[5]

The Autistic Adolescent

The normal developmental changes of adolescence can be absent or aberrant in the presence of autism, a behavioral disorder syndrome defined below:

> Autism is a severely incapacitating and lifelong developmental disability that typically appears during the first three years of life. It occurs in approximately 15 out of every 10,000 births and is four times more prevalent in boys than girls. There appears to be several causes, each with distinct neurological effects.... The most common symptoms of autism include:
>
> a. disturbances in the rate of appearance of physical, social, and language skills;

b. abnormal responses to sensations. Any one or a combination of sight, hearing, touch, pain, balance, smell, taste, and the way a child holds his/her body are affected.

c. speech and language are absent or delayed while specific thinking capabilities may be present;

d. abnormal ways of relating to people, objects and events.[6]

Infantile Autism by definition has an onset prior to age 30 months. However, if families refuse or cannot recognize their child's condition, initial diagnosis may not occur until early childhood when there is contact with external institutions.

While some adolescents possess autistic characteristics that are mild while other areas of functioning are normal, this paper is concerned with adolescents who possess the complete symptomology of autism defined above.

Physical appearance of autistic adolescents would not readily distinguish them from their peers. Yet, it is usually immediately apparent that these young people are deviant in some way because of physical behaviors, stereotypic of autism. The self-stimulation of hand flapping, rocking, head banging, or what appears to be over-involvement in a particular object quickly trigger, even to the untrained observer, that something is wrong. Adolescents with severe self-punishing behaviors may bear scars of past punishments that would set them apart physically from their peers.

Activities of daily living (ADL) for the autistic adolescent require minimum to maximum supervision depending on two major factors: (a) previous training in early and late childhood, and (b) innate capacity (e.g., the ability to plan for motor movements and actual motor control). Typically, with good skills training, and sufficient innate abilities, dressing, bathing, and kitchen skills can be done with minimal supervision in the form of verbal cueing for initiation of tasks or activities. Autistic adolescents with poor training or inadequate capacity require verbal cueing plus varying degrees of physical assistance for task completion. It is not uncommon, for example, for autistic persons with severe deficits and insufficient training to require physical assistance with toileting to ensure adequate hygiene.

Interpersonal relationships are atypical for the autistic adolescent. "The failure to develop interpersonal relationships is characterized by a lack of responsiveness to and a lack of interest in people, with a concomitant failure to develop normal attachment behavior".[p. 87,7] Adolescents who are autistic have missed the bonding with parents in infancy, the cooperative play necessary to establish and maintain friendships in childhood, and are typically severely retarded in their relationship with peers in adolescence. It is not uncommon for facial expressions to be socially inappropriate and for nonverbal cues to distance the autistic child from his/her peers. Contributing to the autistic adolescent's inability to maintain relationships with peers are the difficulties experienced in the realm of communication. Language can be nonexistent or inadequate in its development when present.[7] When language is present and verbal skills are developed, this might mislead others in that they attribute to the autistic adolescent emotional skills on the same level as his language skills when the two do not necessarily coexist. Table 1 is presented as a summary and reference guide to developmental tasks of adolescence contrasted for normal and autistic adolescents.

TABLE 1
A COMPARISON OF DEVELOPMENTAL ISSUES BETWEEN NORMAL AND AUSTISTIC ADOLESCENTS

Normal Adolescent	*Autistic Adolescent
Peer relations of major importance.	No
Move toward functional independence (caretaking) from parents	No
Sexual identity matures	May be an issue and mature outlets often lacking.
Self concept expands to include adult possibilities	Not usually, but with support can move into work roles, etc.
Abstract thinking emerges and idealism is prevalent. Focus on "what if."	Variable, usually not communicated.
Move toward self-sufficiency.	Variable, but usually self-sufficiency is not a realistic goal.
Continued financial dependence on parents while earning some on their own.	Yes, possibly could earn some monies.

* These are statements about typical autistic adolescents and their families. Severity of symptoms should be considered in specific case examples.

The Family of the Autistic Adolescent

By the time an autistic child has reached adolescence, the family has had much experience in dealing with the disease. The functional family has passed the stages of surprise, hope for a swift cure, and acute mourning for what could have been. Doubtless, the family has been exposed to bureaucracy, red tape, inadequacy of "trained experts," and ignorance and insensitivity of the general public to the reality of their lives. The family has learned to expect that their child will continue to need their support and assistance (both physically and financially) beyond his/her childhood and adolescence. Assistance might be in the form of financial support for institutional care and emotional support in the monitoring of care provided externally from the family setting. The family cannot look forward to the normal launching of their child into adult roles and full independence, nor to changing their own roles from parent to peer with the continuing development of their offspring.

In families with adolescent members who are not autistic, adolescence typically triggers developmental crises for both generations of family members: The youth is to leave home and establish an individual identity. The older generation is to refocus on the marital relationship and facilitate the youth's leaving. If marital problems or role confusion exist in the older generation, exiting of the younger generation may be hindered. Parents may decide to keep their child young and in the nest to avoid developmental issues of their own. When these family transitions are successful however, the adolescent moves on to more adult-like behaviors and the parents focus on their emerging developmental needs.

Parents of autistic adolescents do not realize these normal developmental demands—these requirements for shifting roles. Both generations are forced to maintain their respective roles of parent and child. Parents may at this time fully experience the realization that these major transitions are never to be made. Typical life events experienced by other families may trigger the mourning process of "what might have been." For example, the autistic adolescent's family may experience a stage of disequilibrium when a normal milestone such as high school graduation is experienced by the peers of their teen. The contrast with their child's functioning is once again accentuated.

Table 2 is presented as a summary and reference guide to developmental tasks of families with normal and autistic adolescents.

Many families having autistic adolescents have not resolved their hope for a swift cure, remorse over what could have been and guilt or anger over the autistic nature of their child. In such cases, the family's capacity to realistically acknowledge and assess the needs, ability, and future of the autistic adolescent is compromised, as is the healthy functioning of the parent generation.

TABLE 2

A COMPARISON OF DEVELOPMENTAL ISSUES BETWEEN NORMAL AND AUTISTIC ADOLESCENTS AND THEIR FAMILIES

Families of Normal Adolescents	Families of Autistic Adolescents
Need to increasingly let go of parenting roles.	No, not usually.
Need to shift relationship style to allow, encourage adult behaviors in adolescents.	Not to extent of normal family adolescents.
Need to develop individual pursuits to fill parenting void.	Not for that reason.
Refocus on marital relationship to fill gap. Reevaluate marital satisfaction.	Possibly triggered by other stimuli.
Parents are faced with their own aging process and possible alterations in physical functioning.	May be accentuated in families with autistic symptoms.
Parents often experience serious illness and/or death of their own parents at this stage.	Parents worry about continued care of offspring as they become physically less capable.
Final reconciliation with one's own parents may be required.	Yes.
Shifts in careers and/or retirement may alter finances.	Similar decisions face parents of autistic adolescents.
Because of stresses related to the aging process and the loss of parental roles, extramarital affairs often surface as a mode of coping.	May occur but stimulated by lack of relief from parenting roles.

A Model Treatment Program for Autistic Adolescents

Traditionally, autistic adolescents and their families have had few specialized services available to them. However, in 1979 the Community Services for Autistic Adults and Children (CSAAC) was created. CSAAC is a private, nonprofit agency dedicated to the education, training and wellness of persons disabled with autism.[8] It developed out of the need for services specifically designed for autistic adolescents and adults in the State of Maryland. The CSAAC services "have been described by experts in the field as among the 'most innovative' in the United States, and mental health researchers from across this country—as well as a team from Spain—have been visiting Bethesda to learn about the operation."[p. C4,9]

The program of services for autistic adolescents is twofold, yet well integrated. *The Preiser School* is one part of the program of services. The school is designed to serve profoundly handicapped autistic adolescents within a community-based setting, paying special attention to the developmental needs and crises of the autistic adolescent and the family. The school is located in Bethesda, Maryland, and offers classes of individualized and group instruction to autistic adolescents. *Residential homes* are the other part of the program of service, i.e., each autistic adolescent attending Preiser School lives in a residential home. The various homes are scattered throughout the community with four students living in each home along with fulltime residential staff. The residential staff is comprised of counselors who live in the homes on a rotating basis. For both the school and residential program, there is at least a one-to-two staff-to-student ratio at all times. Many students go to their parental homes on weekends, but return to the residential home during the week. If the students do return to parental homes on the weekend, the professional staff are available to counsel the parents on behavioral management techniques or for any specific problems the parents have regarding their child. Counseling focuses on skill development so that the weekend visits can be a positive experience for both the family and the autistic adolescent, and to maintain consistency with the school and residential programs.

PROGRAM FUNDING

The Preiser School and the residential homes are funded by CSAAC which, in turn, is funded by the Maryland State Department of Mental Hygiene and State Department of Education. In addition, the U.S. Department of Housing and Urban Development, state and local governments, private foundations and private donations financially support the programs. Each student attending the programs pays according to financial ability.

PROGRAM JUSTIFICATION

There were no programs designed for autistic adolescents in the State of Maryland when CSAAC began. Thus, prior to the onset of CSAAC, approximately 95% of the autistic adolescents faced lifelong institutionalization.[9] With the advent of the CSAAC program services, many autistic adolescents now can learn to live and work in the community, and thus relieve their families of the financial and psychological hardships of institutionalization.

TREATMENT PROGRAMS

In addition to the educational services offered at Preiser School, numerous related services are available. Occupational therapy, speech therapy, and psychological therapy are all available according to the needs of the individual student and family. Individual services are provided as well as a cross-disciplinary approach with all team members having input on programming so that teachers, parents and residential staff can better understand and serve the autistic adolescent. This team approach encourages a consistent environment across geographic locations.

In addition to these related services, fulltime professional staff members are employed to contact and set up employment positions for students within community businesses, so that the autistic adolescent can be placed within a community job once his work skills are sufficiently developed.

GOALS OF THE PROGRAM OF SERVICES

The three primary goals of students in the residential and school programs are (a) to achieve schooling and living experiences for the autistic adolescent within the community setting, (b) to achieve vocational readiness, and (c) to achieve maximal independence in living within group home settings. The ideal end product of these three goals is to have the autistic adolescent working at a job within the community and living as independently as possible within a group home. These primary goals are achieved by specifying skills, abilities, or behaviors needing attention on the Individualized Educational Program (IEP). The IEP is generated by input from all professionals working with an autistic student and subjected to approval by his parents or guardians.

The IEP goals are carried out within both the school and residential settings. Typical content areas of IEP goals for the school and residential settings are summarized below.

School	**Residential Home**
Communication	Homemaking Skills
Self Care	Activities of Daily Living
Functional Academics	Money Management
Fine and Gross Motor Skills	Leisure Activities
Socialization	Banking, Shopping, etc.
Recreation	

OCCUPATIONAL THERAPY SERVICES

Occupational therapy is one of the related services offered at Preiser School. Occupational therapy services consist of (a) evaluation of the autistic adolescent, (b) direct therapy services (if appropriate),[10] and (c) communication with other professionals, parents and staff members (including residential home staff) regarding the functional abilities of the autistic adolescent. Both occupational roles (student, homemaker, family member, employee, etc.) and developmental levels are discussed.

The occupational therapy evaluation consists of the following: first, overall sensory and motor functioning are evaluated using ADL (activities of daily living) tasks, gross and fine motor activities, and observation; second, reflex developments are assessed, especially bilateral motor coordination and ATNR (Asymetric Tonic Neck Reflex) since these can have such adverse effects on midline activity required for most prevocational tasks; third, sensory histories are taken using interviews with teachers, caretakers and other professionals as well as observations of free play in a playground setting. Special attention is given to behaviors associated with tactile defensiveness and gravitational insecurity.[10] Fourth and finally, motor planning ability is specifically assessed using mazes, ADL tasks, observation, and interviews with parents and teachers. Motor planning assessment is important due to its role in communication with sign language as well as ADL and vocational tasks. Each evaluation period lasts approximately two to three hours and individual reports describing the autistic adolescents' strengths and weaknesses related to developmental levels, occupational behaviors in the classroom, home and at play are presented to parents, professionals and staff members of the Preiser School and residential home.

If severe deficits in reflex development, motor planning, gravitational insecurity or tactile defensiveness are found, the students are assigned to individual therapy sessions on a weekly basis. Direct therapy services offer one-to-one treatment designed to enhance sensory integrative organization and prevocational skills. Therapeutic activities for the residential home and classroom are also prescribed and carried out by staff members under the supervision of the occupational therapists.

Summary

In summary, the current paper has identified developmental tasks of adolescents and their families and contrasted them with levels of functioning and areas of concern for autistic adolescents and their families. Awareness of developmental issues of normal adolescents and families that trigger crises and growth to a new stage of development, is quite beneficial for occupational therapists treating autism. Strong knowledge of developmental theory on both individual and family levels enables the therapist to better understand the adolescents and families with whom they deal. Such information (a) allows the therapist to assess how far their patients deviate from what typically occurs in these developmental stages; (b) can be used to help families with autistic teens to normalize some of the experiences, feelings, thoughts they might otherwise label 'crazy' or aberrant. For example, it can be quite reassuring to know that parents of teens struggle with their own developmental issues regardless of the functioning of their children; and (c) might provide clues to sources of depression and grief experienced by parents as they grapple with what is and what might have been.

Further, a program of services specifically designed for autistic adolescents, that includes occupational therapy services, was presented. The program of services for autistic adolescents has recently received national recognition in two ways. First, CSAAC has become the first community program designed for those with autism to be accredited by the Accreditation Council for Services for Mentally Retarded and Other Developmentally Disabled Persons (AC-MRDD). Second, CSAAC has received "model program" status from the U.S. Department of Education and funding was granted for refinement, training and replication of the CSAAC model. Occupational therapists working in the field of autism may find components of the program, herein described, applicable for their settings.

References

1. Schnell, R.E. and Hall, E. *Developmental Psychology Today.* New York: Random House, 1979.

2. McCandless, B.R. *Adolescents: Behavior & Development.* Hinsdale, Illinois: The Dryden Press, Inc., 1980.

3. Dunphy, D.C.: The social structure of urban adolescent peer groups. Sociometry 26: 230–246, 1963.

4. Schenk, Q.F., & Schenk, E.L. *Pulling Up Roots: For Young Adults And Their Parents Letting Go and Getting Free.* Englewood Cliffs, New Jersey: Prentice-Hall, Inc., 1978.

5. McCullough, P.: "Launching Children and Moving On." In E.A. Carter and M. McGoldrick, *The Family Life Cycle: A Framework for Family Therapy.* New York: Gardner Press, Inc., 1980, 171–195.

6. "People with autism are working." *Newsletter of Community Services for Autistic Adults and Children,* Jan. 1984, 5.

7. *Diagnostic and Statistical Manual of Mental Disorders.* DSM-III (3rd Ed.). American Psychiatric Association, 1980.

8. *Community Services for Autistic Adults and Children.* Descriptive Brochure. CSAAC, 751 Twinbrook Parkway, Rockville, MD 20851.

9. Nugent T: "Autistic—And Thriving." *The Sun* (Baltimore), January 1982, C1, C4.

10. Ayres, A.J. and Tickle, L: Hyper-responsivity to touch and vestibular stimuli as a predictor of positive response to sensory integration procedures by autistic children. *Am J Occ Ther* 34: 375–381, 1980.

ACTION PLAN 10: DOMAIN SPECIFICATION

Many of the constructs with which we deal have not been adequately defined or discussed, either as constructs or operational variables. For example, if someone wants to develop a new test on intelligence, they do not have to backtrack and define intelligence. However, if we want to develop a test for gravitational insecurity, functional mobility, and so on, we first have to better define that domain. We have to identify those behaviors and anything else we can think of that is related to it. That is the first step in research.

In 1986 I published "Domain Specification of the Construct Tactile Defensiveness," presented here as an example of **domain specification**.

During the process of peer review, one of the reviewers commented that the article should not be published, because no other discipline publishes domain specifications—only the instrument itself. My counterargument on this peer review was that such domain specification needs to be published because other disciplines are not dealing with new constructs.

As therapists we are dealing with new constructs that we must further define and specify. For example, what are gravitational insecurity, occupational performance, quality of life, functional movement, and occupational health? Description of these domains of interest is the foundation of subsequent measurement.

ILLUSTRATIVE EXAMPLE 13–5

Reprinted from *American Journal of Occupational Therapy*, Vol. 39, Number 9, September, 1985, pp. 596–599. Used with permission.

Domain Specifications of the Construct Tactile Defensiveness

Charlotte Brasic Royeen

Key words: pediatrics • research • sensory integration

Tactile defensiveness is a sensory integrative disorder that results in a syndrome or collection of behaviors, which includes "...excessive emotional reactions, hyperactivity, or other behavioral problems" (1, p. 184). It can also be considered a construct, which is a postulated attribute of some children, assumed to be reflected in their behavior (2). Behavioral manifestations of tactile defensiveness can be excessive fighting, an inability to sit quietly at a school desk, or an inability to enjoy "contact comfort" with a significant other. Although tactile defensiveness is a sensory integrative disorder, it also appears in children who have problems other than sensory integrative dysfunction. The condition has been documented in mentally retarded children (3), autistic children (4), and developmentally delayed children (5).

Larson (5) and Bauer (6) have both elaborated on the pioneering work of Ayres (1, 7, 8) in the delineation of behaviors that are characteristic of tactile defensiveness. But a more extensive specification of behaviors associated with tactile defensiveness is necessary for continued empirical study to implement the psychometric measurement of the construct (9). Thus, the purpose of this study is to specify "the domain of observables" (9, p. 141); that is, to describe tactile defensiveness in elementary schoolchildren by developing a comprehensive list of descriptors of behaviors associated with the condition.

Statement of the Problem

Currently, tactile defensiveness is inferred when a child responds adversely to being touched during the Southern California Sensory Integration Tests or at another time (8). Consequently, therapists depend on behavioral observations to determine tactile defensiveness. Development of an empirically derived list of descriptors associated with tactile defensiveness serves as an "explicit, public exhibition" of the specification of the domain of tactile defensiveness (9, p. 66). Such specification, built on subjective judgments of specialists regarding the degree to which certain descriptions of behavior are associated with tactile defensiveness, serves to build construct validity into any tests that might subsequently be constructed from those descriptors (2, 9, 10). Construct validity is the degree to which a test measures the construct or attribute it purports to measure (10).

Research Plan

This descriptive study is also the first phase of a larger study to construct a standardized instrument that will measure tactile defensiveness. Therefore, the research plan is based on scaling methodology. Scaling is a process for developing a set of items empirically designed to reveal the characteristics of the variable or construct under consideration. A description of how scaling techniques were modified for use with children can be found elsewhere (11). Accordingly, specification of the domain of the construct of tactile defensiveness was accomplished by following guidelines for the first phase of scale development, which is an eight-step process (12).

Procedure

Step One: Definition of the Construct

A constitutive definition of tactile defensiveness was generated: aversive reactions to touch, manifested in atypical psychological or motor behavior.

Step Two: Collection of a Variety of Behaviors Related to the Domain of the Construct

Behaviors were collected in two ways: (a) examples of behaviors thought to be characteristic of tactile defensiveness were gleaned from a literature review, and (b) members of the Greater Washington DC Area Sensory Integration Study Group listed all behaviors they felt were characteristic of tactually defensive children. This step yielded a list of approximately 80 behaviors associated with tactile defensiveness.

Step Three: Submission of a List of Behaviors for Review

To check the content of the items and enhance the construct validity of the 80-item list, the list was submitted to A. J. Ayres for review. A revised list of approximately the same number of items was generated.

Step Four: Generation of the Descriptors

Once the list of behaviors was completed, a list of statements a tactually defensive child might make based on the behaviors (descriptors) was generated.

Step Five: Editing

The list of descriptors was edited to reduce ambiguity and enhance clarity.

Step Six: Elimination

Redundant items were eliminated. The result was a revised list of 73 descriptors.

Step Seven: Rating by a Panel of Experts

The 73 descriptors were then rated by a panel of experts. Each expert gave his or her view of the extent to which each descriptor, if stated or felt by a child, was associated with tactile defensiveness. This panel of experts consisted of 13 faculty members and 1 assistant faculty member of Sensory Integration International (formerly the Center for the Study of Sensory Integration International). Each descriptor was rated on a scale of 1 to 12: a rating of 1 meant that the descriptor had no association with tactile defensiveness, a rating of 6 meant it had some degree of association with tactile defensiveness, and a rating of 12 meant the descriptor was strongly associated with tactile defensiveness.

Step Eight: Data Analysis

The ratings by the panel were analyzed using the program Condescriptive from the Statistical Package for the Social Sciences (13).

Results

Descriptors that had a mean score of 6 or better were included in the compilation of descriptors associated with tactile defensiveness: descriptors that had a mean score of 5 or less (24 of 73) were eliminated. Two other descriptors were dropped because they contained a cultural and sexual bias. The resulting 47 descriptors are presented in Table 1.

Discussion

When the mean scores of the descriptors were reviewed, it became apparent that descriptors 26, 27, 33, 37, 41, and 42 were rated the highest, with scores of 9 or 10. These descriptors dealt with either intrusions into body-centered space (e.g., unexpected touch) or the need to extinguish touch input by rubbing or scratching. Larson (5) found that the most discriminating items for distinguishing between tactually defensive and non-tactually defensive children were those related to the child's response to touch. Similarly, the present study found that the panel of experts rated items based on response to touch as most highly associated with tactile defensiveness. Thus, it can be concluded that there is a growing body of evidence suggesting that children's reactions to touch can be used to validly measure the presence or absence of tactile defensiveness.

Furthermore, the highest rated descriptors also have the smallest standard deviations (under 2). This suggests that there is a high degree of agreement among the experts regarding the significance of these descriptors as behaviors associated with tactile defensiveness.

The standard deviations of the rest of the descriptors range from under 2 to over 4, suggesting less agreement among the raters regarding the significance of

TABLE 1
COMPILATION OF DESCRIPTORS ASSOCIATED WITH TACTILE DEFENSIVENESS IN CHILDREN

Item No.	Mean	SD	*N*	Descriptor
1	6.28	2.201	14	I like wearing shoes better than going barefoot.
2	6.143	1.834	14	I like to wear long sleeves.
3	7.077	1.977	13	I like to wear long pants better than short pants.
4	7.857	2.316	14	It bothers me to go barefoot.
5	6.929	1.817	14	The feel of new clothes bothers me.
6	6.5	2.312	14	I like new clothes to be washed before I wear them.
7	6.5	2.345	14	It bothers me to have my socks pulled up after they have slipped down.
8	7.071	2.586	14	Fuzzy shirts bother me.
9	6.786	3.043	14	Fuzzy socks bother me.
10	6.429	2.954	14	If I had my way, I would like to wear my coat all the time.
11	7.357	2.872	14	Turtleneck shirts bother me.
12	7.429	1.910	14	Tags in shirts and blouses bother me.
13	6.857	1.916	14	Tags in shirts bother me, unless I wear a T-shirt underneath.
14	7.786	2.007	14	Tags in shirts bother me, especially if they are at my neck.
15	6.5	2.929	14	Lace on clothing bothers me.
16	6.143	3.134	14	Embroidery on clothes bothers my skin.
17	8.571	2.277	14	It bothers me to have my face washed.
18	7.429	2.377	14	It bothers me to brush my teeth.
19	6.214	2.636	14	It bothers me to have my nails cut.
20	8.071	2.303	14	It bothers me to have my hair combed by someone else.
21	8.643	2.405	14	It bothers me to have my hair cut.
22	7.286	3.667	14	After I get my hair cut, the hair left on my neck bothers me.
23	6.769	3.032	14	It bothers me if my hands are dirty.
24	6.857	2.070	14	It bothers me to play on a carpet.
25	6.5	2.442	14	I like to play on a smooth floor.
26	9.786	1.251	14	After someone touches me, I feel like scratching that spot.
27	9.714	1.267	14	After someone touches me, I feel like rubbing that spot.
28	8.851	1.351	14	It bothers me to walk barefoot in the grass and sand.
29	8.786	1.528	14	It bothers me to play in a sandbox.
30	7.357	2.405	14	Going to the beach bothers me.
31	6.385	2.219	13	Getting dirty bothers me.
32	6.857	3.325	14	I find it hard to pay attention.
33	9.786	1.477	14	It bothers me if I cannot see who is touching me.
34	8.857	1.834	14	Finger painting bothers me.
35	8.929	1.817	14	Rough bed sheets bother me.
36	7.857	2.797	14	I like to touch people, but it bothers me if they touch me back.
37	9.286	1.541	14	It bothers me when people approach me from behind.
38	6.786	2.940	14	It bothers me to be kissed by someone other than my parents.
39	7.643	2.045	14	It bothers me to be hugged or held.
40	7.857	2.381	14	It bothers me to play games with bare feet.
41	9	1.840	14	It bothers me to have my face touched.
42	10	1.301	14	It bothers me to be touched if I don't expect it.
43	7.21	4.35	14	I am ticklish.
44	7.786	3.423	14	It bothers me when someone tickles me.
45	6.077	3.303	13	I have difficulty making friends.
46	6.5	2.902	14	I get in fights.
47	6.786	3.068	14	It bothers me when someone is close by.

SD, standard deviation.

those descriptors for tactile defensiveness. This finding suggests that although the mean score reflects a strong association between the descriptors and the tactile defensiveness on part of the reviewers, there is less agreement among reviewers on these items. These descriptors can be grouped into the following four categories: a) activities of daily living (ADL), b) play, c) clothing, and d) social/behavioral interactions. Thus, it appears that while there is a fair degree of consistency in how experts rate behaviors such as touch responses to people when they are associated with tactile defensiveness, there is apparently no such consistency in how experts rate behaviors such as ADL activities, play, clothing, and social/behavioral interactions when they are associated with tactile defensiveness. Thus, these latter behaviors should be associated with tactile defensiveness in a more cautious manner than touch responses to people. However, there is ample evidence to consider all of the behaviors identified as potentially associated with tactually defensive behavior.

Conclusions

Specification of the domain of observables for the construct of tactile defensiveness provides evidence of construct validity for subsequent test development (10). Thus, the current specification in children is important in terms of how it can be used in subsequent research. There are two different methodologies that such research can employ: a) scaling techniques for which the current study is preliminary or b) more traditional psychophysical measures, such as observations of responses to activities specified within the domain. The current list of behaviors associated with tactile defensiveness can serve as a foundation for either methodology: construction of either a scaling instrument or a psychophysical test measuring tactile defensiveness. Once such assessments have been developed, a comparison of the performances of normal children to the tactilely defensive children can be made, and the assessments can then be refined.

In addition, domain specification of tactile defensiveness can be used as another piece of information in the continued development of sensory integrative theory and practice. Theory has been advanced by further delineating the domain of one of the constructs within the theory. This is important because the construct tactile defensiveness is fairly new and relatively undefined compared with other more established constructs, such as "intelligence" or "creativity."

Practice can be advanced by cautiously using the specified behaviors as additional areas to be investigated via interview format when conducting a comprehensive sensory integration evaluation or when evaluating a change during treatment.

Delimitations of the Study

The domain of the construct tactile defensiveness has been specified only for elementary school children. Therefore, it cannot be related to infants, adults, or the aged. Furthermore, because specification was accomplished through empirically deriving a list of behaviors associated with tactile defensiveness, it deals only with observable behaviors and does not include the neurophysiological processes underlying the construct. Finally, the list of behaviors of the domain do not constitute a clinically useful diagnostic test and therefore should not be used as such.

Acknowledgments

The author thanks the members of the Greater Washington DC Area Sensory Integration Study Group and the faculty of Sensory Integration International for participating in this study and Dr. James Starr, Psychology Department of Howard University, for giving procedural advice.

This study was made possible through funding from the American Occupational Therapy Foundation (Grant No. 1502-462) and computer time from the Academic Computer Services of Howard University.

References

1. Ayres AJ: *Sensory Integration and the Child.* Los Angeles: Western Psychological Services, 1979
2. Jackson DN, Messick S: *Problems in Human Assessment.* New York: McGraw-Hill, 1967
3. Kinnealey M: Aversive and non-aversive responses to sensory stimulation in mentally retarded children. In *Research in Sensory Integrative Development.* A Price, E Gilfoyle, C Meyers, Editors. Rockville, MD: AOTA, 1976
4. Ayres AJ, & Tickle LS: Hyper-responsivity to touch and vestibular stimulation as a predictor of positive responses to sensory integrative procedures by autistic children. *Am J Occup Ther* 34:375–381, 1980
5. Larson KA: The sensory history of developmentally delayed children with and without tactile defensiveness. *Am J Occup Ther* 36:590–596, 1982
6. Bauer BA: Tactile sensitivity: Development of a behavioral response checklist. *Am J Occup Ther* 31:357–361, 1977
7. Ayres AJ: *Sensory Integration and Learning Disorders.* Los Angeles: Western Psychological Services, 1973
8. Ayres AJ: *Southern California Sensory Integration Tests Manual.* Los Angeles: Western Psychological Services, 1973
9. Nunnally JC: *Introduction to Psychological Measurement.* New York: McGraw-Hill, 1970
10. Wormer FB: *Basic Concepts in Testing.* Boston: Houghton Mifflin, 1968
11. Royeen CB: Adaptation of Likert scaling for use with children. *J Occup Ther Res* 5:59–69, 1985
12. Summers GF: *Attitude Measurement.* Chicago: Rand McNally, 1970
13. Nie NH, Hull CH, Jenkins JG, Steinbrenner K, & Bent DH: *Statistical Package for the Social Services.* New York: McGraw-Hill, 1975

ACTION PLAN 11: EVALUATE INSTRUMENTS FOR CLINICAL AND RESEARCH USE

Review a test for use from the clinical perspective, considering the psychometric principles of the test. It is important to look at tests with a critical eye—not to aspire to unduly criticize them. By analyzing tests we can better understand how to use them appropriately in our practice. Thus, it is a valuable contribution to read, analyze, and write up a criticism of a published measurement tool. The following analysis of the DeGangi-Berk Test of Sensory Integration is an example of such a criticism (Royeen, 1988).

ILLUSTRATIVE REVIEW 13–6

Reprinted from *Physical and Occupational Therapy in Pediatrics,* Vol. 8, Number 2/3, 1988, pp. 71–75. Used with permission.

Review of the DeGangi-Berk Test of Sensory Integration

Charlotte Brasic Royeen

Test Description

Title of Test: DeGangi-Berk Test of Sensory Integration.

Authors: Ronald A. Berk and Georgia DeGangi.

Publisher and Source: Western Psychological Services, 12031 Wilshire Boulevard, Los Angeles, CA 90025.

Purpose of Test: Identification of sensory integrative dysfunction in preschool aged children. It should not be used independently if employed for diagnostic purposes.

Intended Population: The test is intended for use with preschool children aged three to five.

Category of Test: Criterion referenced.

Time Required: Approximately a half hour. The test is meant to be administered in one session.

Who Can Give the Test: This test is designed for occupational and physical therapists to administer. It can also be used by special educators and other professionals and paraprofessionals, however, the test can be used for diagnostic purposes only if administered by occupational and physical therapists. The test is meant to be used only for screening purposes if administered by other professionals or paraprofessionals.

Test Manual: The test manual is clearly written and well presented.

Test Standardization

Sample: This test is primarily locally normed, that is, subjects upon whom the normative data are based are from the greater Washington, D.C., area and a few are from Indiana. The manual can get a bit confusing because different studies are referred to for different types of information. The test appears to be based primarily upon information obtained from a sample of 139 subjects. Of these, 38 were delayed and 101 were "normal" children. The sample was predominately black and more three- and four-year-old children were used than five-year-old children. No information on the socioeconomic status of the subjects was provided.

Comment: Traditional psychometric standards would suggest that the normative sample is too small, too geographically restricted, and that the test is therefore more appropriate as a pilot edition than for national use. Three considerations, however, mitigate application of strict testing standards for evaluation of the test. First, given the dire need for instrumentation in this area, a test with restricted standardization is preferable to no test at all. Second, precedent has been set with prevalent use of a geographically normed test, i.e., the Denver Developmental Screening Test. Third, the authors instruct that this test is not to be used for diagnostic purposes without additional information and test data; therefore, this test can probably be appropriately employed by occupational and physical therapists who are specifically trained in pediatrics.

Test Administration

Training Required: The manual states that approximately two hours of training are necessary in order to administer the test. That is, an individual would need to review and become familiar with the protocol of test administration and scoring; however, he or she would most probably wish to practice actual test administration at least five times and be observed by a therapist competent in administration of the test. Also, test interpretation should probably be discussed with an experienced therapist for the first five to ten administrations.

Scoring: The scoring procedures are clearly explained and presented. Each test item has clear instructions for scoring that ranges from either 0 to 4 or 0 to 3 for each item. Items can then be summed for subdomains (bilateral motor integration, postural control and reflex integration) and summed for all test items combined.

Equipment: Relatively inexpensive items are required for administration of this test, and most can be obtained through Western Psychological Services.

Setting: The test must be administered in a space at least 10 × 15 feet in order to allow for standardized execution of test items requiring a child to move over distances.

Instructions: Test instructions for administration are clearly presented. These include specification of what to say to the child during test administration.

Test Validity

Construct Validity: The test is presented as a test of sensory integrative function and dysfunction in children aged three to five. In the section of the manual, "Theoretical Background," the authors discuss sensory integrative processing and identify the foundations thereof, i.e., tactile, proprioceptive and vestibular sensory systems and interactions. The authors further discuss "vestibular based functions" as being the most easily measured aspects of sensory integration and therefore identify why they have chosen bilateral motor integration, postural control and reflex integration as the domains for test. The reviewer believes that bilateral motor integration, postural control and reflex integration are "end product" motor functions which are related, in part, to vestibular system processing; therefore, to call these functions "vestibularly based" may not be the most precise terminology. In addition, since the entire domain of sensory integration is much broader than just motor functions related to vestibular processing, to call this test a test of sensory integration may be somewhat misleading. This is, more precisely, a test of three areas of brain stem and spinal cord level motor functions which are related to sensory processing generally, and vestibular system processing specifically.

Source of Test Items: The test is concentrated on the domains of bilateral motor integration, postural control and reflex integration. Given these domains, the item development within each is clearly presented and justified. Test items are generated according to accepted psychometric practices. The test consists of 36 items which were selected from a larger pool of items based upon their ability to discriminate between normal and delayed children.

Classification Accuracy: The test developers made a conscious decision to "minimize the false normal error rate." That is, they wished to develop a test most likely to identify dysfunction. The classification accuracy of identifying dysfunction is reported to be 81% for total test scores.

Comment: Due to the greater number of three- and four-year-old children in the sample upon which the test is based and as discussed by the authors of the test, it is probably more valid for these ages than for five-year-old children. In addition, because of the predominance of blacks in the normative sample, the test may contain some degree of cultural bias.

Test Reliability

Test Stability: Based upon a sample of 29 subjects, reliability coefficients of .85 to .96 were obtained for the total test score.

Reliability of Classification: Screening classification of a child into "normal" or "dysfunction" may be considered 83% to 100% accurate, based upon investigation of the 29 subjects.

Comment: Reliability indices for Reflex Integration tend to be lower overall. The total test scores are the most reliable and this reviewer does not recommend using subdomain scores independently except as clinical observations.

Summary

The authors are to be commended for developing a test in an area in great need of more and better measurements. It is a most difficult area and they should be considered as leaders in this field. This reviewer would suggest, however, that a more accurate name be provided for the test, one that better reflects what it actually measures, i.e., a limited subdomain of motor functions related to sensory integrative processing.

Reference

Stangler SR: *Screening Growth and Development of Preschool Children: A Guide for Test Selection.* New York: McGraw-Hill, 1980.

ACTION PLAN 12: ADAPT EXISTING INSTRUMENTS OR METHODOLOGY

This is where therapists excel. We can adapt anything. There is considerable existing methodology around that someone who knows a particular subject group can adapt for use with that group. Or one can take an existing instrument and adapt it for use with another group, obtaining new normative data. By building on existing methods or instruments in this way, one is efficiently and effectively using previous work to generate new knowledge and procedures.

That is what I did with "Adaptation of Likert Scaling for Use with Children" (Royeen, 1989). Recall from chapter 7, on measurement, that Likert scaling is based on the response format of agree, neutral, disagree, and so on.

This methodology is used with adults all the time. It was a challenge, and yet fun, to adapt and validate this methodology for use with children. Adapting methodology underlies subsequent development of an instrument to assess tactile defensiveness. The adaptation process is presented in the following example.

So sometimes, rather than reinventing the wheel by developing a new instrument or process, the best thing to do is to adapt or revise an instrument or process.

Reprinted from *Occupational Therapy Journal of Research,* Vol. 23, Number 1, January, 1989, pp. 23–26. Used with permission.

ILLUSTRATIVE EXAMPLE 13–7

Adaptation of Likert Scaling For Use With Children

Charlotte Brasic Royeen

Key words: research • test construction • pediatrics

Quantitative measurement of qualitative variables has traditionally been accomplished by using the research methodology of scaling. The most widely used and reliable scaling procedure, the Likert scale or summated rating scale, was investigated in order to adapt the research methodology for use with children. Adaptation of the Likert methodology would enable occupational therapists to begin to measure qualitative variables in children in a quantitative way. Five questions germane to the adaptation of Likert scaling in children were investigated by means of pilot studies using children aged 6 to 10: 1) Will graphic representation help children better understand scale items? 2) What is the optimal response format for scale items used with children? 3) How can one ascertain appropriate language levels of items for children? 4) What directions are necessary in order to administer such a scale to children? and 5) What is the validity of employing modified Likert methodology with children? The results of the pilot studies suggest that items composed of simple sentences can be used with children, providing that such items are reviewed by a speech and language pathologist and pretested with children for comprehension. It was found that graphic representation of items was not necessary and, in fact, was confounding. In addition, it was found that a three response format ("No," "A little," "A lot") with the responses inscribed on the blocks worked best. Moreover, the pilot studies revealed that children need to be taught how to participate in responding to a scale procedure and that anxiety was reduced when they were told it was a game and not a test. Scale items worked best when posed in an interrogative format rather than the traditional Likert statement format. Finally, preliminary results indicate the modified Likert methodology is valid to use with children. Suggested directions to use when administering a modified Likert scale to children are presented.

According to Benson and Clark (1982), within the field of occupational therapy "the paucity of adequate instrumentation available for documenting therapeutic effectiveness surfaces as a major problem area" (p. 789). Additionally, the areas of occupational therapy evaluation and theory development are hindered by the lack of a sufficient number of standardized, reliable, and valid instruments for measuring factors germane to the domains of psychiatric, pediatric, gerontologic, and physical dysfunction occupational therapy.

The reasons for the current dilemma regarding instrumentation are twofold. First, in the past there have been few occupational therapists trained in the content areas (research design, statistics, grant writing) necessary for the successful development of standardized instruments. Second, and perhaps more important, is the fundamental problem of attempting to measure factors or variables such as "functional performance" or "psychological processes," which are intrinsically qualitative. Essentially, the measurement problem for occupational therapy, evaluation, documentation of treatment effectiveness, and continued theory development is to render qualitative data in quantitative form. That is, how does one develop instrumentation to measure qualitative variables in a quantitative manner? In the fields of psychology and sociology, this problem has been addressed by the development of methodology that attempts to represent the variable in question on a continuum that can be subdivided and measured numerically. By example, Benson and Clark (1982) imply that the same type of methodology of measurement is appropriate for occupational therapy. This methodology is scaling.

Scaling Defined

Scaling is a general term referring to a collection of methodologies for developing a set of items empirically designed to reveal the characteristics of the variable under consideration. McIver and Carmene (1981) propose three purposes for which scaling models are appropriate:

1. Confirmatory: testing a specific hypothesis.
2. Exploratory: describing the manifestations of a variable.
3. Evaluate: developing a test on which subjects can be given scores.

Given these purposes, scaling techniques can be used by researchers to address each problem area in occupational therapy affected by the lack of sufficient instrumentation. It is also postulated that scaling techniques can help occupational therapy researchers solve the problem of rendering qualitative data in quantitative form and develop much-needed screening and assessment tools.

Scaling methodologies that have been developed and refined by researchers in other disciplines can be modified to meet the specific instrumentation needs of the occupational therapy profession. Such modification of existing research methodologies to meet the specific needs of a discipline or profession is a long-standing research practice. For example, the need to improve agricultural techniques led to the development of systematic research designs (systematic ways for assigning particular types of crops to plots of land) by agricultural scientists, which have subsequently been modified by behavioral scientists to create randomized designs (randomized assignment of treatments to individuals or groups) (Kirk, 1982).

The three most common scaling techniques are the Likert or summated scales, the Thurstone or equal-appearing intervals, and the Guttman or scale analyses. This paper reports on the most commonly used scale methodology, the Likert scale.

Likert Scaling

Traditionally, Likert scales have been used for attitude measurement. Gorden (1977) describes the Likert method:

> In the method of summated ratings, items are selected by a criterion of internal consistency. Subjects check whether they strongly agree, agree, or undecided, disagree, or strongly disagree with each item. Numerical weights are assigned to these categories of response using the successive integers from 0 to 4, the highest weight being consistently assigned to the category which would indicate the most favorable attitude. A high and low group are selected in terms of total scores based upon the sum of the item weighed. The responses of these two groups are then compared on the individual items and the 20 or so most discriminating items are selected on the attitude test. A subject's score on this test is determined by summing the weights assigned to his responses to the 2 items. (p. 112)

Examples of Likert scale items follow:

Strongly Agree	Agree	Undecided	Disagree	Strongly Disagree
1	2	3	4	5

"It is very important to be able to grocery shop without the assistance of friends or relatives."

Strongly Agree	Agree	Undecided	Disagree	Strongly Disagree
1	2	3	4	5

"All adults should bathe and dress by themselves."

Subjects respond to each sample item according to the degree to which they agree or disagree with the statement by checking a particular number.

Statement of the Problem

Of all scaling techniques, the Likert methodology is widely recognized as the easiest and most reliable (Maranell, 1974). Likert scaling has long been used for measuring traits in adults. It was the purpose of the current study to investigate the use of Likert scaling with children to adapt it for appropriate use in pediatrics. Given the existing research methodology for Likert scaling, the following questions were investigated via a series of pilot studies:

1. Will pictures representing the content of the individual scale items help the children understand the items?
2. Given that the adult Likert-type response format is usually 5 to 12 categories, ranging on a continuum of strongly disagree to strongly agree, what is the optimal response format for children aged 6 to 10?
3. What kind of directions do children need in order to participate in a study using a modification of Likert scaling?
4. Is the language and writing style of adult-oriented Likert items too complex for children? If so, how can one ascertain appropriate language levels of items for use with children?
5. What is the validity of employing a modified Likert methodology with children?

Investigation of these questions was accomplished by conducting a series of pilot studies. These are reported seriatim.

PILOT STUDY 1: ASSESSING THE NEED FOR GRAPHIC REPRESENTATION

The Likert type of scoring requires subjects to read a statement and respond to it. Since the methodology is being adapted for use with children, the subject's reading of the items was discounted because it would require too much skill of most children. Therefore, it was decided that a research assistant would read each descriptor to a child. Whether or not graphic representation of the descriptors would help the child comprehend the meaning conveyed by each descriptor was questioned. Thus, the items were pretested using graphic representation. Graphic representation consisted of two black-and-white line drawings on a 21.6 cm x 27.9 cm (8 1/2 by 11 in.) white page, illustrating the two different situations described in each item. These items were generated as part of a larger study (Royeen, 1984) and are shown below.

- I like wearing shoes better than going barefooted.
- I like to wear long pants better than short pants.
- It bothers me to go barefooted.
- It bothers me to stand in line.

Subjects

The characteristics of the children who served as subjects for this pretest are presented in Table 1. The children for this particular pretest were enrolled in a small, private elementary school in a suburb of Washington, DC. Subjects were selected for participation by the school principal. Since the adaptation of Likert scaling was being developed for children aged 6 to 10, most of the children serving as subjects in the pretests were 6 years old. It was assumed that a 6-year-old's performance would represent a baseline and that older children would perform as well or better.

Procedure

The descriptor was read to the subject, and the subject was asked to respond. Subsequently, the descriptor was read to the child while simultaneously presenting a graphic depiction of the content of the descriptor. The subject was then

TABLE 1
CHARACTERISTICS OF CHILDREN IN PILOT STUDY 1

Subject	Sex	Chronological Age	Race
1	Male	6 yr 11 mo. 5 days	Black
2	Male	6 yr. 10 mo. 5 days	Taiwanese
3	Female	6 yr. 11 mo. 19 days	Caucasian
4	Female	6 yr. 11 mo. 1 day	Caucasian
5	Male	8 yr. 9 mo. 22 days	Caucasian

questioned regarding his or her understanding of the descriptor with and without graphic representation.

Results and Conclusions

Four of the five subjects preferred a verbal presentation of the descriptors without graphic representation. Some of the subjects' statements were, "I can think better without the pictures," and "It is confusing with the pictures." Therefore, use of graphic representation was not deemed necessary. The pictures did not seem to help the children and, in fact, appeared to confuse them. This consideration, coupled with the practical fact that use of pictures would introduce new and possibly confounding factors in any study, not to mention added expense, indicated that it was prudent to deem pictures unnecessary.

PILOT STUDY 2: DETERMINING THE OPTIMAL RESPONSE FORMAT AND SCALE ADMINISTRATION

A test was conducted to determine whether the usual five types of response patterns—strongly agree (5), agree (4), undecided (3), disagree (2), and strongly disagree (1)—are appropriate for use with children. In addition, the nature of the items and directions for children taking the "test" were explored. Thus, the children were administered a 49-item instrument on an exploratory basis (Royeen, 1984). The items in the scale were all similar to the items used in the first pilot study.

TABLE 2
CHARACTERISTICS OF CHILDREN IN PILOT STUDY 2

Subject	Sex	Chronological Age	Race
1	Female	8 yr. 9 mo. 27 days	Caucasian
2	Male	8 yr. 8 mo. 7 days	Caucasian
3	Female	6 yr. 2 mo. 19 days	Caucasian
4	Male	7 yr. 2 mo. 2 days	Caucasian
5	Male	6 yr. 9 mo. 5 days	Black
6	Male	6 yr. 10 mo. 5 days	Taiwanese
7	Female	6 yr. 11 mo. 19 days	Caucasian
8	Female	6 yr. 11 mo. 18 days	Caucasian
9	Male	8 yr. 9 mo. 22 days	Caucasian

Subjects

Table 2 presents the characteristics of the children in pilot study 2. Subjects were from two small private schools in the suburbs of Washington, DC, and they were again selected for participation by the principal.

Procedures, Results, and Conclusion

Sample Likert items were administered to each child individually. The children were asked about how they responded and why. Also, different response formats were implemented, and, using interview techniques, the children were asked to explain what they felt about the items. The children found the 5-item response format too confusing, and they were confused by the rather abstract notion of how much the item was like them. Also, the children reported less anxiety during the interview when told this was a game to learn more about themselves and not a test.

Based on this particular pilot, four conclusions were drawn which answer the second question, what is the optimal response format for children. First, a 3-item response format seemed optimal; that is, "No" (1), "A little" (2), and "A lot" (3). The children preferred to have the responses printed on three corresponding blocks, which were 2 × 2 in., 2 × 3 in., and 2 × 4 in. Even those children who could not read what was printed on the blocks preferred their use. Children reported, "Different sizes help you to remember different choices," and "It would be a lot harder without them."

Second, the children needed to be taught how to participate. With no directions or teaching, the children were confused and did not orient to the task. They should be told it is a game and not that it is a test, since they reported less anxiety over a game format. Moreover, they needed a chance to practice responding to sample items before actual scale items were administered. Each child needed only three to four tries to grasp the concept. Also, they needed to be reminded that the items can be repeated and explained if necessary, since the purpose is to obtain their response to an item and not to test them on memory or vocabulary.

Third, rephrasing items from statement format ("Fuzzy socks bother me.") into question format ("Do fuzzy socks bother you?") made the items easier for the children to comprehend. The direct question-answer format is more in line with the children's usual way of giving information. Finally, many children were distracted by the researcher's papers having the list of items. Use of a shield to block such distracting materials solved the problem.

PILOT STUDY 3: LANGUAGE ASSESSMENT

Any scale designed for children must ensure the appropriateness of the vocabulary and sentence structure, and it must be determined whether children really understand the items.

Subjects

Eight subjects from the same two schools as in pilot study 2 served as subjects; their characteristics are presented in Table 3.

TABLE 3
CHARACTERISTICS OF CHILDREN IN PILOT STUDY 3

Subject	Sex	Chronological Age	Race
1	Female	6 yr. 0 mo. 0 days	Black
2	Male	7 yr. 0 mo. 12 days	Caucasian
3	Male	7 yr. 0 mo. 24 days	Black
4	Female	7 yr. 2 mo. 19 days	Caucasian
5	Female	6 yr. 0 mo. 9 days	Caucasian
6	Female	6 yr. 0 mo. 22 days	Caucasian
7	Female	6 yr. 4 mo. 16 days	Caucasian
8	Female	6 yr. 6 mo. 8 days	Caucasian

Procedure

The children were individually administered the same scale items as used in pilot study 2. All items had previously been reviewed by a speech pathologist to ensure appropriateness of the vocabulary. Thus, the question of how one can ascertain appropriate language levels of Likert items for use with children was addressed. A review of scale items by a speech pathologist before actually testing items helped to establish appropriate vocabulary levels. Most items were clearly understood by the children, except for those items having two parts. For example, a statement like "Does it bother you to have your socks pulled up, after they have fallen down?" was confusing since it has two concepts that are related sequentially. It is suggested that two-part items are unnecessarily confusing for children. Rather, all statements should be straightforward, simple sentences with no dependent clauses.

Discussion

A compilation of suggested directions to use when administering a modified Likert scale to children as developed from these pilot studies is included in the appendix.

The final question that prompted the current study—what is the validity of employing a Likert-type methodology with children—needs to be addressed. In a related study to develop a scale measuring tactile defensiveness in children (Royeen, 1984), 102 children, aged 6 to 10 years, were administered a modified Likert scale. Of those 102 children, only 3 had tests that were somewhat questionable in terms of attentiveness or vigilance. Comparatively, in one study 50 out of 350 adults had tests that were questionable due to distractibility, random answers, and the like (Gorden, 1977). Thus, evidence suggests that children were more conscientious in responding to a modified Likert scale. One can surmise that the findings of a study employing modified Likert methodology with children has an excellent chance for valid results.

It should be noted that methodology (question-response format) may interact with question content. Consequently, the proposed modified Likert methodology might work with some, but not all, types of content. Caution should be exercised when applying the revised methodology to different content domains.

Subsequent research studies employing the modified Likert scale methodology developed in the current study can further investigate the validity as well as determine the reliability of this methodology when used with children. The methodology may have promise as a way to expand occupational therapy assessment of qualitative variables in children. However, continued development and refinement of the methodology is needed if that promise is to be fulfilled.

APPENDIX

Suggested Directions for Administering a Modified Likert Scale to Children

The subject (S) and the examiner (EX) sit at a table with the S across from the EX. EX uses a shield to cover the instrument. EX orients S to the task. EX explains that they will be playing a game in which there are no "right" answers and there are no "wrong" answers. They are playing a game just so that the EX can learn more about the S. EX explains the response format to the S. EX states:

"I will ask you questions and you are to answer them by saying either 'no,' 'a little,'or 'a lot.'"

EX simultaneously points to each of the three blocks inscribed with these phrases while saying them out loud. EX continues, saying:

"Let's practice the game for you to learn how to play it. I will ask you a question: Do you like ice cream? You answer saying either 'no,' 'a little,' or 'a lot.'"

EX again points to the blocks when stating choices for response. EX continues:

"Remember to point to the block or state the one that is your choice."

S may point to the block that is his or her choice or state the answer out loud. The purpose of the block is to aid the S in remembering the response items. It is the purpose of the practice session to teach the child the response format. Thus, this procedure should be repeated until the EX is certain that the S understands how to answer the questions. Suggested questions to use if further practice is required are:

- Do you like snakes?
- Do you like vegetables?
- Do you like school?
- Do you like turtles?

Once the S understands the task and required response style, EX states: "Now we will play the game." The EX may restate or explain any item until the S understands the item or if the S asks the EX to repeat an item or states that he does not understand the question. EX should read the question and wait for the S to respond. If the S does not respond and needs prompting, EX may ask:

Which answer do you want? [Gesturing] "No," "a little," or "a lot"?

EX records the S's answer and notes any observations that are pertinent. Upon completion of the session, the EX praises the S for his participation.

Acknowledgments

This study was supported in part by Grant #1502-462 from the American Occupational Therapy Foundation, Inc. The author wishes to acknowledge Dr. G. Cline of VPI&SU as a source for some of the concepts expressed herein.

References

Benson, J., & Clark, F. (1982). A guide for instrument development and validation. *American Journal of Occupational Therapy, 36,* 789–800.

Gorden, R. L. (1977). *Unidimensional scaling of social variables.* New York: Free Press.

Kirk, R. E. (1982). *Experimental design: Procedures for the behavioral sciences.* Belmont, CA: Brooks/Cole Publishing Co.

Maranell, G. M. (1974). *Scaling: A sourcebook for behavioral scientists.* Chicago: Aldine Publishing Company.

McIver, J. P., & Carmene, E. G. (1981). *Unidimensional scaling.* Beverly Hills: Sage Publications.

Royeen, C. B. (1984). Development of a scale measuring tactile defensiveness in children. Manuscript submitted for publication.

ACTION PLAN 13: INVESTIGATE CONCURRENT VALIDITY OF TESTS

Theory drives test development and an individual should perform certain ways on tests as predicted by theory. You can give an individual two different tests and according to some theory, predict that the individual should perform either the same or differently on the tests. For example, if you gave a child an intelligence test and the child scores poorly, theory would predict that on any visual perception test the same child would not score terribly high as these constructs are related.

You can do this kind of research with instruments in occupational therapy based on what you know about sensory integration, occupational behavior, and neurodevelopmental treatment theory, or based on your clinical experiences. You can select instruments and use your knowledge of theory to predict subject performance. Then, measure and see what happens. Thus, how one test relates to another based on another is investigation of **concurrent validity**. Review the following example of such an investigation.

ILLUSTRATIVE EXAMPLE 13–8

Reprinted from *Occupational Therapy Journal of Research,* Vol. 9, Number 1, January/February, 1989, pp. 3–15. Used with permission.

Tactile Functions in Learning-Disabled and Normal Children: Reliability and Validity Considerations

Moya Kinnealey

Key Words: sensory integration • sensory integrative dysfunction • touch

Touch is a primary sensation and is basic to early learning. Child development theories of Piaget (Ginsburg & Opper, 1979), Kulka, Fry, and Goldstein (1960), and Bruner (1973) emphasize the primacy of the sense of touch or sensory motor systems in cognitive as well as in motor development. Touch has been one of the predominating senses throughout evolution. It is present at and before birth and probably continues to be more critical to human functioning throughout life than is generally recognized (Ayres, 1972). The sense of touch begins to affect humans even when they are in the womb and is one of the first systems to become myelinated and thus to become functional in the fetus (Huss, 1977). The integration of touch sensation can be observed in the newborn in the early rooting reflex whereby a baby, when touched on the cheek, will turn his or her head toward the stimulus (Ayres, 1979).

The association of tactile dysfunction with academic problems in relatively normal children can be traced to Gerstmann, a German neurologist who described and named a syndrome of neurological signs (Gerstmann, 1927). The classical tetrad was as follows: right-left disorientation, finger agnosia (indicative of tactile problems), agraphia, and acalculia. Kinsbourne and Warrington (1973) and Benson and

Geshwind (1970) studied children with Gerstmann syndrome and related their findings to children with dyslexia and academic difficulty. They also noted that the children were clumsy. Henderson and Hall (1982) and others studying clumsy children, found that a large proportion of children labeled "clumsy" have normal intelligence but experience learning difficulties in aspects of their school work such as reading and arithmetic (Dare & Gordon, 1970; Gordon & McKinley, 1980; Gubbay, 1975). The tactile problems of these children are described as loss of proprioception, loss of discriminatory abilities, agnosia for touch sensation, defects in finger localization, and a disorder of body image characterized by an inability to relate the parts of the body to extrapersonal space (Lesny, 1980; Walton, Ellis, & Court, 1969).

Hyperactivity is often linked to learning disabilities (Nelson, 1984; Strauss & Lehtinen, 1947) and is characterized by excessive gross motor activity, developmentally inappropriate inattention, and impulsivity (American Psychiatric Association, 1980). One theory of hyperactivity in learning-disabled children is that it is the result of a tactile system deficit—that is, tactile defensiveness (Ayres, 1964, 1972). The basic postulates of this theory are that there are two functional tactile systems—a protective system, which responds to stimuli with movement, alertness, and a high degree of affect; and a discriminative system, which enables interpretation of the temporal and spatial nature of stimuli. Under certain circumstances, the two systems lose (or never attain) their natural balance, and the protective system predominates. When the protective system predominates, the hyperactivity syndrome is aggravated, affect and somatic discomfort is heightened, and perceptual motor development is retarded (Ayres, 1964).

Bauer (1977b) studied the relationship between tactile defensiveness and hyperactivity, first developing a behavioral response checklist to help identify the clinically determined phenomena of tactile defensiveness. In a second study (1977a), she found that boys with hyperactive behaviors displayed a greater frequency of the behaviors defined as evidence of tactile sensitivity, or tactile defensiveness.

Sears (1981) identified the tactilely defensive child for the special educator working with learning-disabled students. In this study, the children's behavior is described as hyperactive and distractible, and the tactile problems described influence school relationships, activities, and academics as well as the adaptive teaching techniques used. Although the definition of *learning disability* and the criteria to identify learning-disabled children for services have been continually refined over the past years, the literature suggests that the clinical symptoms exhibited by the population most likely to be classified as learning disabled extend beyond academic problems and include clumsiness, hyperactivity, and tactile dysfunction (Ayres, 1964, 1972; Bauer, 1977a, 1977b; Benson & Geshwind, 1970; Dare & Gordon, 1970; Gordon & McKinley, 1980; Gubbay, 1975; Henderson & Hall, 1982; Kinsbourne & Warrington, 1973; Lesny, 1980; Nelson, 1984; Sears, 1981; Strauss & Lehtinen, 1947; Walton et al., 1969).

Despite the importance of tactile functions in development, few tests of tactile functions exist. Those that do exist have been criticized as being unreliable and lacking in demonstrated validity (Adams, 1985; Kephart, 1972; Westman, 1978). For example, the Southern California Sensory Integration Tests (Ayres, 1980), which were developed in the early 1960s to assess the biological substrates that underlie learning, have been used to evaluate children with learning disabilities, minimal brain damage, or perceptual impairments. The three major areas tested are visual perception, perceptual motor ability, and tactile perception. As the Southern California tests grew in popularity and the sophistication of psychometric testing advanced, they were continually criticized for low reliability and lack of demonstrated validity, although their unique contributions were also recognized (Kephart, 1972; Westman, 1978). The kinesthesia and tactile tests of the battery have been of particular concern, with test–retest reliability ranging from .01 to .75 (Kephart, 1972).

One recently published set of tests that claims to measure similar functions, that is, the neurological substrated of behavior, is the Luria-Nebraska Neuropsychological Battery (Golden, Hammeke, & Purisch, 1980). Although developed for adults, the children's battery that appeared later is designed for children as young as age 8. There are 11 separate scales: Motor Functions, Rhythm, Tactile Functions, Visual Functions, Receptive Speech, Expressive Speech, Writing, Reading, Arithmetic, Memory, and Intellectual Processes.

The adult version of the Luria-Nebraska battery has been criticized for the questionable statistical methodology used to validate the tests and establish their reliability (Adams, 1985). Reliability, as reported in the manual, is satisfactory for the battery as a whole, but the tactile section is less reliable at .78 for test–retest (Golden, Hammeke, & Purisch, 1980). However, several studies of the children's version, which has not yet been published, have shown that the children's battery is also reliable as a whole—that is, that it discriminates between normal and brain-damaged children (Gustavson, Golden, & Leark, 1982; Leark, Gustavson, & Golden, 1982; Wilkening, Golden, MacInnes, Plaistead, & Hermann, 1981). In these studies, the judgment of brain damage was based on the external criterion of presence of hard neurological signs as revealed by a neurosurgical report, an abnormal computerized axial tomography (CAT) scan, an abnormal electroencephalogram, or a neurological evaluation. Learning-disabled children or children with minimal brain dysfunction who did not meet the criterion were not included in the samples used in these studies.

Because the sensitivity and reliability of the Southern California tactile tests developed for children diminish at the older age range of the test, that is, at 8 years (Westman, 1978), and the children's version of the Luria-Nebraska battery is given only experimentally to children as young as 7 or 8 (R. A. Leark, personal communication, November 9, 1981), reliability must be established for the tactile sections of these two batteries on 8-year-old children. Given adequate reliability, the question of validity arises. Can the tactile sections of these two batteries discriminate between the normal and learning-disabled populations as currently defined,[1] especially in light of their intended use, that is, for the organically brain-damaged population?

1. "The term 'children with specific learning disabilities' means those children who have a disorder in one or more of the basic psychological processes involved in understanding or in using language, spoken or written, which disorder may manifest itself in imperfect ability to listen, think, speak, read, write, spell, or do mathematical calculations. Such disorders include such conditions as perceptual handicaps, brain injury, minimal brain dysfunction, dyslexia, and developmental aphasia. The term does not include children who have learning problems which are primarily the result of visual, hearing, or motor handicaps, of mental retardation, of emotional disturbances, or of environmental, cultural, or economic disadvantage." (Education for All Handicapped Children Act of 1975, 20 U.S.C. §1401[15])

Finally, since the two batteries are unique among psychoeducational tests in that they claim to assess the biological substrates of behavior, is there, in fact, concurrent validity between them in the assessment of tactile functions?

The purpose of this study was to compare tactile functions in learning-disabled and normal children as measured by the Southern California and Luria-Nebraska tactile tests and to evaluate the reliability and validity of the two measurement tools on 8-year-old children. A secondary purpose was to explore the reliability and validity of the individual Southern California tactile tests and the tactile subsections of the Luria-Nebraska battery to determine if subsections of the somatosensory domain could be reliably tested. (For the purposes of this study, the tactile section of the Luria-Nebraska battery was artificially separated into 8 subsections.)

Method

SUBJECTS

The subjects were 30 normal 8-year-old children from public schools and 30 learning-disabled 8-year-old children who had been placed in special classes by the public schools. All children were from middle-class families and lived in southern New Jersey towns. In each group there were 24 boys and 6 girls, and of this number 29 were Caucasian and 1 was black. The mean age in months was 100.7 for the normal group and 100 for the learning-disabled group. A *t* test of mean age differences of the normal and learning-disabled subjects indicated there was no significant difference in age as calculated by months.

Learning disability had been determined for each child through referral of the child by a classroom teacher for a team evaluation of his or her learning problems. Each child had been determined by the team to require special placement for these problems and fit the legal definition of learning disability accepted by the U.S. Congress in 1975 (Education for All Handicapped Children Act of 1975). All learning-disabled children were receiving educational and related services in special classes. Since neither the normal nor the learning-disabled population was large enough to allow for random selection, all children who met the stated criteria were tested.

PROCEDURE

The tactile tests of the Southern California battery and the tactile section of the Luria-Nebraska battery were administered individually to the children in 45-min sessions. The first administration of the tests was on Tuesday, and the retest was on Friday of the same week. The short interval between test and retest was designed to limit threats to external validity from each child's individual history, maturation, and treatment, as well as from the interaction of these factors. Short intervals between tests and retests are discouraged in psychoeducational testing to limit the subject's possible acquisition of insight into problems posed in the tests. This is believed to be less of a problem in sensory or motor testing, however. All children were tested both times by the primary researcher in the same setting. The tactile tests of the Southern California required about 25 minutes to administer; the tactile section of the Luria-Nebraska, about 15 minutes. The sequence of the two tests was alternated with each successive subject, but the same sequence was maintained per subject across administrations.

Results

Two types of reliability analyses are presented—coefficients of internal consistency and the test–retest coefficients of temporal stability. Analyses of validity include construct validity determined by *t* tests and discriminant analyses, and concurrent validity.

Internal consistency is a form of reliability that determines to what extent the items in the test are drawn from a relatively homogeneous universe of items. Traditionally, this is done by computing Cronbach's alpha.

The Southern California tactile tests were analyzed together. Data from the total group of subjects were used in the analysis. Correlations between the individual tests and the tactile battery total score ranged from .55 to .67, with an average of .59. Cronbach's alpha was .82. Alpha could not be increased by removal of any items. The Southern California tactile battery was therefore found to be internally consistent in describing the single, underlying dimension of touch.

Internal consistency for the tactile functions section of the Luria-Nebraska battery ranged from .08 to .76, with an average of .41. The correlation between individual items and the total score ranged from .35 to .69, with an average of .53. Cronbach's alpha was .80.

To determine temporal stability, Pearson product-moment correlations were computed between the test and retest scores of both tests for the total group. Coefficients were .86 for both tests.

For exploratory purposes, reliability coefficients using the Pearson product-moment correlation were next calculated for the six individual tactile tests of the Southern California and for the eight artificially created subsections of the tactile section of the Luria-Nebraska. As can be seen in *Table 1,* reliability in both cases was below .80.

To determine to what extent the two tests discriminated between the normal and the learning-disabled children, two procedures were used. First, a *t* test was computed on the means of the two measures to determine whether the subjects represented the same or different populations.

To do this, the *z* scores on the six Southern California tactile tests were summed to achieve a total score, creating a feasible range of scores from –18.0 to +18.0 with a mean of 0.0. The *t* scores on the tactile section of the Luria-Nebraska ranged from 40 to 133, with a low score indicating *no error* or *better functioning*. Results shown in *Table 2* indicate that the difference between groups was significant and that learning-disabled children scored substantially lower than the normal children ($p < .001$).

A *t* test was also done on each subsection of the Luria-Nebraska tactile section and on each test in the Southern California tactile battery to determine how well they discriminated between normal and learning-disabled children. Multivariate analyses, although generally preferable over multiple *t* tests, were not used as the

TABLE 1
TEST–RETEST RELIABILITY COEFFICIENTS FOR THE SIX TACTILE TESTS OF THE SCSIT AND THE EIGHT TACTILE SUBSECTIONS OF THE LNNB ($N = 60$)

SCSIT	r	LNNB	r
Kinesthesia	.57*	Tactile Localization	.51*
Manual Form Perception	.56*	Tactile Discrimination	.49*
Finger Identification	.77*	Intensity	.70*
Graphesthesia	.78*	Tactile Spatial Discrimination	.61*
Localization of Tactile Stimuli	.53*	Direction of Movement	.11
Double Tactile Stimuli	.47*	Identification of Traced Shapes	.58*
		Identification of Traced Numbers	.41*
		Identification of Objects	.69*

Note: SCSIT = Southern California Sensory Integration Tests. LNNB = Luria-Nebraska Neuropsychological Battery.
* $p < .001$.

TABLE 2
***t* TESTS COMPARING NORMAL AND LEARNING-DISABLED CHILDREN TESTED WITH THE SCSIT AND LNNB TACTILE BATTERIES**

	N	$\overline{X}$	SD	t
Southern California				
Normal	30	0.5	3.7	7.13*
Learning disabled	30	–9.8	6.2	
Luria-Nebraska				
Normal	30	51.0	8.4	7.44*
Learning disabled	30	83.7	22.5	

Note: SCSIT = Southern California Sensory Integration Tests. LNNB = Luria-Nebraska Neuropsychological Battery.
* $p < .001$.

subtests are highly intercorrelated and thus violate a basic assumption of the multivariate procedure. To diminish the chance of a Type I error occurring in the performance of the multiple t tests, the Bonferroni Correction, a variation of the Bonferroni t procedure (Kirk, 1982), was adopted. An alpha level of .007 was employed for the individual tests of significance of the Southern California data to preserve an error-in-procedure rate of .05. In a similar design, an alpha level of .006 was used for the individual tests of significance of the Luria-Nebraska data, thus allowing the error-in-procedure rate to be no greater than .05.

As is shown in *Table 3,* all tactile subsections of the Luria-Nebraska tactile section and all tests of the Southern California tactile battery differentiated between normal and learning-disabled children at the .01 level with the exception of Direction of Movement and Sharp–Dull Discrimination on the Luria-Nebraska.

TABLE 3

***t* TESTS COMPARING NORMAL AND LEARNING-DISABLED CHILDREN'S SCORES ON THE INDIVIDUAL SCSIT TACTILE TESTS AND THE TACTILE SUBSECTIONS OF THE LNNB**

Tests	*M*	*SD*	*t*
	Southern California		
Kinesthesia			
Normal	+0.5	0.9	4.52*
Learning disabled	−0.9	1.4	
Manual Form Perception			
Normal	−0.3	1.2	3.21*
Learning disabled	−1.4	1.5	
Finger Identification			
Normal	−0.1	1.2	4.70*
Learning disabled	−1.6	1.2	
Graphesthesia			
Normal	−0.2	1.3	5.79*
Learning disabled	−2.3	1.5	
Localization of Tactile Stimuli			
Normal	−0.4	1.4	3.42*
Learning disabled	−1.7	1.6	
Double Tactile Stimuli			
Normal	0.2	0.6	4.97*
Learning disabled	−2.0	2.1	
	Luria-Nebraska		
Light Touch			
Normal	0.0	0.2	3.54**
Learning disabled	1.0	1.4	
Sharp–Dull Discrimination			
Normal	0.1	0.7	2.65
Learning disabled	0.9	1.3	
Hard and Soft Discrimination			
Normal	0.1	0.3	5.17**
Learning disabled	1.5	1.4	
Two Point Discrimination			
Normal	0.6	1.0	4.00**
Learning disabled	2.0	1.7	
Direction of Movement			
Normal	0.0	0.0	2.34
Learning disabled	0.3	0.7	
Identification of Design			
Normal	0.8	1.0	2.95**
Learning disabled	1.8	1.4	
Number Identification			
Normal	0.2	0.8	6.02**
Learning disabled	2.3	1.6	
Object Identification			
Normal	1.0	1.1	
Learning disabled	2.4	1.4	4.34**

Note: SCSIT = Southern California Sensory Integration Tests. LNNB = Luria-Nebraska Neuropsychological Battery.

* $p < .001$. ** $p < .006$.

TABLE 4
F TEST OF DISCRIMINANT FUNCTIONS FOR THE SOUTHERN CALIFORNIA SENSORY INTEGRATION TESTS AND THE LURIA-NEBRASKA NEUROPSYCHOLOGICAL BATTERY

Variable	Wilk's Lambda	F
Southern California	.53	50.85*
Luria-Nebraska	.51	55.32*

* $p < .00001$.

A discriminant functions analysis was the second procedure used to determine to what extent the total scores on the Southern California and the Luria-Nebraska would correctly predict group membership.The Southern California cutoff score between groups was –.52; the Luria-Nebraska cutoff score between groups was 67.38.

An F test of discriminant functions was computed to determine whether the discriminant function prediction equation derived from both batteries facilitated more accurate prediction than would be achieved by chance alone. The results shown in *Table 4* indicate that the prediction equation was significant ($p < .00001$) in both cases. Furthermore, 90% of the children were correctly classified as either normal or learning disabled; all normal children were correctly classified, and 80% of the learning-disabled children were correctly classified. Prediction by the Southern California equation alone resulted in the correct classification of 82% of the children, and prediction by the Luria-Nebraska equation alone resulted in the correct classification of 85%.

The concurrent validity of the two measures was shown by a Pearson product-moment correlation of .73, which was computed on the test scores of the first testing session for all 60 children.

Discussion

The study was done on a small sample of limited age range, and the learning-disabled children had disabilities severe enough to require placement in a special class. Therefore, generalizations of all results must be done with extreme caution. However, a number of interesting trends emerge that warrant further exploration.

The tactile functions of normal and learning-disabled children were found to be significantly different. In fact, a cutoff score was identified in the prediction equation of both tests that differentiated learning-disabled from normal children. For the Southern California the cutoff score was –.52, attained by summing all the individual tactile scores. For the Luria-Nebraska the cutoff score was 67.3.

Both the Southern California and the Luria-Nebraska tactile tests were found to be more reliable as a whole than previously reported in the testing manuals. Internal consistency was .82 and .80, respectively, and test–retest reliability was .86

for both measures. The test–retest reliability of the individual tests of both the Southern California and the Luria-Nebraska tactile sections are less reliable and suggest that all tactile tests of the Southern California should be given together as standardized and are most reliable when so administered. Although the tactile section of the Luria-Nebraska was artificially separated into subsections in this study for exploratory purposes, this procedure is not recommended as it lowers reliability. The authors of both tests recommend that the entire battery be given as a whole. The results of this study suggest that although formal testing of the tactile domain is reliable for both measures, in both cases testing of individual aspects of the tactile domain is much less so and should be used cautiously.

The construct and concurrent validity results were of particular interest. Significant differences were found between the means of the learning-disabled and normal groups on all aspects of tactile function as tested by these measures. Discriminant analysis applied to the scores indicated that 90% of those tested were correctly classified as learning disabled or normal. All those who were misclassified were learning disabled. This result suggests that caution must be taken in oversimplifying evaluation techniques or in overgeneralizing limited test results from this population. Concurrent validity between the two tests was .73, indicating that knowledge of test scores of one test could explain 53% of the score variance of the other test.

Finally, this study has implications for understanding the nature of children with learning disabilities. Although learning-disabled children are identified in the educational system by their lack of academic success, the results of this study support the theory that other problems exist, specifically, poor tactile functioning. Poor tactile functioning may be a specific problem, but more likely it is only one aspect of a heterogeneous problem, of which learning disability is itself only one aspect. Disordered tactile perception may be both a causative and a complicating factor in some of the heterogeneous problems found in the learning-disabled population. These problems might include interference with discriminative aspects of tactile exploration and sensorimotor learning, since accurate sensory feedback is so important to motor responses. Poor tactile functioning may be a major contributor to clumsiness or to developmental apraxia (Ayres, 1985). Tactile problems in the form of tactile defensiveness may contribute significantly to the hyperactivity, the poor ability to attend, and the emotional instability frequently found in this population.

Acknowledgments

I gratefully acknowledge the inspiration and support of the late A. J. Ayres, PhD, and thank Sensory Integration International of Torrance, California, for providing a grant for the pilot project; Nancy Kauffman, EdM, OTR/L. and Carol Petrokonis, OTR/L, for their assistance with testing on the pilot project; Mary Rita Mahlman for her technical assistance throughout the pilot project and the dissertation research; my doctoral committee at Temple University School of Special Education, chaired by Diane Bryen, PhD, for its guidance; and the staff and students of Kingsway Learning Center and the public schools of Bellmawr, New Jersey, for their cooperation and for providing children for both the pilot project and the dissertation research.

References

Adams, R. L. (1985). Review of the Luria-Nebraska Neuropsychological Battery. In J. V. Mitchell (Ed.), *Ninth mental measurement yearbook* (pp. 878–881). Lincoln, NE: University of Nebraska Press.

American Psychiatric Association. (1980). *Diagnostic and statistical manual of mental disorders* (3rd ed.). Washington, DC: Author.

Ayres, A. J. (1964). Tactile functions: Their relation to hyperactive and perceptual motor behavior. *American Journal of Occupational Therapy, 18,* 6–11.

Ayres, A. J. (1972). *Sensory integration and learning disabilities.* Los Angeles: Western Psychological Services.

Ayres, A. J. (1979). *Sensory integration and the child.* Los Angeles: Western Psychological Services.

Ayres, A. J. (1980). *Southern California Sensory Integration Tests: Manual* (rev. ed.). Los Angeles: Western Psychological Services.

Ayres, A. J. (1985). *Developmental Dyspraxia and adult onset apraxia.* Torrance, CA: Sensory Integration International.

Bauer, B. A. (1977a). Tactile-sensitive behavior in hyperactive and nonhyperactive children. *American Journal of Occupational Therapy, 31,* 447–453.

Bauer, B. A. (1977b). Tactile sensitivity: Development of a behavioral responses checklist. *American Journal of Occupational Therapy, 31,* 357–361.

Benson, D. F., & Geshwind, N. (1970). Developmental Gerstmann syndrome. *Neurology, 20,* 3–11.

Bruner, J. S. (1973). Organization of early skilled action. *Child Development, 44,* 1–11.

Dare, M. T., & Gordon, N. (1970). Clumsy children: A disorder of perception and motor organization. *Developmental Medicine and Child Neurology, 12,* 178–185.

Education for All Handicapped Children Act of 1975 (Public Law 94–142), 20 U.S.C. § 1401.

Gerstmann, J. (1927). Fingeragnosie und isolierte agraphie, ein neues syndrom [Finger agnosia and isolated agraphia, a new syndrome]. *Zeitschrift fur die Gesamte Neurologie und Psychiatrie, 108,* 152–177.

Ginsburg, H., & Opper, S. (1979). *Theory of intellectual development.* Englewood Cliffs, NJ: Prentice-Hall.

Golden, C. J., Hammeke, T. A., & Purisch, A. D. (1980). *The Luria-Nebraska Neuropsychological Battery and manual.* Los Angeles: Western Psychological Services.

Gordon, W., & McKinley, I. (Eds.) (1980). *Helping clumsy children.* Edinburgh: Churchill Livingstone.

Gubbay, S. S. (1975). *The clumsy child.* New York: Saunders.

Gustavson, J. L., Golden, C. J., & Leark, R. A. (1982). *The Luria-Nebraska Neuropsychological Battery—Children's revision.* Paper presented at the annual convention of the American Psychological Association, Washington, DC.

Henderson, S. E., & Hall, D. (1982). Concomitants of clumsiness in young school children. *Developmental Medicine and Child Neurology, 24,* 448–460.

Huss, A. J. (1977). Touch with care or a caring touch? 1976 Eleanor Clarke Slagle lecture. *American Journal of Occupational Therapy, 31,* 11–18.

Kephart, N. C. (1972). Review of Southern California Kinesthesia and Tactile Perception tests. In O. K. Boros (Ed.), *Seventh mental measurement yearbook* (pp. 1288–1289). Highland Park, NJ: Gryphon Press.

Kinsbourne, M., & Warrington, E. K. (1973). The developmental Gerstmann syndrome. *Archives of Neurology, 8,* 40–51.

Kirk, R. E. (1982). Experimental design: Procedures for the behavioral sciences. Belmont, CA: Brooks-Cole.

Kulka, A., Fry, C., & Goldstein, F. J. (1960). Kinesthetic needs in infancy. *American Journal of Osteopsychiatry, 30,* 562–571.

Leark, R. A., Gustavson, J. L., & Golden, C. J. (1982, October). *Relationship of the Luria-Nebraska children's battery to intelligence as assessed by the WISC-R.* Paper presented at the annual meeting of the National Academy of Neuropsychologists, Atlanta, Georgia.

Lesny, I. A. (1980). Developmental dyspraxia-dysagnosia as a cause of congenital children's clumsiness. *Brain Development, 2,* 69–71.

Nelson, D. L. (1984). *Children with autism and other pervasive disorders of development and behavior.* Thorofare, NJ: Slack.

Sears, C. J. (1981). The tactilely defensive child. *Academic Therapy, 16,* 563–569.

Strauss, A., & Lehtinen, L. (1947). *Psychopathology and education in the brain-injured child.* New York: Grune & Stratton.

Walton, J. N., Ellis, E., & Court, S. D. M. (1969). Clumsy children: Developmental apraxia and agnosia. *Brain, 85,* 603–612.

Westman, A. S. (1978). Review of the Southern California Sensory Integration Tests. In O. K. Boros (Ed.), *Eighth mental measurement yearbook* (pp. 1406–1409). Highland Park, NJ: Gryphon Press.

Wilkening, G. N., Golden, C. J., MacInnes, W. D., Plaistead, J. R., & Hermann, B. (1981). *The Luria-Nebraska Neuropsychological Battery—Children's revision: A preliminary report.* Unpublished manuscript.

ACTION PLAN 14: REPLICATE A STUDY

The test-retest reliability of the Southern California Postrotary Nystagmus Test (Ayres, 1989) is probably the single most researched piece or test in the therapy literature because, in part, it is so easy to give. Many investigators have replicated this test with different groups and norms, usually varying the procedures in some slight manner. It is relatively easy to do replication studies, particularly if you do not have access to methodological consultation. Replication of findings is a key to the scientific process and is important. It is only through repeated demonstration, that is, through replication, that a body of knowledge develops. Look back in chapter 3 at the article "Test–Retest Reliability of the Southern California Postrotary Nystagmus Test" for an example of a replication study.

Conclusion

Are you committed to your profession? Are you committed to being a professional? If so, you are automatically committed to being a research consumer and perhaps even to becoming a research practitioner. This chapter has given you an array of action plans that you can implement to continue on your path of research participation.

By completing this book, you have taken an important step in your professional growth and in your participation in the research process. Some of you will continue to take part in the process as research consumers. Some of you will join in the process of being a research practitioner. Whichever path you choose, remember the goal of this struggle with the meaning and process of research: to better serve and work with those who can benefit from our services. It is indeed a humbling and noble endeavor we undertake.

References

Bohannon, R. W., & LeVeau, B. F. (1986). Clinician's use of research findings: A review of the literature with implications for physical therapists. *Physical Therapy, 66,* 45–50.

Cermak, S. A. (1991). [Review of the book Children's psychological testing. A Guide for nonpsychologists (2nd ed.)]. *Physical & Occupational Therapy in Pediatrics, 11(2),* 83–85.

Domholdt, E. A., & Malone, R. T. (1985). Evaluating research literature: The educated clinician. *Physical Therapy, 65,* 487–491.

Hanft, B., & Royeen, C. B. (1991). Commentary. *Infants and Young Children, 4,* 8–10.

Harris, S. R. (1991). Commentary. *Infants and Young Children, 4,* 11–13.

Kaplan, C. (1992). [Review of the book Marketing Techniques for Physical Therapists]. *Physical Therapy, 72,* 93.

Kinnealey, M. (1989). Tactile functions in learning-disabled and normal children: Reliability and validity considerations. *Occupational Therapy Journal of Research, 9(1),* 3–15

Parette, H. P., Jr., Hendricks, M. D., & Rock, S. L. (1991). Efficacy of therapuetic intervention intensity with infants and young children with cerebral palsy. *Infants and Young Children, 4,* 1–8.

Royeen, C. B. (1985). Domain specifications of the construct tactile defensiveness. *American Journal of Occupational Therapy, 39(9),* 596–599.

Royeen, C. B. (1988). Review of the DeGangi-Berk test of sensory integration. *Physical and Occupational Therapy in Pediatrics, 8(2/3),* 71–75.

Royeen, C. B. (1989). Adaption of Likert scaling for use with children. *Occupational Therapy Journal of Research, 5,* 59–69.

Royeen, C. B., & DeGangi, G. A. (1992). Use of neurodevelopmental treatment as an intervention: Annotated listing of studies 1980-1990. *Physical Therapy, 66,* 45–50.

Royeen, C. B., & Little, L. F. (1985). Autistic adolescents: Developmental milestones and a model treatment program. *Occupational Therapy in Health Care, 2(3),* 59–68.

Smith, J. P. (1975). Is the nursing professional really research-based? *Journal of Advances in Nursing, 4,* 319–325.

Index

Page references in bold type refer to tables or figures.

F

G

H

I

N

O

P

R

S

T

U

V

W

X

Y